D1717066

Carrier-Based Drug Delivery

ACS SYMPOSIUM SERIES **879**

Carrier-Based Drug Delivery

Sönke Svenson, Editor
Dendritic Nanotechnologies, Inc.

**Sponsored by the
ACS Division of Colloid and Surface Chemistry**

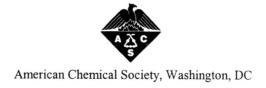

American Chemical Society, Washington, DC

Library of Congress Cataloging-in-Publication Data

Carrier-based drug delivery / Sönke Svenson, editor.

p. cm.—(ACS symposium series ; 879)

Includes bibliographical references and index.

ISBN 0–8412–3839–1

1. Drug carriers (Pharmacy)—Congresses.

I. Svenson, Sönke, 1956- II. Series.

RS201 V43C37   2004
615′.7—dc22   2003063742

PRINTED IN THE UNITED STATES OF AMERICA

Foreword

The ACS Symposium Series was first published in 1974 to provide a mechanism for publishing symposia quickly in book form. The purpose of the series is to publish timely, comprehensive books developed from ACS sponsored symposia based on current scientific research. Occasionally, books are developed from symposia sponsored by other organizations when the topic is of keen interest to the chemistry audience.

Before agreeing to publish a book, the proposed table of contents is reviewed for appropriate and comprehensive coverage and for interest to the audience. Some papers may be excluded to better focus the book; others may be added to provide comprehensiveness. When appropriate, overview or introductory chapters are added. Drafts of chapters are peer-reviewed prior to final acceptance or rejection, and manuscripts are prepared in camera-ready format.

As a rule, only original research papers and original review papers are included in the volumes. Verbatim reproductions of previously published papers are not accepted.

ACS Books Department

Contents

Overview

Liposomes and Tubules as Carrier Systems

Polymeric Micelles as Carriers in Drug and Gene Delivery

Micro- and Nanoparticulate Carriers

Indexes

Preface

The development of successful drug delivery technologies requires an intense interdisciplinary research effort, spanning the range from materials development to pharmacology and toxicology. Materials useable for drug delivery have, of course, to be biocompatible. Furthermore, these materials must interact with the many different active pharmaceutical ingredients (API) to be delivered, such as hydrophilic and hydrophobic small organic molecules, peptides, proteins, oligonucleotides, and DNA, in a well-defined, predictable, and reproducible way. The purpose of these interactions is very different as well, involving encapsulation, protection, local delivery, and various release modes, such as controlled, sustained, and burst release, as well as release triggered by an internal or external event. The delivery of API follows many routes, for example, oral, intravenous, subcutaneous, intramuscular, transdermal or topical. Each delivery route involves special challenges and requirements for the delivery material.

These challenges require a thorough understanding of material properties, interactions among carriers and API, and interactions of both of the preceeding within the human body. This understanding is rarely combined within one research group. It is, therefore, surprising how little communication takes place between researchers in chemistry, chemical engineering, and materials science, the experts in the synthesis and characterization of drug delivery materials; and researchers from pharmaceutical and medical sciences, the experts in the application and evaluation of delivery systems to medical problems. Both communities are attending their specific conferences and symposia with little cross over activity.

Thus the main motivation for organizing the *Carrier-Based Drug Delivery* symposium during the 223rd National Meeting of the American Chemical Society (ACS) in Orlando, Florida, in April 2002 was to provide a forum for discussion for both communities involved in drug delivery and to trigger a more intense cooperation between members of these two groups. Twenty-two well recognized international experts, almost equally representing both communities, had been invited to present research being conducted in the United States, Canada, Japan, Germany, the United Kingdom, Switzerland, and the Netherlands. This ACS Symposium Series book presents highlights from this symposium.

The content of the book is divided into three main sections, covering the major carrier systems. The first section describes the use of liposomes and tubules as carriers. Seven chapters report the use of stimuli-responsive liposomes and liposome–polymer complexes in drug and DNA delivery, the application of neutral liposomes in gene transfer, and the use of niosomes in the delivery of poorly soluble drugs. The role of vesicle shape in delivery is dis-cussed, followed by the use of microtubules and templated nanotubes for the delivery and separation of bioactives.

The second section is devoted to the use of polymeric micelles as targetable pharmaceutical carriers, novel therapeutics in drug delivery, and endosomolytic agents for gene delivery. The section concludes with a chapter on the use of ultrasound to improve the efficiency of polymeric micelles as carriers.

The third section details the use of micro- and nanoparticulate carriers in drug delivery. These chapters address methods to prepare precise micro- and nanoparticles, the utilization of lipids in peptide and protein release, and the construction of nanocontainers, either by stabilization of liposomal templates or by layer-by-layer deposition of polymers around colloidal templates. The reduction or prevention of burst release from matrices are discussed, as well as the use of muco-adhesion and mechanical adhesion for localized nasal and peroral delivery of pharmaceutical actives.

This book is intended for readers in the chemical and pharmaceutical industry and academia who are interested or involved in drug delivery research as well as advanced students who are interested in this active and rapidly developing research area.

I deeply appreciate the willingness of the authors to contribute to this im-portant overview of drug delivery technologies. I also appreciate the help of my colleagues at The Dow Chemical Company to review these contributions, not only ensuring clarity and technical accuracy of the manuscripts but also providing an industrial point of view. I thank the ACS Division of Colloid and Surface Chemistry (COLL) for the opportunity to hold the symposium as a part of their program. I appreciate the patience and support of the ACS Symposium Series acquisitions and production team during the production of this book. Last but not least I thank The Dow Chemical Company for financial support and the COLL division for their matching contribution.

Sönke Svenson
Dendritic NanoTechnologies, Inc.
2625 Denison Drive
Mount Pleasant, MI 48858
(989) 774–1179 (telephone)
(989) 774–1194 (fax)
Svenson@dnanotech.com (email)

Overview

Chapter 1

Carrier-Based Drug Delivery

Sőnke Svenson

Dendritic NanoTechnologies, Inc., 2625 Denison Drive, Mount Pleasant, MI 48858 (email: Svenson@dnanotech.com)

A steadily growing number of active pharmaceutical ingredients (API) exhibits low bioavailability and requires protection from enzymatic and acid-catalyzed degradation in the body. Therefore, the development of efficient carrier-based delivery systems is of increasing importance. Carrier systems based on liposomes, polymeric micelles, and micro- and nanoparticles and capsules are presented. Methods to prepare the carriers as well as routes of drug encapsulation, delivery, and release are reviewed. The advantages and disadvantages of each carrier type are mentioned. As one can reasonably expect, there is no one carrier that fits all requirements but carriers have been developed that will address the needs of a specific API.

Introduction

In 2002, advanced delivery products generated $38 billion in revenue. This amount is expected to grow twenty-eight percent per year over the next five years. By 2007 these products are expected to account for thirty-nine percent of all pharmaceutical sales. A thorough understanding of advanced delivery technologies is, therefore, of essential importance. The bioavailability of active pharmaceutical ingredients (API) is an important factor in development and application of these actives. About forty percent of newly developed API are rejected by the pharmaceutical industry and will never benefit a patient because of low bioavailability. In addition, about seventeen percent of launched API exhibit a suboptimal performance for the same reason. The bioavailability of these drugs is limited due to their low water solubility and/or low membrane permeability. Sixty-five percent of the human body is made up of water, therefore, a drug must have a certain hydrophilicity or polarity to be water-soluble. At the same time, these drugs must exhibit a certain lipophilicity or apolarity to be able to cross lipophilic cell membranes. These requirements have led to the biopharmaceutical qualification system of drugs shown in Figure 1. Class I drugs have a high bioavailability and provide no challenge. On the other end, Class IV drugs are pharmaceutical bricks that will never make it to the market. Class II and Class III drugs have a reduced bioavailability because of their low solubility and low membrane permeability, respectively.

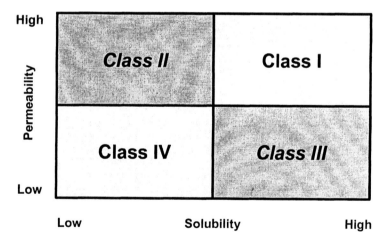

Figure 1. Biopharmaceutical Classification System of Drugs. The bioavailability of Class II and Class III drugs is reduced because of their low solubility and low permeability.

An increasing number of drugs are based on biomolecules such as peptides, proteins, oligonucleotides, and DNA. These molecules often show low bio-availability and the need for protection against enzymatic or acid-catalyzed breakdown in the human body. The common approach to increase the bio-availability of API involves increasing the surface area per particle by reducing the particle size. This approach, however, often subjects the API to some form of aggressive processing such as milling, mixing, extrusion, or organic solvent exchange, which can reduce the performance of the API especially in case of biomolecules. In addition, there is a limit to particle size reduction from a prac-tical point of view during the production of large drug quantities. Drug particles in the nanometer size, for example, are extremely difficult to stabilize and isolate. Furthermore, this approach does not provide protection of biomolecules against enzymatic and acid-catalyzed degradation.

Carrier-based drug delivery is an alternative approach to improve the bioavailability of drugs while at the same time providing the necessary protection of drug molecules. As an additional benefit, the release profile of encapsulated drugs can be tailored to the respective medical needs by choosing an appropriate encapsulation material. The most often studied carrier systems are liposomes and niosomes, formed by self-assembly of phospholipids and non-ionic lipids and surfactants; polymeric micelles formed by self-assembly of charged or neutral block copolymers; and nano- and microparticulate carriers formed by various processes. While most particulate drug delivery vectors are spherical, there are some exceptions in which tubular carriers have been studied. In this overview, some basic information concerning these carrier systems will be given to facilitate the understanding of the more specialized research topics discussed in the following chapters of this book.

Results and Discussion

Carrier-Based Drug Delivery Pathways

In general, carrier-based drug delivery can be broken down into four major steps: (i) encapsulation/adsorption of a drug into/onto a carrier, (ii) delivery of the drug-carrier construct to the desired location within the human body, (iii) uptake of the construct by a cell membrane, and (iv) release of the drug from the carrier. In Figure 2, these steps are illustrated for oral and intracellular delivery of an API. Depending on the actual delivery technology, there are variations to this general scheme. For example, drug delivery can be passive through accu-mulation of the drug in inflammatory tissues and tumors as a result of the enhanced permeability and retention (EPR) effect caused by leaky vasculature at these sites; or the delivery can be active (targeted) using cell-specific receptors

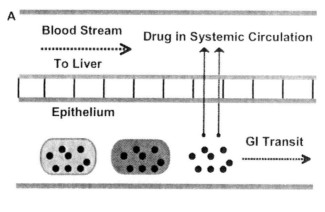

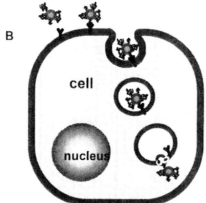

Figure 2. (A) Gastrointestinal drug delivery. A drug encapsulated into a carrier is delivered to the GI tract, released through biodegradation of the carrier, and enters the systemic circulation by passing through the epithelium. (B) Intracellular drug delivery. A drug encapsulated into a carrier containing cell-specific ligands at its surface attaches to a cell membrane, gets internalized through endocytosis, and is released from both endosome and carrier through various release mechanisms.

as shown in Figure 2B. *(1-8)* Furthermore, the drug can be released from the carrier prior to reaching the final location or after reaching its target.

Liposomes and Related Drug Carriers

Initially, liposomes were utilized as a model system for biological membranes. Phospholipids and other amphiphilic molecules self-assemble in water to form bilayer lipid membranes (BLM), separating the aqueous inner core of the

6

liposome from the bulk aqueous phase (Figure 3). This lipid bilayer structure mimics the barrier properties of biomembranes and, therefore, offers the possibility of examining the behavior of these membranes. Membrane models have facilitated the study of membrane structure and function and of lipid-protein interactions within biomembranes.

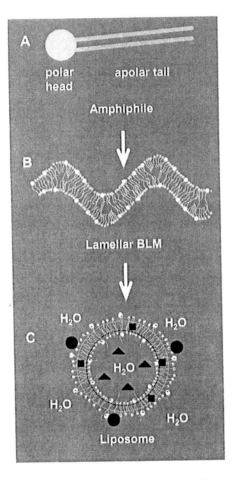

Figure 3. (A) Amphiphilic monomers and polymers self-aggregate in water to form lamellar bimolecular lipid membranes (BLM), reducing the interphase between lipophilic hydrocarbon tails and water. (B) BLM rearrange to spherical liposomes either spontaneously or assisted (i.e., by shear or ultrasonication) to further reduce the tail/water interphase. (C) Hydrophilic API can either be adsorbed onto the liposome surface (●) or encapsulated into the inner aqueous core (π), while lipophilic API insert into the lipid membrane (■).

This type of carrier is often characterized by its composition as a liposome (zwitterionic/amphiphilic phospholipids), niosome (neutral lipids and surfactants), and vesicle (non-phospholipids); and by its morphology as a small or large unilamellar vesicle (SUV, LUV) or multilamellar vesicle (MLV). Long circulating or "stealth" liposomes are surface-modified using minor proportions (0.5-10 mol%) of a biocompatible polymer, most often poly(ethylene glycols) or PEG with molecular weights of 1000-5000 Da. These liposomes are not immediately recognized by the body's defense system and can avoid or delay uptake by the reticuloendothelial system (RES) because the inert polymer brush on their surface prevents or delays opsonization. *(9-13)* In addition, one can construct targeted liposomes or immunoliposomes, which contain ligands on their surface that interact with specific cell membrane receptors, i.e., low-density lipoprotein (LDL) or folate receptors. *(6-10,14-16)*

There are many ways to produce liposomes. The most common approach includes (i) dissolving a phospholipid into a volatile organic solvent, (ii) removing the solvent under vacuum so that the lipid forms a dry film onto the container glass wall, and (iii) mechanically agitating the dry film in the presence of water. This last step of forming an aqueous lipid dispersion can be improved by applying several freeze-thaw cycles to the dispersion. However, the multilamellar liposomes formed during this process usually are heterogeneous in size but can be converted into uniform unilamellar liposomes by extrusion under pressure through a membrane of known pore size. *(17)* Other approaches include application of ultrasound via a probe sonicator to an aqueous lipid dispersion, dialysis of a lipid dispersion, and liposome formation by injection of an organic solution containing the lipid into water as the anti-solvent.

API molecules can either be encapsulated into the aqueous core of a liposome, inserted into the lipid part of the bilayer membrane, or attached to the liposome surface (Figure 3). Passive encapsulation is the most basic approach of loading an API into a liposome. The API sample is prepared in the presence of a high lipid concentration (>200mM or 15 wt%) where the internal volume after liposome formation exceeds the external one. Non-encapsulated material is removed by size-exclusion chromatography. Hydrophilic API will concentrate within the aqueous core while hydrophobic drugs accumulate within the bilayer lipid membrane. However, the encapsulation yields are usually small, especially when the API possesses some membrane permeability and leaks out from the liposome either during storage of the sample or dilution of the liposome formulation after application to a patient. The encapsulation yield can be improved by active encapsulation, a process in which the API is forced into the liposome using some gradient across the membrane, i.e., a gradient in pH or the chemical potential. *(18)* For example, the anticancer drug doxorubicin has been loaded into liposomes by producing the liposomes in water at pH 4.0, then raising the pH of the external bulk water phase to 7.5, followed by the addition of small aliquots of a doxorubicin solution to the liposome dispersion. The internal drug concentration can several-fold surpass its aqueous solubility if the drug precipitates within the liposome.

Release of the API from the carrier is often a challenge. Once the liposomes have been optimized for *in vivo* stability, they are typically incapable of rapidly releasing the encapsulated API. Release either relies on passive mechanisms such as liposome disintegration or diffusion-driven leakage through the membrane or active release mechanisms triggered by a change in acidity or temperature, phototriggering, or enzymatic degradation. *(10)* The use of pH-sensitive phospholipids or other membrane constituents such as co-surfactants is the most common triggering mechanism employed. The low pH within endosomal compartments (pH 4.5-6.5), tumor interstitial fluids, and sites of inflammation (pH 6.2-6.9) leads to destabilization of the liposome followed by release of the encapsulated API. *(10,19-21)* Thermally induced release systems are based on either a gel-to-liquid crystalline phase transition of the bilayer lipid membrane, where the encapsulated content leaks from the liposome due to an increased permeability of the bilayer at higher temperatures, or a liquid crystalline-to-hexagonal phase transition that results in the collapse of the bilayer with release of contents from the inner liposome. Three different heating technologies have been used, (i) bulk heating, where the tissue temperature is raised above body temperature usually by immersion in a water bath, (ii) microwave heating, where microwave coils are used for localized tissue heating, and (iii) photophysical heating, where intense laser excitation of a chromophore encapsulated within the liposome or the nearby extraliposomal environment produces large thermo-acoustic pertubations, triggering the content release by a combined effect of thermally accelerated transmembrane diffusion and shear-induced membrane rupture. *(10,22-25)* Phototriggering is an excellent method to initiate content release since light activation provides a broad range of parameters that can be optimized to suit a given application. It can be applied to surface and remote sites via fiber optic endoscopy with continuous or pulsed excitation of various intensity and wavelength. *(26,27)* Finally, the incorporation of building blocks into the liposome membrane that can be accessed and hydrolyzed by enzymes provides another route of triggered release. For example, phospholipase C has been utilized to hydrolyze the head groups of liposomes containing phosphatidylcholine/phosphatidylethanolamine/cholesterol (2:1:1) as membrane constituents. *(10,28)* Various applications of liposome technology have been reviewed recently. *(29-32)* Some examples of marketed products based on liposome formulations are shown in Table I.

Table I. Examples of marketed products based on liposomes. (Reproduced with permission. Copyright 2002 Northern Lipids, Inc.)

Name	Company	Drug Class	Structure	Indication
Epaxal Berna	Swiss Serum and Vaccine Institute Berne	Vaccine	Liposome	hepatitis A
AmBisome®	Gilead (NeXstar)	Amphotericin B	Liposome	antifungal
ABELCET®	Elan (TLC)	Amphotericin B	Complex	antifungal
DaunoXome®	Gilead (NeXstar)	Daunorubicin	Liposome	kaposi's sarcoma (KS)
Doxil®	Alza (Sequus)	Doxorubicin	Liposome	kaposi's sarcoma (KS)
Myocet®	Elan (TLC)	Doxorubicin	Liposome	metastatic breast cancer
Visudyne®	QLT PhotoTherapeutics	Verteporfin	liposome	age-related macular degeneration

Drug Carriers Based on Polymeric Micelles

The second important class of drug carriers consists of polymeric micelles. Amphiphilic molecules, i.e., molecules containing hydrophilic and hydrophobic (lipophilic) parts, self-assemble in water above a certain, molecule-specific concentration to form micelles, in which the hydrophobic moieties of the monomers aggregate with each other to reduce the interphase with water as described for liposomes, while the hydrophilic moieties are directed towards the bulk water phase (Figure 4). This specific aggregation concentration is called the critical micelle concentration (CMC). The disintegration of micelles into monomers when diluted below the CMC, i.e., after injection of a micelle formulation into the blood stream, is the major obstacle for this carrier class. However, by using amphiphilic block copolymers it is possible to keep the CMC very low and, at the same time, reduce the exchange kinetics of the monomers between micelles and the bulk water phase, resulting in micelles that are stable enough for drug delivery applications. Different types of copolymers have been used for micelle formation; AB diblock and ABA triblock copolymers, with A being the hydrophilic and B the hydrophobic moiety of the molecules, as well as grafted copolymers in which hydrophobic side chains are grafted onto a hydrophilic polymeric backbone. (33-38) Depending on the lengths of the A and B blocks, copolymers with molecular weights between 1000 and 10,000 Da and different hydrophilic-lipophilic balances (HLB) have been synthesized. The hydrophilic block A most often consists of poly(ethylene glycol) (PEG), also referred to as poly(ethylene oxide) (PEO), for the same reasons as in case of liposomes, i.e., good water solubility, biocompatibility, and steric protection of the micelles. The hydrophobic block B can be formed by various molecules, such as propylene glycol, L-lysine, aspartic acid, β-benzyl-L-aspartate, γ-benzyl-L-glutamate, caprolactone, D,L-lactic acid, and spermine, to name a few examples. (33,39-49) The block copolymers can be neutral or charged, depending on the molecular subunits. Another approach to create micelles with defined size is based on the interaction of diblock copolymers containing a charged and a neutral block (i.e., poly(ethylene glycol)-b-poly(sodium methacrylate) with single, double, or triple tail surfactants. In such complexes, the surfactants are bound to the oppositely charged blocks of the copolymers and form the core, while the PEG blocks form the shell. Depending on the length of the charged and nonionic blocks and the structure of the surfactants, micelles or small liposomes form in water. (50,51) The size of polymeric micelles is largely determined by the size of their constituent molecules, covering the range from approximately 5 to 100 nm.

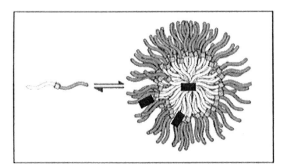

Figure 4. Self-assembly of AB diblock copolymers to form a polymeric micelle. The hydrophilic block A is shown in dark grey, the hydrophobic block B in light grey. Hydrophilic drugs can attach to the hydrophilic block A or partially insert into the micellar core, while hydrophobic drugs completely insert into the hydrophobic core as shown schematically (black rectangles). (Adapted from Ref. 52. Reproduced by permission of The Royal Society of Chemistry.)

The formation of polymeric micelles is straightforward because it is based on self-assembly. The copolymers are dissolved in water at ambient or elevated temperature at concentrations well above the CMC. Copolymers with very low water solubility are converted into micelles by first dissolving the monomers into a water-miscible organic solvent such as dimethylsulfoxide, dimethylformamide, acetonitrile, and tetrahydrofuran, followed by dialysis against water. *(33)* The ideal micelle for pharmaceutical applications should possess a size in the range of 10 to 100 nm, demonstrate sufficiently high stability both *in vitro* and *in vivo*, i.e., have a combination of low CMC and high kinetic stability, and carry a substantial quantity of API but eventually disintegrate into bioinert and non-toxic monomers that can easily be cleared from the body. The CMC value of a polymeric micelle can be estimated by a few "rules of thumb", (i) increasing the length of the hydrophobic block at constant hydrophilic block length causes a noticeable decrease in CMC and increase in micelle stability, while the inverse situation results in an only minor CMC increase, (ii) increasing the molecular weight of a copolymer while keeping the HLB constant causes some decrease in CMC, and (iii) the CMC of ABA triblock copolymers is generally higher than the CMC of AB diblock copolymers with the same molecular weight and HLB. *(33,55)*

Micelles can be surface-modified with biodegradable polymers and cell-specific ligands such as antibodies or sugar moieties in the same way as liposomes. These ligands are usually attached to the end of some of the hydrophilic blocks of the copolymers to reduce steric hindrance. The main morphological difference compared to liposomes is the lack of an aqueous core. Hydrophilic API, therefore, can only attach to the micelle surface or partially insert into the core, depending on the hydrophilicity of the respective drug, while hydrophobic API insert into the micellar core (Figure 4). In some instances, the hydrophobic drug itself is utilized as the lipophilic component of micelle-forming molecules. Self-assembly of these amphiphilic polymer-drug conjugates or prodrugs then creates the micellar drug carrier. The linker between drug and polymer in these conjugates is of essential importance because in case of an unstable linker the conjugate will be hydrolyzed before the drug reaches its target within the body. On the other hand, a non-biodegradable polymer-drug linker may yield an inactive conjugate. Even if the drug-polymer conjugate shows pharmacological activity, each conjugate would be considered a new entity by the FDA and would require extensive clinical testing. Nevertheless, at least seven drug-polymer conjugates were in phase I/II clinical trials by 2001, including drugs such as doxorubicin, paclitaxel, and camptothecin linked to polymeric N-(2-hydroxy-propyl)methacrylamide (HPMA). *(53,54)*

Loading of an API into the micelles follows different protocols. In case of drug-polymer conjugates, loading and micelle formation occur simultaneously. In the direct dissolution protocol of micelle formation, a copolymer solution is

12

added to a drug dried from organic solution or, alternatively, a drug dissolved in a volatile organic solvent is added to the preformed micelles in water, followed by removal of the organic solvent. In case of the dialysis approach, drug and copolymer are dissolved in an organic solvent and dialyzed against water. Here again, drug encapsulation and micelle formation occur simultaneously. Regardless of the loading mechanism, the partition coefficient P of the API between micelle and bulk solution determines the entrapment efficacy. The better the compatibility between loaded drug and core-forming block the higher are log P and the amount of encapsulated drug. This compatibility is based on drug characteristics such as polarity, hydrophobicity (HLB), and charge but also on the size of the micellar core. *(55)*

Release of an API from a polymeric micelle is either passive, caused by diffusion of the drug from the intact micelle, disintegration of the micelle due to dilution, or biodegradation of the copolymeric constituents; or the release is active, triggered by changes of external pH or temperature (stimuli-responsive micelles), similar to the release mechanisms described for liposomes. *(56-60)* The potential of polymeric micelle-based drug delivery can be exemplarily shown for taxol encapsulated into poly(ethylene glycol)-b-poly(D,L-lactic acid) micelles. The solubility of taxol increased from less than 0.1 to 20 mg/ml. Furthermore, the taxol-micelle complex was less toxic against normal organs and tissues than the free drug but had the same anti-tumor activity. *(61,62)* Examples of polymeric micelles used in drug delivery applications are listed in Table II.

Table II. Examples of polymeric micelles used in drug delivery applications. (Adapted from Ref. 33.)

Block copolymer	Drug
Pluronics®	doxorubicin, cisplatin, haloperidol
polycaprolactone-b-PEG	FK506, L-685,818
polycaprolactone-b-methoxy-PEG	Indomethacin
poly(aspartic acid)-b-PEG	doxorubicin, cisplatin, lysozyme
Poly(γ-benzyl-L-glutamate)-b-PEG	clonazepam
Poly(D,L-lactide)-b-methoxy-PEG	paclitaxel, testosterone
poly(β-benzyl-L-aspartate)-b-PEG	indomethacin, amphotericin B
poly(L-lysine)-b-PEG	DNA

As mentioned earlier, a main obstacle for the use of polymeric micelles in medical applications is their instability upon dilution below the CMC. Cross-linking the copolymers is a promising approach to increase micelle stability. This can be done either by direct reaction between adjacent chain segments or via addition of multifunctional crosslinking reagents. There are several potential locations to crosslink copolymers within micelles, (i) at the core chain ends, (ii) within the core domain, (iii) at the core-shell interface, (iv) throughout the shell, and (v) at the shell surface. Crosslinks within the core will increase the glass transition temperature of the core and, therefore, reduce its encapsulation capacity for drug molecules and lower the diffusion rate of their release. Crosslinks within the hydrated shell could affect its function as a steric stabilizer. Furthermore, the presence of water molecules, longer distances between the shell blocks, and their higher mobility might reduce the degree of polymerization. It could be anticipated that crosslinking the interphase between hydrophilic and hydrophobic blocks would provide stability while not adversely affecting the encapsulation and carrier properties of polymeric micelles. *(52,63)* These shell crosslinked (SCK) micelles are one approach to fabricate nanoparticles with defined dimensions. Hydrolysis of the linker between hydrophilic and hydrophobic blocks after crosslinking the interface, and removal of the hydrophobic moieties will create nanocapsules with dimensions that are determined by the dimensions of the micellar template (Figure 5). Other approaches to construct micro- and nanoparticles and capsules for delivery applications will be discussed in the next section.

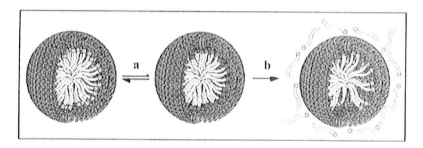

Figure 5. Crosslinking polymeric micelles at the core-shell interface creates shell crosslinked (SCK) nanoparticles (a). Hydrolysis and removal of the hydrophobic blocks transforms nanoparticles into nanocapsules (b). (Adapted from Ref. 52. Reproduced by permission of The Royal Society of Chemistry.)

Micro- and Nanoparticulate Drug Carriers

While the carriers discussed so far generally form through self-assembly of the constituent molecules, the formation of micro- and nanoparticles and containers strongly depends on the respective processing conditions. The fabrication of these carriers follows two major routes, one consists of the formation and stabilization of small particles, while the other route consists of the formation of a stabilized shell around a preexisting template that either remains a part of the construct (particle formation) or is removed in the final processing step (capsule formation). The diversity of the systems under investigation and the processes applied to fabricate these carriers make it quite challenging to provide a general overview of this research area.

Microparticles. Biodegradable microparticles used for drug delivery applications can be divided into natural and synthetic materials. Natural materials include polypeptides and proteins such as albumin, fibrinogen, gelatin, and collagen; polysaccharides such as hyaluronic acid, alginic acid, starch, and chitosan; virus envelopes and living cells, such as erythrocytes, genetically engineered fibroblasts and myoblasts. However, natural polymers usually vary in purity depending on their natural sources, and often require crosslinking in the microencapsulation process, which can lead to denaturalization of the polymer. This can result in product quality variations and potential immunogenic adverse reactions. Synthetic polymers, therefore, are preferable for the development of commercial products. These polymers include aliphatic polyesters of hydroxy acids such as poly(lactic acid) (PLA), poly(lactic-*co*-glycolic acid) (PLGA), poly (hydroxybutyric acid), poly(ε-caprolactone); poly(orthoesters); poly(alkylcarbonates); poly(amino acids); polyanhydrides; polyacrylamides; poly(alkyl-α-cyanoacrylates), and polyphosphates, to name a few examples. PLA and PLGA have received particular attention as microparticle materials because these polymers are biocompatible and currently being used as surgical sutures. Drug-containing microparticles can be divided into two categories, (i) homogeneous or monolithic particles, in which the drug is dissolved or dispersed throughout the polymer matrix (solid dispersion) and (ii) reservoir-type particles, in which drug monomers or small aggregates are surrounded by a polymer matrix. *(64-68)*

There are four main routes to prepare microparticles, (i) emulsion solvent evaporation, using oil-in-water (O/W) and water-in-oil (W/O) emulsions, and water-in-oil-in-water (W/O/W) double emulsions, (ii) phase separation processes, in which particle formation is triggered by addition of an anti-solvent to a solution, (iii) milling, and (iv) spray-drying, in which a solution stream breaks up into droplets while passing through a nozzle, followed by drying of the droplets prior to their collection. *(69-78)* The API is usually added at some point during the particle fabrication process and is encapsulated *in situ* while the particles form. The release of an API occurs via diffusion through aqueous channels or pores within the polymer matrix or during surface or bulk erosion of the carrier.

Trigger-mediated release mechanisms such as temperature and pH changes have been studied as well to improve control over the release process. *(64,80-88)*

Nanoparticles. The motivation to develop an alternative drug delivery system using nanoparticles instead of microparticles is based on several assumptions and observations. First, from a physical point of view the larger surface area-to-volume ratio of nanoparticles compared to microparticles should result in faster polymer degradation and drug release. However, this effect might not be as pronounced as expected, especially in the presence of components within a pharmaceutical formulation that could counteract this physical phenomenon. *(89)* Second, particles having a size below 100 nm can evade mechanical filtration from the blood stream and accumulation in liver, spleen and kidneys, resulting in longer blood circulation times. Third, nanoparticles are able to deliver API across a number of biological barriers, i.e., the blood-brain barrier (BBB), different types of mucosae and epithelia, and cell membranes for transfection applications. Fourth, nanoparticles show excellent adhesion to biological surfaces such as the epithelial gut wall, an advantage for sustained drug delivery. *(90-92)*

Preparation methods of nanoparticles are broadly divided into two categories, those based on physicochemical properties such as phase separation and solvent evaporation, and those based on chemical reactions such as polymerization and polycondensation. The first route is normally been used to produce nanoparticles from hydrophobic or crosslinked water-insoluble hydrophilic polymers, i.e., polylactic acid and its derivatives, cellulose derivatives, polyacrylate and polymethacrylate derivatives. For the second route, emulsion polymerization and precipitation polymerization have been applied as well as the preparation of nanoparticles from graft copolymers having a hydrophobic backbone and hydrophilic branches. *(93-99)* Alternative approaches include the preparation of nanoparticles via nanoemulsions, and the use of solid lipid nanoparticles (SLN) dispersed in water. *(100-102)* Drug encapsulation into and drug release from nanoparticles essentially follow the same protocols as discussed for microparticles.

Micro- and Nanocapsules. The last carrier types presented in this overview are micro- and nanocapsules. These carriers can be produced by crosslinking a preformed liposome or micelle and removal of the core molecules as described earlier (Figure 5). Alternatively, capsules can be made by encapsulation of a spherical template, i.e., a colloidal particle, oil droplet, liposome, or micelle by a polymer, stabilization of the shell by crosslinking and removal of the template, or by layer-by-layer deposition of oppositely charged polyelectrolytes around a template, followed by removal of the template. *(103-106)* Another approach to produce capsules involves an emulsion-diffusion method, in which oil droplets are fabricated using a high-speed stirrer and coated with a polymer. The oil core is removed by diffusion from the nanoparticle into the bulk solvent phase. *(107)*

Approaches to fabricate capsules, as well as encapsulation and release studies are discussed in detail in the chapters authored by Meier and coworker, Panzner and coworkers, and Sukhorukov.

Conclusions

This overview presents basic information about carrier systems utilized in the delivery of active pharmaceutical ingredients, i.e., liposomes, polymeric micelles, and micro- and nanoparticles. Methods to prepare the carriers as well as routes of drug encapsulation and release are discussed. The advantages and disadvantages of each carrier type are mentioned. As one can reasonably expect, there is no one carrier that fits all requirements but carriers have been developed that will address the needs of a specific API. The development of delivery systems is becoming more and more important and requires an interdisciplinary approach. The goal of this overview is to facilitate the understanding of the following, more specialized chapters for the non-specialized reader.

References

1. Greish, K.; Fang, J.; Inutsuka, T.; Nagamitsu, A.; Maeda, H. Macromolecular therapeutics – Advantages and prospects with special emphasis on solid tumor targeting. *Clinical Pharmacokinetics* **2003**, *42*, 1089-1105.
2. Maeda, H.; Fang, J.; Inutsuka, T.; Kitamoto, Y. Vascular permeability enhancement in solid tumor: Various factors, mechanisms involved and its implications. *Int. Immunopharm.* **2003**, *3*, 319-328.
3. Maeda, H.; Wu, J.; Sawa, T.; Matsumura, Y.; Hori, K. Tumor vascular permeability and the EPR effect in macromolecular therapeutics: A review. *J. Contr. Rel.* **2000**, *65(1-2)*, 271-284.
4. Park, J.W. Liposome-based drug delivery in breast cancer treatment. *Breast Cancer Res.* **2002**, *4*, 93-97.
5. Duncan, R. Polymer conjugates for tumor targeting and intracytoplasmic delivery. The EPR effect as a common gateway? *Pharm. Sci. Technol. Today* **1999**, *2*, 441-449.
6. Sapra, P.; Allen, T.M. Ligand-targeted liposomal anticancer drugs. *Progress in Lipid Res.* **2003**, *42*, 439-462.
7. Allen, T.M.; Sapra, P.; Moase, E.; Moreira, J.; Iden, D. Adventures in targeting. *J. Liposome Res.* **2002**, *12*, 5-12.
8. Torchilin, V.P. Drug targeting. *Europ. J. Pharm. Sci.* **2000**, *11*, S81-S91.
9. Lasic, D.D. Liposomes in drug delivery. In: *Vesicles*, Rosoff, M. Ed.; Marcel Dekker: New York, Basel, Hong Kong; Surfactant Science Series; Vol. 62, 1996, pp 447-476.

10. Gerasimov, O.V.; Rui, Y.; Thompson, D.H. Triggered release from liposomes mediated by physically and chemically induced phase transitions. In: *Vesicles*, Rosoff, M. Ed.; Marcel Dekker: New York, Basel, Hong Kong; Surfactant Science Series; Vol. 62, 1996, pp 679-746.

11. Allen, C.; Dos Santos, N.; .Gallagher, R.; Chiu, G.N.C.; Shu, Y.; Li, W.M.; Johnstone, S.A.; Janoff, A.S.; Mayer, L.D.; Webb, M.S.; Bally, M.B. Controlling the physical behavior and biological performance of liposome formulations through use of surface grafted poly(ethylene glycol). *Bioscience Reports*, **2002**, *22*, 225-250.

12. Lukyanov, A.N.; Gao, Z.G.; Mazzola, L.; Torchilin, V.P. Polyethylene glycol-diacyllipid micelles demonstrate increased accumulation in subcutaneous tumors in mice. *Pharm. Res.* **2002**, *19*, 1424-1429.

13. Guo, X.; Szoka, F.C. Steric stabilization of fusogenic liposomes by a low pH-sensitive PEG-diorthoester-lipid conjugate. *Bioconj. Chem.* **2001**, *12*, 291-300.

14. Koning, G.A.; Morselt, H.W.M.; Gorter, A.; Allen, T.M.; Zalipsky, S.; Scherphof, G.L.; Kamps, J.A.A.M. Interaction of differently designed immunoliposomes with colon cancer cells and Kupffer cels. An *in vitro* comparison. *Pharm. Res.* **2003**, *20*, 1249-1257.

15. Wang, S.; Lee, R.J.; Cauchon, G.; Gorenstein, D.G.; Low, P.S. Delivery of antisense oligodeoxyribonucleotides against the human epidermal growth-factor receptor into cultured KB cells with liposomes conjugated to folate via poly(ethylene glycol). *Proc. Natl. Acad. Sci. USA* **1995**, *92*, 3318-3322.

16. Reddy, J.A.; Low, P.S. Enhanced folate receptor mediated gene therapy using a novel pH-sensitive lipid formulation. *J. Contr. Rel.* **2000**, *64*, 27-37.

17. Hope, M.J.; Bally, M.B.; Webb, G.; Cullis, P.R. Production of large uni-lamellar vesicles by a rapid extrusion procedure – characterization of size distribution, trapped volume and ability to maintain a membrane potential. *Biochim. Biophys. Acta* **1985**, *812*, 55-65.

18. Mayer, L.D.; Reamer, J.; Bally, M.B. Intravenous pretreatment with empty pH-gradient liposomes alters the pharmacokinetics and toxicity of doxo-rubicin through *in vivo* active drug encapsulation. *J. Pharm. Sci.* **1999**, *88*, 96-102.

19. Guo, X.; MacKay, J.A.; Szoka, F.C. Mechanism of pH-triggered collapse of phosphatidylethanolamine liposomes stabilized by an ortho ester poly-(ethylene glycol) lipid. *Biophys. J.* **2003**, *84*, 1784-1795.

20. Li, S.; Huang, L. Targeted delivery of antisense oligodeoxynucleotides formulated in a novel lipid vector. *J. Liposome Res.* **1998**, *8*, 239-250.

21. For further references on pH-triggered release see chapters by Thompson and coworkers and Leroux and coworkers.

22. Needham, D.; Dewhirst, M.W. The development and testing of a new temperature-sensitive drug delivery system for the treatment of solid tumors. *Adv. Drug. Del. Rev.* **2001**, *53*, 285-305.

23. Huang, S.K.; Stauffer, P.R.; Hong, K.; Guo, J.W.H.; Phillips, T.L.; Huang, A.; Papahadjopoulos, D. Liposomes and hyperthermia in mice – increased tumor uptake and therapeutic efficacy of doxorubicin in sterically stabilized liposomes. *Cancer Res.* **1994**, *54*, 2186-2191.

24. Unezaki, S.; Maruyama, K.; Takahashi, N.; Koyama, M.; Yuda, T.; Suginaka, A.; Iwatsuru, M. Enhanced delivery and antitumor activity of doxorubicin using long-circulating thermosensitive liposomes containing amphipathic poly(ethylene glycol) in combination with local hyperthermia. *Pharm. Res.* **1994**, *11*, 1180-1185.

25. VanderMeulen, D.L.; Misra, P.; Michael, J.; Spears, K.G.; Khoka, M. Laser mediated release of dye from liposomes. *Photochem. Photobiol.* **1992**, *56*, 325-332.

26. Mueller, A.; Bondurant, B.; O'Brien, D.F. Visible light-stimulated destabilization of PEG-liposomes. *Macromol.* **2000**, *33*, 4799-4804.

27. Spratt, T.; Bondurant, B.; O'Brien, D.F. Rapid release of liposomal contents upon photoinitiated destabilization with UV exposure. *Biochim. Biophys. Acta-Biomembranes* **2003**, *1611*, 35-43.

28. Meers, P. Enzyme-activated targeting of liposomes. *Adv. Drug Deliv. Rev.* **2001**, *53*, 265-272.

29. Lasic, D.D. Ed.; *Liposomes: Physics to Applications*, Elsevier: Amsterdam, 1993.

30. Gregoriades, G. Ed.; *Liposome Technology*, CRC Press: Boca Raton, FL, 1993, Vol. I-III.

31. Lasic, D.D.; Martin, F.J. Eds.; *Stealth® Liposomes*, CRS Press: Boca Raton, FL, 1995.

32. Schreier, H.; Bouwstra, J. Liposomes and niosomes as topical drug carriers – dermal and transdermal drug delivery. *J. Contr. Rel.* **1994**, *30*, 1-15.

33. Torchilin, V.P. Structure and design of polymeric surfactant-based drug delivery systems. *J. Contr. Rel.* **2001**, *73*, 137-172.

34. Kwon, G.S.; Kataoka, K. Block copolymer micelles as long-circulating drug vehicles. *Adv. Drug Deliv. Rev.* **1995**, *16*, 295-309.

35. Yokoyama, M. Block copolymers as drug carriers. *Crit. Rev. Ther. Drug Carrier Syst.* **1992**, *9*, 213-248.

36. Alakhov, V.Y.; Kabanov, A.V. Block copolymeric biotransport carriers as versatile vehicles for drug delivery. *Expert. Op. Invest. Drugs* **1998**, *7*, 1453-1473.

37. Kwon, G.S. Diblock copolymer nanoparticles for drug delivery. *Crit. Rev. Ther. Drug Carrier Syst.* **1998**, *15*, 481-512.

38. For further references on polymeric micelles see chapters by Kabanov and coworkers and Torchilin and coworkers.

39. Rapoport, N. Stabilization and activation of Pluronic® micelles for tumor-targeted drug delivery. *Coll. Surf. B: Biointerf.* **1999**, *16*, 93-111.

40. Katayose, S.; Kataoka, K. Remarkable increase in nuclease resistance of plasmid DNA through supramolecular assembly with poly(ethylene glycol)-poly(L-lysine) block copolymer. *J. Pharm. Sci.* **1998**, *87*, 160-163.

41. Harada, A.; Kataoka, K. Novel polyion complex micelles entrapping enzyme molecules in the core. Preparation of narrowly-distributed micelles from lysozyme and poly(ethylene glycol)-poly(aspartic acid) block copolymer in aqueous medium. *Macromol.* **1998**, *31*, 288-294.

42. Kwon, G.S.; Naito, M.; Yokoyama, M.; Okano, T.; Sakurai, Y.; Kataoka, K. Block copolymer micelles for drug delivery: loading and release of doxorubicin. *J. Contr. Rel.* **1997**, *48*, 195-201.

43. Kataoka, K.; Matsumoto, T.; Yokoyama, M.; Okano, T.; Sakurai, Y.; Fukushima, S.; Okamoto, K.; Kwon, G.S. Doxorubicin-loaded poly(ethylene glycol)-poly(β-benzyl-L-aspartate) copolymer micelles: their pharmaceutical characteristics and biological significance. *J. Contr. Rel.* **2000**, *64*, 143-153.

44. Jeong, Y.I.; Cheon, J.B.; Kim, S.H.; Nah, J.W.; Lee, Y.M.; Sung, Y.K.; Akaike, T.; Cho, C.S. Clonazepam release from core-shell type nanoparticles *in vitro*. *J. Contr. Rel.* **1998**, *51*, 169-178.

45. Kim, S.Y.; Shin, I.G.; Lee, Y.M.; Cho, C.G.; Sung, Y.K. Methoxy poly(ethylene glycol) and ε-caprolactone amphiphilic block copolymeric micelle containing indomethacin. II. Micelle formation and drug release behaviors. *J. Contr. Rel.* **1998**, *51*, 13-22.

46. Allen, C.; Yu, Y.; Maysinger, D.; Eisenberg, A. Polycaprolactone-b-poly(ethylene oxide) block copolymer micelles as a novel drug delivery vehicle for neurotrophic agents FK506 and L-685,818. *Biocon. Chem.* **1998**, *9*, 564-572.

47. Hagan, S.A.; Coombes, A.G.A.; Garnett, M.C.; Dunn, S.E.; Davies, M.C.; Illum, L.; Davis, S.S. Polylactide-poly(ethylene glycol) copolymers as drug delivery systems. 1. Characterization of water-dispersible micelle-forming systems. *Langmuir* **1996**, *12*, 2153-2161.

48. Yasugi, K.; Nagasaki, Y.; Kato, M.; Kataoka, K. Preparation and characterization of polymer micelles from poly(ethylene glycol)-poly(D,L-lactide) block copolymers as potential drug carrier. *J. Contr. Rel.* **1999**, *62*, 89-100.

49. Kabanov, A.V.; Kabanov, V.A. Interpolyelectrolyte and block ionomer complexes for gene delivery: physico-chemical aspects. *Adv. Drug Deliv. Rev.* **1998**, *30*, 49-60.

50. Bronich, T.K.; Cherry, T.; Vinogradov, S.V.; Eisenberg, A.; Kabanov, V.A.; Kabanov, A.V. Self-assembly in mixtures of poly(ethylene oxide)-graft-poly(ethyleneimine) and alkyl sulfates. *Langmuir* **1998**, *14*, 6101-6106.

51. Bronich, T.K.; Popov, A.M.; Eisenberg, A.; Kabanov, V.A.; Kabanov, A.V. Effects of block length and structure of surfactant on self-assembly and solution behavior of block ionomer complexes. *Langmuir* **2000**, *16*, 481-489.

52. Murthy, K.S.; Ma, Q.G.; Clark, C.G.; Remsen, E.E.; Wooley, K.L. Fundamental design aspects of amphiphilic shell-crosslinked nanoparticles for controlled release applications. *Chem. Commun.* **2001**, 773-774.

53. Duncan, R.; Gac-Breton, S.; Keane, R.; Musila, R.; Sat, Y.N.; Satchi, R.; Searle, F. Polymer-drug conjugates, PDEPT and PELT: basic principles for design and transfer from the laboratory to clinic. *J. Contr. Rel.* **2001**, *74*, 135-146.

54. Harada, M.; Imai, J.; Okuno, S.; Suzuki, T. Macrophage-mediated activation of T-2513-carboxymethyl dextran conjugate (T-0128): possible cellular mechanism for antitumor activity. *J. Contr. Rel.* **2000**, *69*, 389-397.

55. Allen, C.; Maysinger, D.; Eisenberg, A. Nano-engineering block copolymer aggregates for drug delivery. *Coll. Surf. B: Biointerf.* **1999**, *16*, 1-35.

56. Chung, J.E.; Yokoyama, M.; Aoyagi, T.; Sakurai, Y.; Okano, T. Effect of molecular architecture of hydrophobically modified poly(N-isopropyl-acrylamide) on the formation of thermoresponsive core-shell micellar drug carriers. *J. Contr. Rel.* **1998**, *53*, 119-131.

57. Cammas, S.; Suzuki, K.; Sone, C.; Sakurai, Y.; Kataoka, K.; Okano, T. Thermoresponsive polymer nanoparticles with a core-shell micelle structure as site-specific drug carriers. *J. Contr. Rel.* **1997**, *48*, 157-164.

58. Meyer, O.; Papahadjopoulos, D.; Leroux, J.C. Copolymers of N-isopropyl-acrylamide can trigger pH sensitivity to stable liposomes. *FEBS Lett.* **1998**, *41*, 61-64.

59. Cai, Q.X.; Zhu, K.J.; Chen, D.; Gao, L.P. Synthesis, characterization and *in vitro* release of 5-aminosalicylic acid and 5-acetyl aminosalicylic acid of polyanhydride – P(CBFAS). *Eur. J. Pharm. Biopharm.* **2003**, *55*, 203-208.

60. De Jesus, O.L.P.; Ihre, H.R.; Gagne, L.; Frechet, J.M.J.; Szoka, F.C. Polyester dendritic systems for drug delivery applications: *In vitro* and *in vivo* evaluation. *Biocon. Chem.* **2002**, *13*, 453-461.

61. Ramaswamy, M.; Zhang, X.; Burt, H.-M.; Wasan, K.M. Human plasma distribution of free paclitaxel and paclitaxel associated with diblock copolymers. *J. Pharm. Sci.* **1997**, *86*, 460-464.

62. Zhang, X.; Burt, H.-M.; Mangold, G.; Dexter, D.; Von Hoff, D.; Mayer, L.; Hunter, W.L. Anti-tumor efficacy and biodistribution of intravenous polymeric micellar paclitaxel. *Anticancer Drugs* **1997**, *8*, 696-701.

63. Thurmond II, K.B.; Huang, H.; Clark Jr., C.G.; Kowalewski, T.; Wooley, K.L. Shell cross-linked polymer micelles: stabilized assemblies with great versatility and potential. *Coll. Surf. B: Biointerf.* **1999**, *16*, 45-54.

64. Okada, H. Preface. *Adv. Drug Del. Rev.* **1997**, *28*, 1-3.

65. Peniche, C.; ArguellesMonal, W.; Peniche, H.; Acosta, N. Chitosan: An attractive biocompatible polymer for microencapsulation. *Macromol. Biosci.* **2003**, *3*, 511-520.

66. Anderson, J.M.; Shive, M.S. Biodegradation and biocompatibility of PLA and PLGA microspheres. *Adv. Drug Del. Rev.* **1997**, *28*, 5-24.

67. Bernkop-Schnurch, A.; Egger, C.; Imam, M.E.; Krauland, A.H. Preparation and *in vitro* characterization of poly(acrylic acid)-cysteine microparticles. *J. Contr. Rel.* **2003**, *93*, 29-38.

68. Chaubal, M.V.; Sen Gupta, A.; Lopina, S.T.; Bruley, D.F. Polyphosphates and other phosphorus-containing polymers for drug delivery applications. *Crit. Rev. Ther. Drug Carrier Syst.* **2003**, *20*, 295-315.

69. O'Donnell, P.B.; McGinity, J.W. Preparation of microspheres by the solvent evaporation technique. *Adv. Drug Del. Rev.* **1997**, *28*, 25-42.

70. Cleland, J.L. Solvent evaporation processes for the production of controlled release biodegradable microsphere formulations for therapeutics and vaccines. *Biotechnol. Prog.* **1998**, *14*, 102-107.

71. Castellanos, I.J.; Griebenow, K. Improved α-chymotrypsin stability upon encapsulation in PLGA microspheres by solvent replacement. *Pharm. Res.* **2003**, *20*, 1873-1880.

72. Meng, F.T.; Ma, G.H.; Qiu, W.; Su, Z.G. W/O/W double emulsion technique using ethyl acetate as organic solvent: Effects of its diffusion rate on the characteristics of microparticles. *J. Contr. Rel.* **2003**, *91*, 407-416.

73. Couvreur, P.; Blanco-Prieto, M.J.; Puisieux, F.; Roques, B.; Fattal, E. Multiple emulsion technology for the design of microspheres containing peptides and oligopeptides. *Adv. Drug Del. Rev.* **1997**, *28*, 85-96.

74. Sugiura, S.; Nakajima, M.; Iwamoto, S.; Seki, M. Interfacial tension driven monodispersed droplet formation from microfabricated channel array. *Langmuir* **2001**, *17*, 5562-5566.

75. Weidenauer, U.; Bodmer, D.; Kissel, T. Microencapsulation of hydrophilic drug substances using biodegradable polyesters. Part I: Evaluation of different techniques for the encapsulation of pamidronate di-sodium salt. *J. Microencapsulation* **2003**, *20*, 509-524.

76. Ando, S.; Putnam, D.; Pack, D.W.; Langer, R. PLGA microspheres containing plasmid DNA: Preservation of supercoiled DNA via cryopreparation and carbohydrate stabilization. *J. Pharm. Sci.* **1999**, *88*, 126-130.

77. Elkharraz, K.; Dashevsky, A.; Bodmeier, R. Microparticles prepared by grinding of polymeric films. *J. Microencapsulation* **2003**, *20*, 661-673.

78. Cortesi, R.; Menegatti, E.; Esposito, E. Spray-drying production of trypsin-containing microparticles. *STP Pharma Sci.* **2003**, *13*, 329-334.

79. Huang, Y.C.; Yeh, M.K.; Cheng, S.N.; Chiang, C.H. The characteristics of betamethasone-loaded chitosan microparticles by spray-drying method. *J. Microencapsulation* **2003**, *20*, 459-472.

80. Chung, T.-W.; Huang, Y.-Y.; Liu, Y.-Z. Effects of the rate of solvent evaporation on the characteristics of drug-loaded PLLA and PDLLA microspheres. *Int. J. Pharm.* **2001**, *212*, 161-169.

81. Berkland, C.; Kim, K.; Pack, D.W. PLG microsphere size controls drug release rate through several competing factors. *Pharm. Res.* **2003**, *20*, 1055-1062.

82. Mi, F.L.; Shyu, S.S.; Lin, Y.M.; Wu, Y.B.; Peng, C.K.; Tsai, Y.H. Chitin/PLGA blend microspheres as a biodegradable drug delivery system: A new delivery system for protein. *Biomater.* **2003**, *24*, 5023-5036.

83. Jeong, J.C.; Lee, J.; Cho, K. Effects of crystalline microstructure on drug release behavior of poly(ε-caprolactone) microsperes. *J. Contr. Rel.* **2003**, *92*, 249-258.

84. Castelli, F.; Giunchedi, P.; La Camera, O.; Conte, U. A calorimetric study on diflunisal release from poly(lactide-co-glycolide) microspheres by monitoring the drug effect on dipalmitoylphosphatidylcholine liposomes: Temperature and drug loading influence. *Drug Delivery* **2000**, *7*, 45-53.

85. Eichenbaum, G.M.; Kiser, P.F.; Simon, S.A.; Needham, D. pH and ion-triggered volume response of anionic hydrogel microspheres. *Macromol.* **1998**, *31*, 5084-5093.

86. Victor, S.P.; Sharma, C.P. Stimuli-sensitive poly(methacrylic acid) microparticles (PMAA) – Oral insulin delivery. *J. Biomater. Appl.* **2002**, *17*, 125-134.

87. Ko, J.A.; Park, H.J.; Park, Y.S.; Hwang, S.J.; Park, J.B. Chitosan micro-particle preparation for controlled drug release by response surface methodology. *J. Microencapsulation* **2003**, *20*, 791-797.

88. Kohane, D.S.; Anderson, D.G.; Yu, C.; Langer, R. pH-triggered release of macromolecules from spray-dried polymethacrylatemicroparticles. *Pharm. Res.* **2003**, *20*, 1533-1538.

89. Panyam, J.; Dali, M.A.; Sahoo, S.K.; Ma, W.X.; Chakravarthi, S.S.; Amidon, G.L.; Levy, R.J.; Labhasetwa, V. Polymer degradation and *in vitro* release of a model protein from poly(D,L-lactide-*co*-glycolide) nano- and microparticles. *J. Contr. Rel.* **2003**, *92*, 173-187.

90. Kreuter, J. Nanoparticulate systems for brain delivery of drugs. *Adv. Drug Del. Rev.* **2001**, *47*, 65-81.

91. Koziara, J.M.; Lockman, P.R.; Allen, D.D.; Mumper, R.J. In-situ blood-brain barrier transport of nanoparticles. Pharm. Res. 2003, 20, 1772-1778.

92. Takeuchi, H.; Yamamoto, H.; Kawashima, Y. Mucoadhesive nano-particulate systems for peptide drug delivery. *Adv. Drug Del. Rev.* **2001**, *47*, 39-54.

93. Sakuma, S.; Hayashi, M.; Akashi, M. Design of nanoparticles composed of graft copolymers for oral peptide delivery. *Adv. Drug Del. Rev.* **2001**, *47*, 21-37.

94. Rouzes, C.; Leonard, M.; Durand, A.; Dellacherie, E. Influence of poly-meric surfactants on the properties of drug-loaded PLA nanospheres. *Coll. Surf. B: Biointerf.* **2003**, *32*, 125-135.

95. Panoyan, A.; Quesnel, R.; Hildgen, P. Injectable nanospheres from a novel multiblock copolymer: cytocompatibility, degradation, and *in vitro* release studies. *J. Microencapsulation* **2003**, *20*, 745-758.

96. Peltonen, L.; Koistinen, P.; Hirvonen, J. Preparation of nanoparticles by nanoprecipitation of low molecular weight poly(L-lactide). *STP Pharma Sci.* **2003**, *13*, 299-304.

97. Muramatsu, N.; Nakauchi, K. A novel method to prepare monodisperse microcapsules. *J. Microencapsulation* **1998**, *15*, 715-723.

98. Cai, T.; Hu, Z.B.; Ponder, B.; St. John, J.; Moro, D. Synthesis and study of and controlled release from nanoparticles and their networks based on functionalized hydroxypropylcellulose. *Macromol.* **2003**, *36*, 6559-6564.

99. Eerikainen, H.; Kauppinen, E.I. Preparation of polymeric nanoparticles containing corticosteroid by a novel aerosol flow reactor method. *Int. J. Pharm.* **2003**, *263*, 69-83.

100. Müller, R.H.; Jacobs, C.; Kayser, O. Nanosuspensions as particulate drug formulations in therapy: rationale for development and what we can expect for the future. *Adv. Drug Del. Rev.* **2001**, *47*, 3-19.

101. Lippacher, A.; Müller, R.H.; Mäder, K. Semisolid SLN^{TM} dispersions for topical application: Influence of formulation and production parameters on viscoelastic properties. *Eur. J. Pharm. Biopharm.* **2002**, *53*, 155-160.

102. Bondi, M.L.; Fontana, G.; Carlisi, B.; Giammona, G. Preparation and characterization of solid lipid nanoparticles containing cloricromene. *Drug Del.* **2003**, *10*, 245-250.

103. Couvreur, P.; Barratt, G.; Fattal, E.; Legrand, P.; Vauthier, C. Nanocapsule technology: A review. *Crit. Rev. Ther. Drug Carrier Syst.* **2002**, *19*, 99-134.

104. Watnasirichaikul, S.; Rades, T.; Tucker, I.G.; Davies, N.M. Effects of formulation variables on characteristics of poly(ethylcyanoacrylate) nanocapsules from w/o microemulsions. *Int. J. Pharm.* **2002**, *235*, 237-246.

105. Muller, C.R.; Bassani, V.L.; Pohlmann, A.R.; Michalowski, C.B.; Petrovick, P.R.; Guterres, S.S. Preparation and characterization of spray-dried polymeric nanocapsules. *Drug Develop. Ind. Pharm.* **2000**, *26*, 343-347.

106. Sukhorukov, G.B.; Antipov, A.A.; Voigt, A.; Donath, E.; Möhwald, H. pH-controlled macromolecule encapsulation in and release from polyelectrolyte multilayer nanocapsules. *Macromol. Rapid Commun.* **2001**, *22*, 44-46.

107. Guinebretiere, S.; Briancon, S.; Lieto, J.; Mayer, C.; Fessi, H. Study of the emulsion-diffusion of solvent: Preparation and characterization of nanocapsules. *Drug Develop. Res.* **2002**, *57*, 18-33.

Liposomes and Tubules as Carrier Systems

Chapter 2

Stimuli-Responsive Liposome–Polymer Complexes

Toward the Design of Intelligent Drug Carriers

Emmanuelle Roux[1,2], Mira Francis[1,2], Françoise M. Winnik[2,3], and Jean-Christophe Leroux[1,2,*]

[1]Canada Research Chair in Drug Delivery, [2]Faculty of Pharmacy, and [3]Department of Chemistry, Université de Montréal, C.P. 6128 Succ. Centreville, Montréal, Québec H3C 3J7, Canada
*Corresponding author: email: Jean-Christophe.Leroux@unmontreal.ca

Drug delivery systems capable of releasing active compounds in response to stimuli such as pH or temperature changes have attracted increasing interest in recent years. Among these systems, pH-sensitive liposomes have been studied extensively. These vesicles are generally stable at neutral pH and become leaky and/or fusogenic under acidic conditions. In this work, we describe the preparation of pH-sensitive phospholipid (liposomes) and non-phospholipid vesicles (niosomes) through the formation of pH-sensitive polymer/bilayer complexes. The vesicles are characterized with respect to their pH-sensitivity, stability in serum, pharmacokinetics and *in vitro* ability to deliver a model compound to the cytoplasm.

Introduction

Liposomes are widely studied as drug delivery systems in many biomedical applications, such as anticancer and gene/antisense therapies. Liposomes are phospholipid vesicles that can encapsulate either hydrophilic or amphiphilic drugs in their inner core or lipophilic drugs within their bilayers. The encapsulation of drugs in such carriers presents several advantages, among which one can cite sustained delivery, passive accumulation at certain disease sites, and the possibility of active targeting through ligand-mediated systems. Progress in this field has led to the approval of anthracycline liposomal formulations for cancer treatment, such as Doxil®, Evacet™ and DaunoXome®. In these cases, enhanced therapeutic index derives from the reduction of drug distribution volume and passive carrier accumulation at the tumor site by the so-called "enhanced permeation and retention" (EPR) effect. *(1)* However, the development of a more effective liposomal formulation is still needed in order to achieve better drug availability at the target site. While amphiphilic drugs such as anthracyclines are able to cross cell membranes, highly hydrophilic and high molecular weight compounds, which cannot diffuse freely through biological membranes, may benefit from internalization by cells. Specific targeting to cell surface receptors having the ability to trigger the internalization of liposomes by endocytosis has been shown to improve the efficacy of liposomal drugs. *(2)* Such systems could be further improved by targeting specific cell compartments. Genetic material and highly water-soluble drugs remain generally sequestrated in the endocytic compartment and are ultimately delivered to lysosomes, where they can be degraded by different enzymes. *(3)* As the endosomal pH (5.0-6.5) is more acidic than that of extracellular fluids, the control of intracellular drug trafficking can be achieved with pH-responsive carriers. pH-Sensitive liposomes are colloidal vesicles that become destabilized in an acidic environment, releasing their content prior to reaching the lysosomes. In addition, these liposomes may facilitate cytoplasmic delivery of the drug by fusing with and/or destabilizing the endosomal membrane. The fate of pH-sensitive liposomes upon receptor-mediated endocytosis is illustrated in Figure 1.

The first generation of pH-sensitive liposomes was obtained through the use of non-bilayer-forming lipids, such as dioleoylphosphatidylethanolamine (DOPE), that are stabilized in the lamellar phase by the addition of mildly acidic amphiphiles (i.e., oleic acid). Upon protonation of the negatively charged head group of the amphiphile in an acidic environment, DOPE reverts to non-bilayer structures, causing the release of the liposomal content. However, the instability of such vesicles constitutes a major drawback for possible *in vivo* applications, as rapid content leakage or substantial loss of pH-sensitivity has been observed in biological fluids. *(4,5)*

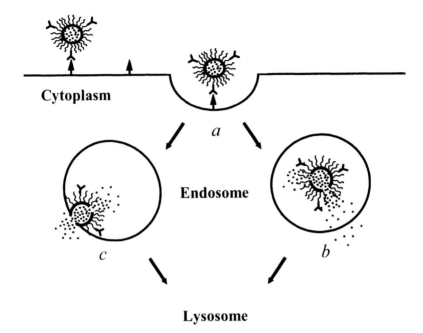

Cytoplasm

a

Endosome

c

b

Lysosome

Figure 1. After receptor-mediated internalization (a), polymer-based, pH-sensitive vesicles are destabilized in the endosome and release their contents (b). Vesicles can also fuse with the endosomal membrane and/or destabilize it (c).

An alternative approach to intrinsically pH-sensitive liposomes consists of coating conventional liposomes with pH-responsive polymers. Such polymers are generally weak acidic polyelectrolytes, and their ability to destabilize liposome membranes depends, among others, on their degree of ionization. One of the advantages of polymer-based systems is that almost any liposomal formulation can acquire pH-sensitive properties. This is an important feature since, in theory, liposomal compositions demonstrating high stability and prolonged circulation times *in vivo* can be rendered pH-sensitive.

We have already shown that copolymers of *N*-isopropylacrylamide (NIPAM) bearing randomly distributed hydrophobic alkyl chains and pH-sensitive units, such as methacrylic acid (MAA) or glycine acrylamide (Gly), can confer pH-sensitivity to intrinsically-stable liposomes. *(6-8)* Indeed, NIPAM copolymer-modified egg phosphatidylcholine (EPC), EPC/cholesterol (Chol), and EPC/Chol/distearoylphosphatidylethanolamine-*N*-methoxy poly(ethylene glycol) (DSPE-PEG) liposomes can efficiently release their content under mildly acidic conditions. *(6,7)* The versatility of NIPAM copolymers has also been exploited to prepare pH-sensitive niosomes. *(9)* Niosomes are vesicles that are structurally related to liposomes but consist mainly of non-ionic surfactants.

They were first introduced for cosmetic applications. *(10)* Because non-ionic surfactants are less susceptible to hydrolysis than phospholipids, the use of niosomes in drug delivery may offer an interesting alternative to liposomes. *(11)* Moreover, some amphiphiles in niosome formulations (i.e., polyoxyethylene alkyl ether) may be involved in hydrogen bonding with the structural units of the polymer chain, a characteristic that can be exploited to strengthen the polymer affinity to the vesicle surface. *(12)*

The ultimate goal of this research is to produce a serum-stable, long-circulating vesicle/polymer complex that will efficiently deliver its content to the cytoplasm after endocytosis. This chapter summarizes some of our recent progress in the design, preparation and assessment of pH-sensitive vesicles (liposomes and niosomes), modified with NIPAM copolymers.

Materials and Methods

Polymer synthesis. Randomly and terminally alkylated NIPAM copolymers were prepared by free radical polymerization as described previously, using MAA or Gly as pH-sensitive moieties. *(13,14)* The selected hydrophobic anchors were octadecylacrylate (ODA), octadecylacrylamide (ODAM) (randomly alkylated polymers), and dioctadecylamide (DODA) (terminally alkylated polymer). *N*-vinylpyrrolidone (VP) was added in some polymers to maintain their water solubility. The chemical structures of the polymers and their composition are shown at the end of this section in Figure 2 and Table I, respectively.

In vitro release. Unilamellar distearoylphosphatidylcholine (DSPC)/Chol and EPC/chol (3:2 molar ratio) liposomes were prepared by mechanical dispersion of lipids in buffer, followed by repeated extrusion through polycarbonate filters of varying pore sizes (50-200 nm). The fluorescent marker trisodium 8-hydroxypyrene trisulfonate (HPTS) and the collisional fluorescence quencher *p*-xylene-bis-pyrimidium bromide were co-encapsulated in the liposomes. The copolymers were incubated overnight at 4°C with the liposomes. Free copolymer was removed by size exclusion chromatography over Sepharose 2B (column i.d. 1 cm, length 23 cm) equilibrated in Hepes-saline buffer (20 mM Hepes, 144 mM NaCl). Release of the entrapped fluorescent dye was measured as described elsewhere. *(6)* The loss of liposomal pH-sensitivity after 1-h incubation in 75% (*v/v*) human serum at 37°C was also investigated after separation of the liposomes from excess serum components, using a Sepharose 2B column.

Cytoplasmic delivery of calcein. J774 murine macrophage-like cells (a generous gift from Professor Alain Petit, Lady Davis Institute for Medical Research, Montréal, Qc, Canada) were grown in RPMI 1640 medium (Invitrogen Corp.) supplemented with 5% heat-inactivated fetal bovine serum (FBS) and containing 100 units/mL penicillin G and 100 µg/mL streptomycin (Invitrogen). J774 cells were plated in 6-well tissue culture plates (1 mL RPMI-FBS containing 3 x 10^5 viable cells) and allowed to adhere and proliferate for 24 h. They were rinsed twice with phosphate-buffered saline (PBS, pH 7.2) and incubated for 1 h in RPMI. Liposomes composed of 1-palmitoyl-2-oleyl-phosphatidylcholine/Chol (POPC/Chol, 3:2 molar ratio) and loaded with 120 mM calcein were prepared as described above. The copolymer was added during the liposome preparation process at a polymer/lipid ratio of 0.3% (w/w). After solvent evaporation, the dried lipid/polymer film was hydrated in an isotonic calcein solution. Untrapped marker was removed by passage over Sephadex G100 column equilibrated with Hepes/Dextrose buffer (20 mM Hepes/5% (w/v) dextrose). The cells were incubated with 0.5 mM liposomes for 4 h at 37 °C, rinsed twice with cold PBS, and viewed with an Axiovert inverted microscope equipped with a fluorescence illuminator (λ_{ex}=435-485 nm, λ_{em}= 515-555 nm, Zeiss). Photographs were obtained with a 1310C DVC digital camera (DVC Company, Inc.).

Pharmacokinetics. *In vivo* studies were performed on male Sprague-Dawley rats (300-350 g, Charles River), which were prepared surgically for intravenous administration and arterial blood sampling. Polyethylene catheters, inserted into the femoral vein and artery, were protected with a tethering system, and the rats were allowed to recover for at least 24 h. Liposomes (30 mM lipids, 180-230 nm, unimodal size distribution) containing ^{67}Ga were prepared by hydrating the lipid film with a ^{67}Ga citrate solution (2 mCi/mL) that was previously neutralized (pH 7.5-8.5). After removal of the free ^{67}Ga, a 400-µL sample (10 µmol lipids/kg) was administered via the venous cannula. Blood samples (400 µL) were collected, and ^{67}Ga levels were measured by γ-counting (Cobra II auto-gamma counting system, Packard Instrument Company). Areas under the curve of blood concentration versus time (AUC_∞) were calculated for the different formulations using PK Solutions 2.0 software (Summit Research Services). These animal studies were approved by the Canadian Council on Animal Care and in-house ethics committee.

Results and Discussion

In vitro pH-triggered release of vesicle/polymer complexes

Liposomes composed of high phase transition lipids. PNIPAM are characterized in water by a lower critical solution temperature (LCST) of about 32°C, at which the polymer solution undergoes phase separation. *(15)* By adding an acidic comonomer, such as MAA or Gly, it is possible to achieve pH-dependency of the LCST. Complexation to vesicles of randomly alkylated NIPAM copolymers containing MAA (Figure 2A) have been shown to trigger the content release of various fluid phase liposomal formulations, and the pH-

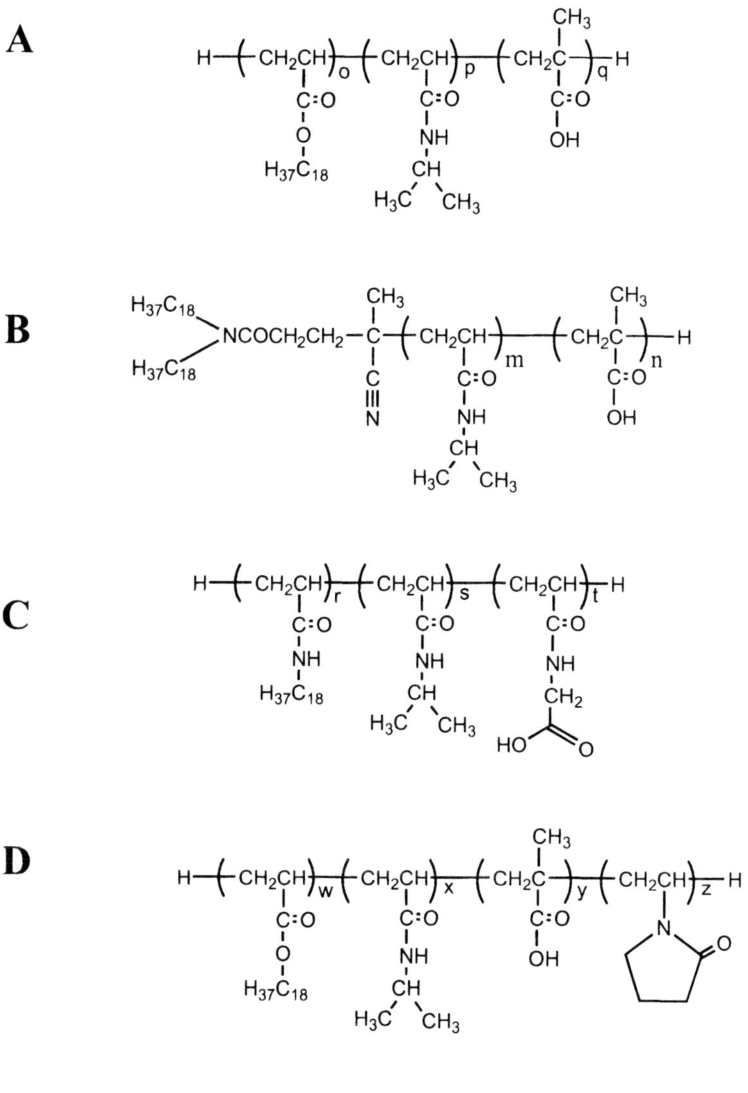

A

B

C

D

Figure 2. Structures of copolymers P(NIPAM-co-MAA-co-ODA) (A), DODA-P(NIPAM-co-MAA) (B), P(NIPAM-co-Gly-co-ODAM) (C), and P(NIPAM-co-MAA-co-ODA-co-VP) (D).

32

Table I. Characteristics of different pH-sensitive formulations and AUC after their i.v. administration in rats.

Entry	Liposome formulation (mol:mol)[a]	Polymer composition[b]	MW[c] [kDa]	AUC$_\infty$ ± SD[d]	Ref.
A	DSPC/Chol (3:2)	-		36 ± 4	
B	DSPC/Chol (3:2)	DODA-P(NIPAM$_{95}$-co-MAA$_5$)	29	37 ± 10	
C	EPC/Chol (3:2)	-		8 ± 3	*(18)*
D	EPC/Chol (3:2)	DODA-P(NIPAM$_{95}$-co-MAA$_5$)	8.2	12 ± 4	*(18)*
E	EPC/Chol (3:2)	P(NIPAM$_{90}$-co-MAA$_4$-co-ODA$_4$-co-VP$_2$)	22.6	15 ± 5	*(19)*
F	EPC/Chol/PEG-PE (3:2:0.3)	P(NIPAM$_{90}$-co-MAA$_4$-co-ODA$_4$-co-VP$_2$)	22.6	50 ± 4	*(19)*
G	EPC/Chol/PEG-PE (3:2:0.15)	P(NIPAM$_{90}$-co-MAA$_4$-co-ODA$_4$-co-VP$_2$)	22.6	20 ± 4	*(19)*

[a] Liposome size: 180-230 nm, unimodal size distribution.

[b] Numbers in subscript refer to the molar proportion of each unit.

[c] The weight-average molecular weight of the polymers was determined by gel permeation chromatography performed in tetrahydrofuran using polystyrene standards for calibration.

[d] ([% injected dose]-h/mL).

content release of such vesicles has been correlated with the phase transition pH of the copolymer. *(6, 7)* However, liposomes constituted of low phase transition lipids, such as EPC, generally have a lower stability in biological fluids than those composed of high phase transition lipids, such as DSPC (T_m = 55°C). *(16)* As serum stability is a prerequisite for the development of a viable liposomal drug delivery system, we attempted to confer pH-sensitivity to DSPC/Chol lipo-somes with a terminally alkylated NIPAM copolymer (Figure 2B and Table 1, B). As shown in Figure 3, it was possible to trigger the release of HPTS from these liposomes coated with copolymer B at pH 4.9. Maximum release (53%) at acidic pH was obtained with the copolymer anchored to 200-nm liposomes. When the liposome size was reduced to 100 nm, the dye release was less pronounced despite faster kinetics. The higher release observed with large liposomes may be explained by a lesser extent of copolymer desorption from liposomes that have a lower degree of curvature. The liposomes were found to be stable in 90% human serum in the presence or absence of the copolymer (data not shown). Some pH-sensitivity was lost after incubation in serum. At pH 4.9, only 15% of HPTS was released from 200-nm liposomes *vs* 53% before incubation in serum. There was a shift in the destabilization pH with 37% of HPTS released at pH 4.3 (Figure 4). These results indicate that part of the polymer may be extracted from the liposome surface by serum components.

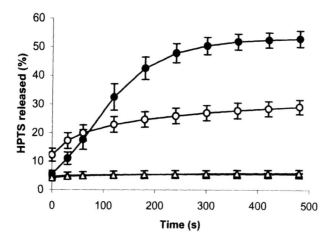

Figure 3. Percent HPTS release from DSPC/Chol liposomes bearing DODA-P(NIPAM$_{95}$-co-MAA$_5$) over time at 37°C at pH 7.4 (triangles) and 4.9 (circles). Solid symbols: 200-nm liposomes; empty symbols: 100-nm liposomes.

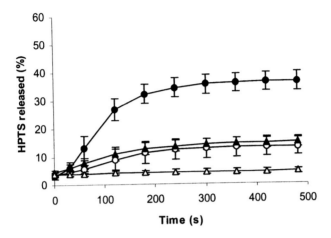

Figure 4. Percent HPTS release from 200-nm liposomes bearing DODA-P(NIPAM₉₅-co-MAA₅) over time at 37°C at pH 7.4 (empty triangles), 4.9 (empty circles), 4.6 (solid triangles), and 4.3 (solid circles) after 1-h (37°C) incubation in human serum.

Niosomes. Since poor retention of the copolymer into the liposome bilayers seems to limit the stability of liposome/polymer complexes, niosomes (*n*-octadecyldiethylene oxide/Chol) were evaluated for the preparation of pH-sensitive vesicles with increased affinity for the copolymer. Indeed, Polozova and Winnik have reported that randomly alkylated NIPAM copolymers interacted differently with non-phospholipid vesicles compared to liposomes. *(12)* It was demonstrated that although the addition of a cationic amphiphile in niosomes (dimethyldioctadecylammonium bromide) increased their affinity to the copolymer by means of attractive electrostatic forces, the main driving force for polymer binding involved hydrogen bonding. Complexation with niosomes also involved the entire surface of the vesicles. The hydroxy and ether groups of the main amphiphile used in the niosome formulation participate in hydrogen bonding with the amide group of NIPAM units. Figure 5 displays possible interactions between a randomly alkylated, pH-sensitive NIPAM copolymer and the niosome bilayer. In contrast, complexation between the copolymer and liposomes was mainly driven by hydrophobic interactions between the alkyl chains (anchor) and the bilayers.

Niosomes (*n*-octadecyltriethylene oxide/Chol) modified with an alkylated NIPAM/Gly copolymer (Figure 2C, NIPAM/Gly/ODAM; 93:5:2 molar ratio) were also shown to release their content under acidic conditions. However, the pH required for destabilization was higher than the pH at which the polymer collapsed in solution in contrast to the case of the polymer-coated liposomes. *(9)*

It is believed that hydrogen bonding with niosomes changed the pH of coil-to-globule transition of the copolymer, presumably by changing its hydration state. The strong interactions that occur between niosomes and the copolymer were expected to provide better anchoring of the polymer in bilayers and, consequently, greater stability of this system in biological fluids. Unfortunately, niosome/polymer complexes were found to be leaky in serum and did not maintain their pH-sensitivity. *(9)*

Liposomes composed of low phase transition lipids. To increase the affinity of the copolymer for the liposome bilayer, its composition was modified

Hydrogen Bonds:

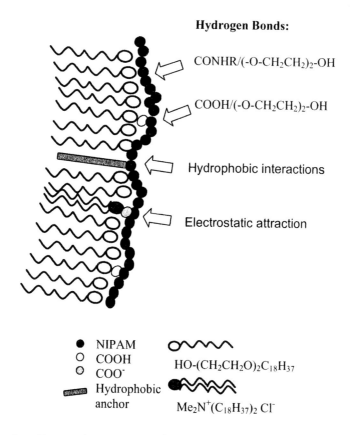

CONHR/(-O-CH$_2$CH$_2$)$_2$-OH

COOH/(-O-CH$_2$CH$_2$)$_2$-OH

Hydrophobic interactions

Electrostatic attraction

- ● NIPAM
- ○ COOH
- ○ COO⁻
- ▨ Hydrophobic anchor

HO-(CH$_2$CH$_2$O)$_2$C$_{18}$H$_{37}$

Me$_2$N$^+$(C$_{18}$H$_{37}$)$_2$ Cl⁻

Figure 5. Proposed interactions between a cationic niosome and a pH-sensitive, randomly alkylated NIPAM copolymer (for clarity only half a bilayer is shown and cholesterol has been omitted). (Reproduced from Polozova and Winnik (12), with permission from the American Chemical Society).

to strengthen anchoring in liposomal membranes. Thus, the proportion of hydrophobic anchoring (ODA) was increased from 2 to 4 mol%. Furthermore, VP was added as a co-monomer in order to increase the water-solubility of the polymer (Figure 2D). When incubated with preformed liposomes, this copolymer (NIPAM/ODA/VP/MAA; 90:4:4:2 molar ratio) did not bind efficiently to the lipid bilayer, as demonstrated indirectly by the low pH-triggered release from vesicles. *(17)* However, higher binding could be achieved by incorporating the polymer during the liposome preparation procedure. In this case, relatively high content release (59%) was obtained at acidic pH (pH 4.9) with EPC/Chol liposomes. Moreover, this formulation has been found to maintain its pH-sensitivity after 1-h incubation in serum, with 46% content release at pH 4.9. *(17)*

In vitro cytoplasmic delivery

Intracellular delivery of calcein encapsulated in liposomes coated with the above-mentioned copolymer was studied using J774 macrophage-like cells. Figure 6 shows that liposomes bearing NIPAM copolymer can increase cytoplasmic delivery of the fluorescent dye as cells treated with pH-sensitive liposomes present a diffuse fluorescence (Figure 6B). However, cells treated with the non-pH-sensitive control formulation display more punctuated fluorescence (Figure 6A), suggesting sequestration of the liposomes in endosomes/lysosomes.

The ability of this polymer to increase the cytoplasmic delivery of liposomal content was also demonstrated with cytosine arabinofuranoside (ara-C), an anticancer drug that is susceptible to degradation by lysosomal enzymes. Rapid release of ara-C in endosomes is expected to enhance its efficiency. *(3)* Indeed, compared to non-pH-sensitive liposomes, ara-C was found to be more toxic toward J774 cells when delivered with EPC/Chol liposomes (4:1 molar ratio) coated with the pH-sensitive copolymer (LD_{50} = 23 *vs* 8 μM, respectively). *(17)*

Pharmacokinetics. Since long circulation time is a prerequisite for the passive accumulation of liposomal carriers at tumoral sites, the pharmacokinetics of different pH-sensitive formulations was investigated. The AUC_∞ obtained are summarized in Table I. Coating of DSPC/Chol liposomes with terminally alkylated NIPAM copolymer did not change their circulation time (Table I, A and B). This might result from fast removal of the polymer in blood, as confirmed by the loss of pH-sensitivity of liposomes observed after incubation in serum (see above section). Fluid phase liposomes are known to be less stable *in vivo*, and this is apparent from the AUC_∞ of EPC/Chol liposomes, which is 4 times lower than DSPC/Chol AUC_∞ (Table 1, A and C). However, the presence of a terminally or randomly alkylated copolymer (Table 1, D and E) on the liposome surface slightly increased the circulation time of EPC/Chol liposomes (50 and 88% increase in the AUC_∞, respectively). In the case of the terminally alkylated copolymer, we have shown that the polymer anchored at the liposomal surface provides a steric barrier below its LCST. *(18)* As NIPAM copolymers had

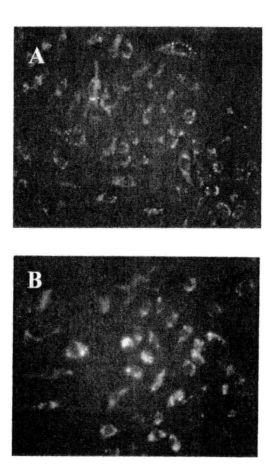

Figure 6. Fluorescence micrographs of J774 macrophage-like cells treated with vesicles containing calcein. (A) Naked POPC/Chol liposomes; (B) POPC/Chol liposomes coated with P(NIPAM$_{90}$-co-VP$_4$-co-MAA$_2$-co-ODA$_4$).

marginal effect on liposome pharmacokinetics, a poly(ethylene glycol)-phosphatidylethanolamine lipid (PEG-PE) was added to the formulation. *(19)* The presence of PEG at the liposome surface is known to slow liposomal clearance by the mononuclear phagocyte system. *(20,21)* PEG efficiently prolonged the liposome circulation time but a significant decrease in the liposome pH-sensitivity was also observed (Table 1, F and G). *(19)* PEG was found to produce a similar effect on DOPE-based liposomes. *(22)*

Conclusions

Studies described in this chapter show that liposomes made with low or high phase transition temperature lipids as well as niosomes can be rendered pH-sensitive by coating with NIPAM copolymers. Binding of the polymer to niosomes probably occurs *via* hydrogen bonding. However, in serum, niosome/polymer complexes were found to be leaky and to lose their pH-sensitivity. NIPAM copolymers could facilitate the cytoplasmic transfer of liposomal contents but alone did not provide liposomes with a circulation time long enough for passive tumor targeting. Future work will consist of modulating the copolymer composition, to design a liposomal formulation with a long half-life and good pH-responsiveness.

Acknowledgements

This work was financially supported by the Canadian Institutes of Health Research (CIHR) (JCL), the Natural Sciences and Engineering Council of Canada (FMW), and the Canada Research Chair Program. JCL acknowledges a scholarship from the Fonds de la Recherche en Santé du Québec.

References

1. Maeda H.; Wu J.; Sawa T.; Matsumura Y.; Hori K. *J. Controlled Release* **2000**, *65*, 271-284.
2. Park J.W.; Hong K.; Kirpotin D.B.; Papahadjopoulos D.; Benz C.C. *Adv. Pharmacol.* **1997**, *40*, 399-435.
3. Huang A.; Kennel S.J.; Huang L. *J. Biol. Chem.* **1983**, *258*, 14034-14040.
4. Senior J.H. *Crit. Rev. Ther. Drug Carrier Syst.* **1987**, *3*, 123-193.
5. Collins D.; Litzinger D.C.; Huang L. *Biochim. Biophys. Acta* **1990**, *1025*, 234-242.
6. Meyer O.; Papahadjopoulos D.; Leroux J.C. *FEBS Lett.* **1998**, *42*, 61-64.
7. Zignani M.; Drummond D.C.; Meyer O.; Hong K.; Leroux J.-C. *Biochim. Biophys. Acta* **2000**, *1463*, 383-394.
8. Winnik F.M.; Principi T. In *Stimuli-responsive water soluble and amphiphilic polymers*; McCormick C.L., Ed.; ACS symposium series 780; American Chemical Society: Washington, DC. 2000 pp. 277-297.
9. Francis M.F.; Dhara G.; Winnik F.M.; Leroux J.-C. *Biomacromolecules* **2001**, *2*, 741-749.
10. Handjani-Vila R.M.; Ribier A.; Rondot B.; Vanlerberghe G. *Int. J. Cos. Sci.* **1979**, *1*, 303-314.
11. Kemps J.M.A.; Crommelin D.J.A. *Pharm. Weekbl.* **1988**, *123*, 355-363.

12. Polozova A.; Winnik F.M. *Langmuir* **1999**, *15*, 4222-4229.
13. Leroux J.-C.; Roux E.; Le Garrec D.; Hong K.; Drummond D.C. *J. Controlled Release* **2001**, *72*, 71-84.
14. Spafford M.; Polozova A.; Winnik F.M. *Macromolecules* **1998**, *31*, 7099-7102.
15. Heskins M.; Guillet J.E. *J. Macromol. Sci. Chem.* **1968**, *A2*, 1441-1455.
16. Senior J.; Gregoriadis G. *Life Sci.* **1982**, *30*, 2123-2136.
17. Roux E.; Francis M.; Winnik F.M.; Leroux J.-C. *Int. J. Pharm.* **2002**, *In press*.
18. Roux E.; Stomp R.; Giasson S.; Pézolet M.; Moreau P.; Leroux J.-C. *J. Pharm. Sci.* **2002**, *91*, 1795-1802.
19. Roux E.; Lafleur M.; Lataste E.; Moreau P.; Leroux J.-C. Canada Research Chair in Drug Delivery; Faculty of Pharmacy; Department of Chemistry. Université de Montréal. *Unpublished data.*
20. Lasic D.; Martin F.J.; Gabizon A.; Huang S.K.; Papahadjopoulos D. *Biochim. Biophys. Acta* **1991**, *1070*, 187-192.
21. Papahadjopoulos D.; Allen T.M.; Gabizon A.; Mayhew E.; Matthay K.; Huang S.K.; Lee K.D.; Woodle M.C.; Lasic D.D.; Redemann C.; Martin F.J. *Proc. Natl. Acad. Sci. USA* **1991**, *88*, 11460-11464.
22. Slepushkin V.A.; Simoes S.; Dazin P.; Newman M.S.; Guo L.K.; Pedroso de Lima M.C.; Düzgünes N. *J. Biol. Chem.* **1997**, *272*, 2382-2388.

Chapter 3

Proniosome-Derived Niosomes for the Delivery of Poorly Soluble Drugs

David G. Rhodes[1,3] and Almira Blazek-Welsh[2]

[1]Lipophile Consulting, 93 Timber Drive, Storrs, CT 06268
[2]University of Connecticut, Storrs, CT 06269
[3]Current address: PowderJect Vaccines, Inc., 585 Science Drive, Madison, WI 53711 (email: David.Rhodes@powderject.com)

A novel approach to delivery of hydrolyzable, poorly soluble drugs is described. The method is based on a liposome production method using "proniosomes." These proniosomes consist of maltodextrin powder coated with surfactant or a surfactant/drug mixture to yield a dry powder. Upon addition of hot water and brief agitation, the maltodextrin dissolves and the surfactant forms a suspension of multilamellar vesicles (niosomes) containing the poorly soluble drug. The niosomes slowly release drug into solution. The proniosome powder can also be mixed with hydrogel powder. Adding hot water to the mixed powders allows formation of a hydrogel in which niosomes spontaneously form. The niosome-containing hydrogel can be formulated as a gel that will degrade and release intact niosomes or as a stable gel, which slowly releases the drug from niosomes that remain in side the gel matrix.

Introduction

Because many pharmaceutical actives are poorly soluble, formulating them has been an ongoing problem for pharmaceutical scientists. Poorly soluble drugs can be formulated as oil-filled capsules or emulsions, for example, or can be chemically modified by conversion to salts or prodrugs. In addition to solubility concerns, some drugs are susceptible to hydrolysis and must be protected from water in their formulation and packaging. One approach to formulating poorly soluble drugs is to use liposomes. *(1)* The number of approved lipid-based drug formulations has been slowly increasing, but there remain certain stability issues. Liposomes are large particles and tend to precipitate out of suspension upon prolonged storage. Depending upon the chemical composition and physical properties of the liposomes, they can also aggregate, thus exacerbating the precipitation problem. In addition to these physical stability issues, liposome suspensions can suffer from chemical instability due to the presence of water. Hydrolysis of the surfactant can result in destabilization of the liposomes and/or alteration of the release properties of the suspension. Hydrolysis of the active can result in inactivation of the product and thus a shortened shelf life.

Liposomes can be produced by any of a number of methods and the properties of the resulting liposomes will be determined by the choice of method. The most common approach involved drying surfactant (lipid) from organic solvent into a thin film (Figure 1). *(2)* The drying is normally performed in a round bottom flask on a rotary evaporator so the surface area available for the film is typically on the order of 10^2 cm^2 and the films are tens of μm thick. Once the film has been thoroughly dried, it can be rehydrated with aqueous medium at a temperature above the phase transition temperature (T_m). The lipid film takes up water and begins to swell. In the absence of agitation, very large unilamellar vesicles can form as large "blebs" before breaking off into solution. *(3)* With agitation, shearing forces result in formation of multilamellar vesicles. The time of agitation required to recover the lipids from the surface of the flask can be significant and the size distribution of the multilamellar vesicles can be broad and poorly reproducible. Further processing of the multilamellar vesicles to form unilamellar vesicles of desired size is possible.

Liposomes can be used to formulate soluble drugs by entrapping the drugs in the aqueous solvent between lipid bilayers or the aqueous volume inside unilamellar vesicles. *(1)* Because the aqueous volume per lipid is smaller in multilamellar vesicles than in unilamellar vesicles, unilamellar vesicle are often preferred for drugs with good solubility. In liposomal formulations of poorly soluble drugs, the drug can be partitioned into the bilayer interior or at the bilayer interfacial region between the aqueous exterior and the hydrophobic core. For uniformly non-polar molecules, x-ray and neutron diffraction experiments have demonstrated that the molecules partition to the bilayer center, while amphiphilic drugs stay near the bilayer surface. *(4)* The association of poorly soluble drugs with liposomes is thus a partitioning process rather than an entrapment per se, but calculations of "entrapment efficiency" do not normally make this distinction.

Vesicles can also be formed using nonionic surfactants such as Span 60, but these are more stable if some ionic surfactant and/or cholesterol is added. Nonionic surfactant liposomes, referred to as "niosomes", have been widely studied and are used in commercial preparations. Niosomes are normally multi-lamellar and are formed using a methodology similar to that used for liposomes. *(5)* The advantages usually cited for using nonionic surfactants include cost of materials, availability, and chemical stability.

The dosage forms described in this chapter were designed to overcome several significant issues encountered in formulating drugs in liposomes. In particular, (a) the formulation allows liposomes or niosomes to be produced "as needed," hydrating the suspension only when ready to use, (b) significantly reduces the agitation time required to form the liposomes, (c) improves the quality and consistency of the resulting liposomes or niosomes, (d) allows for flexibility in the dosing, and (e) provides a platform for new dosage forms based on the proniosome system. The system is suitable for use with nonionic surface-tants or phospholipids, but the data described here are for nonionic surfactants, and the text refers to "niosomes".

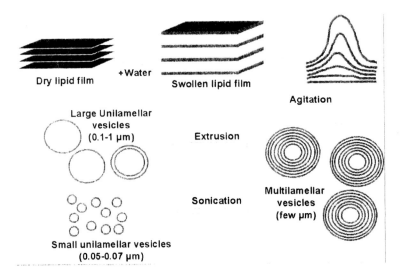

Figure 1. Hydration of a dry lipid film above the phase transition temperature T_m and subsequent agitation yields multilamellar vesicles, which can then be further processed.

Results and Discussion

Proniosome-Based Niosomes

Most proniosome-based niosomes are mixtures of Span 60 (mixture of sorbitan stearate and palmitate), cholesterol, and dicetyl phosphate. These nonionic surfactant-based systems are less expensive than phospholipid-based systems and are generally less susceptible to degradation of the surfactant. Nevertheless, some of the same problems persist. If a suspension is made ahead of time, there is a risk of physical or chemical instability. If the formulation is hydrated "as needed," problems of lengthy rehydration time, inconsistent reconstitution, and lack of flexibility in the dose are still present. Hu and Rhodes demonstrated that niosomes could be produced from a dry, sorbitol-based formulation. *(6)* In this system, a sorbitol powder was sprayed with surfactant in chloroform and dried. Because the sorbitol was soluble in chloroform, however, the process required repeated spray/dry cycles so that the powder morphology was not significantly altered. Compared to the conventional approach, in which surfactant is dried onto the inner surface of a glass container, this approach provided a much higher surface area, and thus a much thinner coating. The niosomes were reconstituted by adding aqueous buffer at 60°C and agitating the mixture (Figure 2). Compared to conventional niosomes, the proniosome-derived niosomes were slightly smaller and more uniform in size (Figure 3). For the model systems tested, hydrophilic drugs were not entrapped efficiently, but hydrophobic drugs could easily be included in these multilamellar niosomes. Release of the entrapped drug was slightly slower than observed for conventional niosomes.

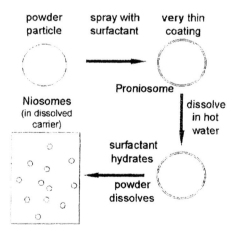

Figure 2. Proniosomes are a dry formulation made by coating a water-soluble "carrier" powder with a thin film of surfactant. Rehydration of the dry proniosome preparation by addition of a hot aqueous phase and brief agitation results in the formation of multilamellar vesicles in a dilute solution of carrier.

44

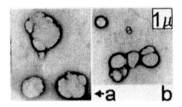

Figure 3. Niosomes produced using conventional methods (a) and derived from proniosomes (b).

Aside from the difficulty of repeated spray/dry cycles, one of the most signifycant problems with this system was the presence of residual carrier. The presence of large amounts of dissolved sorbitol was observed to affect the entrapment of drug. A large number of alternative substrates was explored (see acknowledgements), including soluble and insoluble materials. Eventually, a material was identified that was soluble in water but not in chloroform, the solvent used to dissolve the surfactants. *(7)* Maltodextrin, obtained from GPC, is available as solid particles (Maltrin QD M500) with a bulk density 0.34 g/cm^3 or hollow particles (Maltrin M700) with a bulk density of 0.13 g/cm^3 (Figure 4).

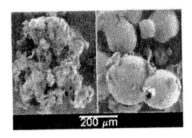

Figure 4. Electron micrographs of maltodextrin powder. The solid powder (M500, left) has a rough texture, while the hollow-blown powder (M700, right) is a thin, smooth shell.

The surface area of the hollow product was estimated to be 8000 cm^2/g, approximately 20 times greater than that of M500. Because the powders were insoluble in chloroform, the preparation was very simple. The desired proportions of surfactant and poorly soluble drug in a chloroform solvent were added to maltodextrin powder in a rotary evaporator flask. The mixture was subjected to agitation and vacuum to remove the solvent, resulting in a dry powder. The powder, surfactant coated maltodextrin, was then kept under vacuum overnight to assure that the solvent was completely removed. Niosomes were made by adding hot (60°C) water to a vial of proniosome powder and shaking the vial for at least one minute. It was important to keep the temperature of the aqueous solvent above the main phase transition temperature T_m, while agitation beyond two minutes did not appear to have an effect on the quality of the niosomes. One parameter which affected the quality of the niosomes was the loading of maltodextrin with surfactant. In the presence of excess surfactant, the maltodextrin surface becomes depleted and the dried film becomes unacceptably thick. Too little surfactant results in good quality niosomes, but the proportion of residual carrier would be higher. Good quality niosomes were easily obtained at 10-15 mM surfactant per gram of maltodextrin carrier, although higher loads (20-25 mM/g) could produce acceptable results. *(8)* At very high loading (>25 mM/g), adhesion of surfactant to carrier could not be maintained. Under these conditions, large surfactant fragments, which appeared to have been "cast" on spherical maltodextrin particles were observed. The resulting niosomes were harder to hydrate and were of very poor quality, similar to niosomes which were obtained from direct hydration of surfactant powder. Based on images of pro-niosomes with different surfactant loading (Figure 5), there appeared to be a correlation between thin, uniform coating and the quality of the niosomes. The advantage of using a carrier to increase the surface area is lost if the surfactant load results in a thick, irregular surface with a texture similar to that of surfactant powder.

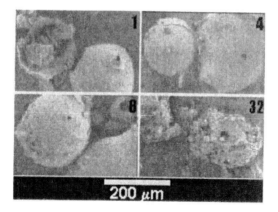

Figure 5. Maltodextrin-based proniosomes. The surfactant loadings shown here are 0.5 mmol/g (1x), 2 mmol/g (4x), 4 mmol/g (8x), and 16 mmol/g (32x).

Proniosome and Hydrogel Powder Mixtures

To extend the potential of this approach, a novel concept was tested in which proniosome powder was mixed with hydrogel powders such as agarose or gellan. The question in these experiments was whether the presence of the hydrogel polymer would compromise the ability of the surfactant to self-assemble into niosomes. Similarly, it was possible that the presence of surface-tant would affect the gelling ability of the hydrogel polymer. To prepare the gels (Figure 6), proniosome powder and hydrogel powder were blended in a test tube by vortex mixing. Hot aqueous phase (buffer or water) was added while vor-texing, and the tubes were maintained at high temperature in a heating block for several minutes. The temperature and the time of continued heating varied with the choice of hydrogel, and initial conditions were determined by manufacturer's recommendations. The tubes were removed frequently and vortexed to assure uniform hydration and swelling and to prevent settling.

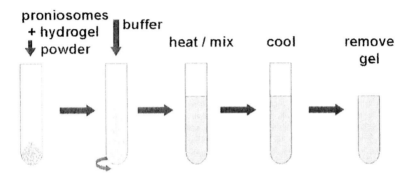

Figure 6. Process for making niosome-containing hydrogels. The aqueous phase is added at elevated temperature (> T_m), while the powder mixture is being agitated. Continued heating of the mixture is required in order to obtain gellation. In some cases, rapid cooling (i.e., on ice) is required in order to avoid settling.

Niosomes formed in the hydrogel in all cases tested. Using light micro-scopy, gel-entrapped proniosome-derived niosomes (GEProDeN) could be directly observed. Using a flourescent dye as a model "drug" allowed direct observation of the drug distribution of using fluorescence microscopy. For dyes with relatively good water solubility, fluorescence was observed in the niosomes and in the surrounding hydrogel. The relative distribution of dye appeared to be consistent with entrapment data determined for free niosomes. Poorly soluble fluorescent dye could be included in the formulation by adding the dye to the solution of surfactact in organic solvent. In this case, the dye was expected to be entrapped in the niosomes and not in the hydrogel. Fluorescence and brightfield microscopy showed that the presence of dye fluorescence correlated with the location of niosomes (Figure 7).

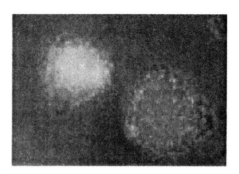

Figure 7. Gel-entrapped-proniosome-derived-niosomes (GEProDeN) stained with Sudan 4 dye. This is an exposure with dual illumination, including brightfield (green) illumination and epifluorescence (orange) illumination. This method shows that the locations of the niosomes and the entrapped dye are correlated. (See page 1 of color insert.)

Experiments were also performed with various types of ionic and zwitter-ionic lipids, including phospholipids. In all cases, proliposomes could be made from these lipids, and the proliposomes were suitable for forming multilamellar liposomes. In most cases, these proniosomes could be used to make gel-entrapped-proliposome-derived-liposomes. Work is ongoing to evaluate appli-cations for these formulations.

Drug release from the hydrogel appears to occur by two mechanisms. Figure 8 shows that for soluble drug, the release is by both free diffusion of drug and by release of niosomes from the hydrogel matrix. For GEProDEN (Figure 8a), the release medium contains free drug in solution similar to that observed for drug-only hydrogels (Figure 8b) and a niosome suspension (as evidenced by light scattering) similar to that observed in control GEProDEN samples with no drug (Figure 8c).

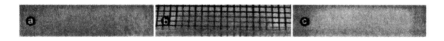

Figure 8. Eosin Yellowish-release from GEProDEN (a) and from hydrogel (b). A blank niosome-containing gel is shown in panel (c). The grid behind the samples is visible only in the sample which does not contain niosomes. These images were obtained after 6 hours. (See page 1 of color insert.)

These observations indicate that if the drug is soluble, direct diffusion of free drug from the hydrogel occurs with a timecourse similar to that observed with drug-only hydrogels. In addition, a later release of drug-containing nio-somes occurs as the hydrogel begins to degrade. Some control over the release

48

rates can be obtained by selection of the hydrogel material and concentration. The distribution of the drug between the niosomes and the hydrogel is passive, and is thus determined largely by the surfactant concentration in the formulation.

For GEProDEN with poorly soluble drug, the only release mechanism is release of drug in niosomes as the hydrogel degrades. The concentation of free drug is negligible and the only significant drug is that associated with the hydrophobic domains of the niosomes. Figure 9 shows that after 6 hours, the drug is visible in the dissolution medium only when it is in the form of niosomes (Figure 9a). In control samples containing only free drug and hydrogel, there is no detectable absorbance characteristic of the drug in the dissolution medium.

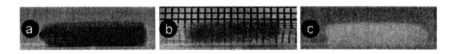

Figure 9. GEProDEN containing Sudan 4, a poorly soluble drug. The drug is only released in niosomes (a), not as free drug (b). As seen in panels (a) and (c), light scattering due to release of niosomes obscures the grid behind the sample. (See page 1 of color insert.)

Conclusions

There are many possible drug delivery applications for niosomes or for GEProDEN. Advantages of proniosome-based or proliposome-based formulations include the ability to solubilize poorly soluble actives, stability enhancement obtained through a dry formulation, which is hydrated only when needed, dose flexibility, and most of the advantages of conventional liposomal formulations. This proniosome formulation has also been tested using phospholipids, and multilamellar liposomes can be produced with this formulation. A large number of carrier powders have been tested, but the maltodextrin carrier is the best choice so far. Because this carrier is not soluble in chloroform, our organic solvent of choice, the process is very straightforward, and it is possible to scale up this method for bulk production. In its present stage of development, this approach appears to be best suited for the formulation of lipophilic drugs, especially in the case where these drugs are susceptible to hydrolysis. *In vivo* experiments are not yet underway, but to appreciate the full potential of the formulation, these experiments will be required in order to determine biodistribution and other properties. Similarly, further testing of the GEProDEN formulation will be required to evaluate its full potential.

Acknowledgements

The authors wish to thank Adeniyi Fisayo, Mary Besl, Camille Persaud, Linh Pham, Phuong Tang, and Jose Cordero, who were all undergraduate research fellows with Dr. Rhodes and contributed to the niosome work. The original work of Chengjiu Hu is also gratefully acknowledged. Material contributions from Grain Products Corporation (Muscatine IA) were greatly appreciated.

References

1. Betageri, G.; Jenkins, S.; Parsons, D. *Liposome Drug Delivery Systems* Technomic Publishing Co. Inc., Lancaster, PA **1993**.
2. Bangham, A.; Standish, M.; Watkins *J. Mol. Biol.* **1965**, *13*, 238-252.
3. Decher, G.; Ringsdorf, H.; Venzmer, J.; Bitter-Suermann, D.; Weisberger, C. *Biochim. Biophys. Acta* **1990**, *1023*, 357-364.
4. Herbette, L.; Rhodes, D.G.; Mason, R. *Drug Design And Delivery* **1991**, *7*, 75-118.
5. Yoshioka T.; Sternberg, B.; Florence, A. *Int. J. Pharmaceutics* **1994**, *105*, 1-6.
6. Hu,C.; Rhodes, D.G. *Int. J. Pharmaceutics* **1999**, *185*, 23 - 35.
7. Blazek-Welsh, A.I.; Rhodes, D. G. *PharmSci* **2001**, *3*, 1-8.
8. Blazek-Welsh, A.I.; Rhodes, D. G. *Pharmaceutical Research* **2001**, *18*, 656-661.

Chapter 4

Intracellular Delivery of DNA and Proteins Using Vinyl Ether-Based Drug Delivery Vehicles

Junhwa Shin and David H. Thompson*

Department of Chemistry, Purdue University, West Lafayette, IN 47907–1393
***Corresponding author: email: davethom@purdue.edu**

Liposomal carriers are an attractive approach for drug delivery due to their biocompatibility and their large loading capacities for either hydrophilic or hydrophobic drugs. Liposomal drug formulations have been slow to penetrate the marketplace because of limited stability and site-specific delivery, and inefficient drug release at the site of action. Our group has developed an efficient drug delivery strategy using acid- or photooxidatively labile plasmenyl-type liposomes. Cleavage of these lipids leads to morphology changes of the liposomal membrane. These phase transitions have been used to promote intracellular drug delivery. For example, cyto-toxic drugs (Ara-C and $AlPcS_4^{4-}$) were successfully delivered via folate-targeted DPPlsC liposomes. The cytotoxicity of these formulations was significantly higher than free drug, non-targeted liposomal drug, or targeted acid-insensitive liposomal drug controls. These results clearly show the synergistic effect of combined targeting and triggering.

Introduction

Liposomal drug delivery has been developed during the last 36 years from Bangham's original discovery of liposomes to a commercially viable delivery vehicle. Liposomal carriers possess good biocompatibility and large drug loading capacities, however, widespread applications of liposomes have been limited by low plasma stability and inefficient drug release at the site of action. Many efforts have focused on solving these limitations, leading to the advent of sterically stabilized liposome that incorporated targeting and triggering strategies. *(1)*

An essential requirement of efficient triggerable liposomes is that they display both compositional and mechanical stability during plasma circulation, yet become unstable upon exposure to an applied stimulus such that they undergo a structural transformation and promote rapid release of contents at the target area. Our work has centered on the development of new efficient triggerable materials using naturally occurring plasmenyl-type lipids con-taining acid- and photooxidatively labile (*Z*)-vinyl ether linkages. The chemical cleavage of these (*Z*)-vinyl ether groups and subsequent physical transformation of the bilayer membrane structure are our essential strategy in the triggered drug delivery. These chemical and physical changes of plasmenyl-type liposomes have been extensively studied in our group. Recent biological studies of these triggerable liposomes show that plasmenyl-type liposomes are very promising drug carriers.

Materials and Methods

Plasmenylcholine (PlsC) and diplasmenylcholine (DPPlsC) were prepared as described in detail elsewhere. *(2,3)* Bacteriochlorophyll (Bchla, Sigma), calcein (Sigma), and chloroaluminium phthalocyanine tetrasulfonate ($AlPcS_4^{4-}$, Porphyrin Products) were used as received. Large unilamellar liposomes were prepared by extrusion, and the rate of contents release monitored using the calcein fluorescence dequenching assay. *(4,5)*. KB cells (a human naso-pharyngeal cancer cell line) were cultured for several weeks in folate-deficient modified Eagle's medium (FDMEM).

Results and Discussion

Triggering Strategy Based On Plasmenylcholine And Diplasmenylcholine

Plasmenylcholines (PlsC) are phospholipids with a (*Z*)-vinyl ether bond in *sn*-1 position and an acyl chain in *sn*-2 position of the glycerol backbone. *(6)* PlsC is predominantly found in electrically active tissues such as brain, heart, and myelin, and is known to be involved in cell signaling, membrane fusion, and lipid peroxidation. *(5,7-11)* Diplasmenylcholine (DPPlsC), having two (Z)-vinyl ether bonds in *sn*-1 and *sn*-2 positions, has only been found in rabbit acrosomal membranes. *(12)* The (Z)-vinyl ether bond is stable at neutral and high pH, however, it is easily cleaved by acid-catalyzed hydrolysis below pH 6.0 or by $^1O_2$-mediated photooxidation (Figure 1). Our group has utilized these chemical transformations as the basis for triggering contents release from plasmenyl-type lipid carrier systems. *(5,13-15)* For example, plasmenyl-cholines form stable lamellar phase liposomes in neutral aqueous solutions, however, after cleaving the vinyl ether bonds the double chain plasmenyl-cholines become single chain lipids. This reaction induces a spontaneous transition from lamellar phase liposomes to micellar phase structures that introduce transient membrane defects, enabling encapsulated contents release.

Plasmenyl-type Lipid Synthesis

Plasmenylcholines are generally obtained as mixtures of alkyl chain lengths at the *sn*-1 and *sn*-2 positions, requiring tedious HPLC separation and/or semi-synthesis to obtain discrete PlsC species. The absence of pure PlsC lipids has greatly limited the study of their biochemical and biophysical properties. We sought to develop a facile synthetic pathway to obtain pure plasmenyl-type lipids. Unfortunately, their synthesis is made difficult because (i) the naturally occurring (Z)-vinyl ether bond must be formed stereoselectively to avoid tedious purification of geometric isomers, and (ii) the vinyl ether bond is unstable toward acidic or oxidative conditions, which limits the choice of reagents and isolation conditions that can be employed. Rui and Thompson developed the first synthetic pathway to pure PlsC and DPPlsC with (Z)-vinyl ether stereospecificity via transformation of acylglycerols to the corresponding vinyl phosphates, followed by reductive cleavage (Figure 2a,b). *(2,3)* Recently, Shin and Thompson have developed more facile synthetic pathways using the reductive cleavage of vinyl acetal as a key step for the stereospecific formation of (Z)-vinyl ether bonds. This approach has also been applied to the synthesis of PlsC (Figure 2c). *(16)*

Photooxidative Triggering

Phototriggering of liposomal contents release is a very attractive approach to drug delivery since a broad range of adjustable parameters (i.e. intensity, wavelength, duration) is available to optimize the drug release. *(17)* In addition, the triggering site can be controlled externally to avoid release of cytotoxic agents in the vicinity of normal cells.

The near infrared (NIR)-absorbing sensitizer bacteriochlorophyll (BChla) has been chosen as the trigger since NIR can penetrate tissue more deeply than short wavelength light (i.e. visible or UV). PlsC liposomes containing BChla within the lipid bilayer were irradiated at 800 nm and the rate of contents release was monitored using the calcein fluorescence dequenching assay. *(5)* The

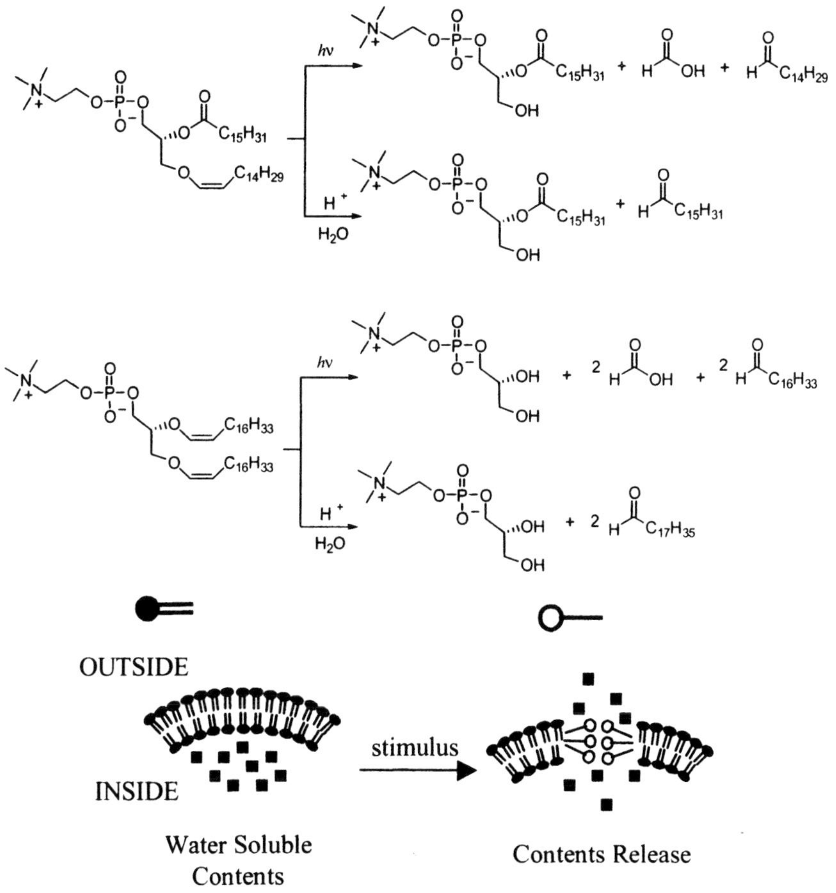

Figure 1. Plasmenylcholine and diplasmenylcholine cleavage pathways under acid- or photooxidative conditions (top), and the resulting L_α-H_I phase change and contents release (bottom).

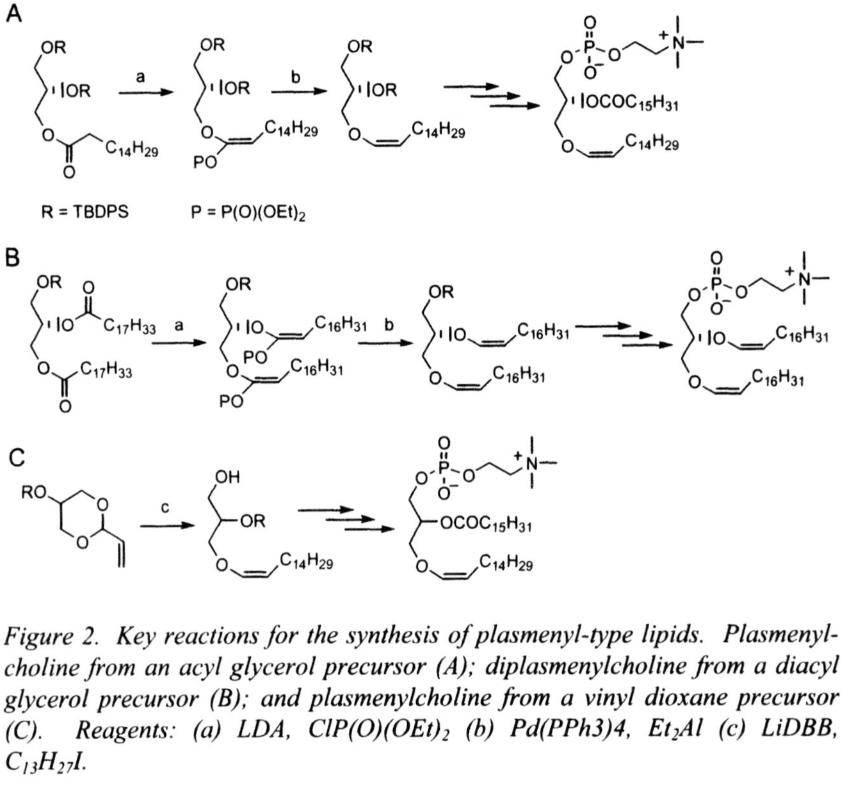

Figure 2. Key reactions for the synthesis of plasmenyl-type lipids. Plasmenyl-choline from an acyl glycerol precursor (A); diplasmenylcholine from a diacyl glycerol precursor (B); and plasmenylcholine from a vinyl dioxane precursor (C). Reagents: (a) LDA, ClP(O)(OEt)$_2$ (b) Pd(PPh3)4, Et$_2$Al (c) LiDBB, C$_{13}$H$_{27}$I.

observed calcein release rates are light-intensity dependent (i.e. at 20 min, 300 mW excitation produced 100% release vs. 60% release at 140 mW). No calcein was release during control studies in the absence of light, sensitizer, or oxygen (Figure 3a). Transmission electron micrographs (TEM) indicated a change of the liposome morphology during the course of photolysis (Figure 3b). Small unilamellar vesicles (SUV; I) fused to form large unilamellar vesicles (LUV; II) and multilamellar vesicles (MLV; II), ultimately leading to the formation of multilamellar structures (III) as a result of continuous membrane-membrane fusion events.

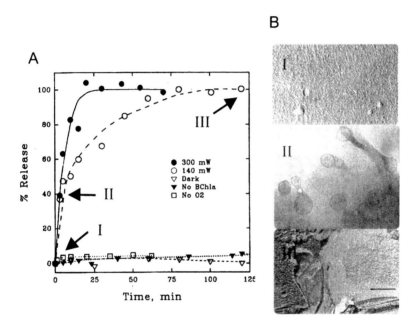

Figure 3. Calcein release from Bchla-PlsC liposomes irradiated at 800 nm excitation under various experimental conditions (A). Freeze-fracture TEM before liposome irradiation (I); cryo-TEM 5 minutes after liposome irradiation (II); freeze-fracture TEM 48 hours after liposome irradiation (III) (B).

Acid-Catalyzed Triggering

Contents release via acid-catalyzed hydrolysis is another important triggering strategy for drug delivery since the pH inside endosomal compartments decreases with time when liposome enter target cells via receptor-mediated endocytosis (RME). We sought to probe the suitability of plasmenyl-type carriers for RME-based delivery by investigating the content release rates of DPPlsC liposomes at low pH using the calcein fluorescence dequenching method. *(14)* Calcein release rates were observed to depend on the pH of the medium and the cholesterol content of the lipid membranes, however, no calcein release was observed at pH 7.4 and 37 °C for 48 h (Figure 4). Our data also indicate that after 76 min at pH 4.5 only 20% of the DPPlsC had been hydrolyzed, yet 50% of the calcein cargo had escaped. We infer from this data that micellar defect structures within the DPPlsC bilayer can form once ≥ 20% of the DPPlsC has been hydrolyzed if the liposome consists of pure DPPlsC. If cholesterol of increasing molar ratios is incorporated within the membrane, more extensive hydrolysis was required to effect contents release due to the membrane stabilizing effect of cholesterol.

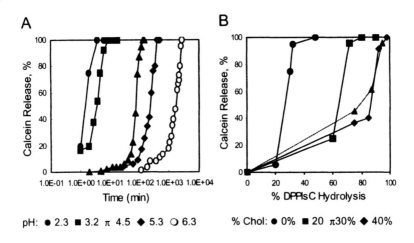

pH: ● 2.3 ■ 3.2 π 4.5 ◆ 5.3 ○ 6.3   % Chol: ● 0% ■ 20 π30% ◆ 40%

Figure 4. Calcein release rates from DPPlsC liposome at 37 °C at various pH (A). Correlation between calcein release and the extent of DPPlsC hydrolysis in the presence of cholesterol at pH 4.5 and 37 °C (B).

Intracellular Drug Delivery

A folate-based RME pathway was chosen as the route of entry into the endosomal compartment for the plasmenyl lipid carriers. Since folate receptors are overexpressed in many cancer cell lines, the attachment of a folate ligand to the liposome surface can selectively target a variety of folate receptor positive cancer cell lines. *(18)* As shown in Figure 5, folate-targeted liposomes enter cells by endocytosis, where the reduction of the endosomal pH with time promotes escape of the liposomal contents into the cytosol. If the drug carrier system lacks an efficient triggering mechanism, the drug cannot effectively escape into the cytoplasm, leading to its degradation after endosome-lysosome fusion. The acid-catalyzed triggering method is designed to efficiently promote contents release to the cytoplasm by destabilizing the liposomal and endosomal membranes at low pH.

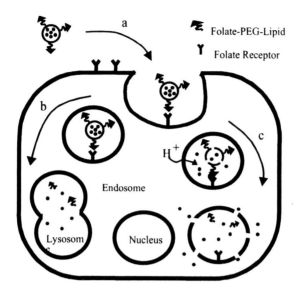

Figure 5. Conceptual drawing of intracellular drug delivery using the targeting and triggering strategy. Receptor-mediated endocytosis (a), lysosomal fusion and content degradation (b), and liposomal and endosomal content release (c).

Cytoplasmic contents release in KB cancer cells following administration of acid-sensitive, folate-targeted DPPlsC liposomes was evaluated by fluoro-metric assay using propidium iodide (PI) as the fluorescent probe. *(14)* Fluorescent microscopy showed intense staining of nuclei and nucleoli, indicating that the released PI had penetrated into the nucleus (Figure 6a). The PI release rate data shown in Figure 6b indicated the escape of 83% of the PI from both the liposomal and endosomal compartments within 8 h, compared to less than 5% escape when an acid-insensitive, folate-targeted egg phosphatidyl-choline (EPC) liposome was used. The cytotoxic antimetabolite drug, $1\text{-}\beta\text{-}$ arabinofuranosylcytosine (Ara-C), was also delivered to the cytoplasm of KB cells using folate-targeted DPPlsC liposomes. In this experiment, the release rates were monitored indirectly using the [³H]thymidine incorporation assay. The results demonstrate a 6000-fold increase in toxicity of Ara-C delivered via acid-sensitive DPPlsC liposome compared to the free drug, and a 100-fold increase in toxicity compared to the same drug concentration delivered via acid-insensitive, folate-targeted EPC liposomes (Figure 6c).

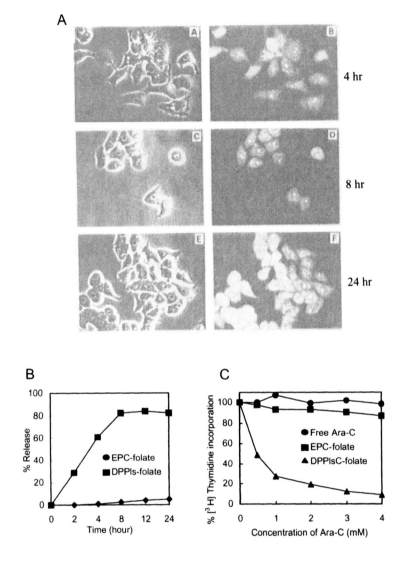

Figure 6. Fluorescent micrographs of KB cancer cells as a function of time after delivery of propidium iodide (PI) via folate-DPPlsC liposome (A). PI release rates in KB cells delivered by pH-sensitive DPPlsC and pH-insensitive EPC liposomes (B). Cytotoxicity of AraC delivered to KB cells by DPPlsC liposomes compared to EPC liposomes and free drug (C).

Chloroaluminium phthalocyanine tetrasulfonate ($AlPcS_4^{4-}$), a water-soluble photosensitizing drug used in photodynamic therapy, was delivered to KB cells using folate-targeted DPPlsC liposome. *(19)* Cytoplasmic distribution via acid-catalyzed triggering was confirmed by confocal microscopy, in contrast to the punctate fluorescence patterns observed when folate-targeted, acid-insensitive liposomes were used. The relative phototoxicity of folate/DPPlsC/$AlPcS_4^{4-}$ liposomes after irradiation (610 nm, 26 mW/cm^2, 30 min), as measured by the MTT and Live/Dead flow cytometry assays, was significantly greater than the relative phototoxicity of controls, i.e. $AlPcS_4^{4-}$ alone and acid-insensitive folate/DPPC/$AlPcS_4^{4-}$ liposomes (Figure 7). These results indicate the most broadly distributed pattern of intracellular $AlPcS_4^{4-}$ fluorescence and the highest phototoxicities for the folate-targeted acid-sensitive DPPlsC liposome system compared to the free drug, and non-targeted liposomal or targeted acid-insensitive liposomal drug delivery.

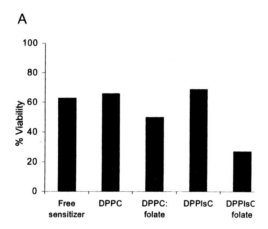

A

B

	Live	Dead	Dual
Free $AlPcS_4^{4-}$	25	57	18
DPPlsC:folate	13	83	4
DPPC:folate	45	43	12

Figure 7. Phototoxicity of commercial $AlPcS_4^{4-}$-treated KB cells obtained by MTT assay after irradiation ($\lambda_{ex} > 610$ nm, 30 min at 26 mW/cm^2) (A), and by flow cytometry (B).

60

Conclusions

Plasmenyl-type liposomes have been demonstrated as a promising intracellular drug delivery vehicle. Activation of these lipid carrier systems can be achieved by cleaving the vinyl ether bond under acidic or photooxidative conditions, which promotes lipid phase transitions and morphology changes. Cytotoxic drugs (Ara-C and $AlPcS_4^{4-}$) were successfully delivered via folate-targeted DPPlsC liposomes. The cytotoxicity of these formulations was significantly higher than free drug, non-targeted liposomal drug, or targeted acid-insensitive liposomal drug controls. These results clearly show that the combination of targeting and triggering provides a synergistic effect to enhance the specificity and efficacy of cytotoxic drug delivery to target cells.

References

1. Gerasimov, O. V.; Boomer, J. A.; Qualls, M. M.; Thompson, D. H. *Adv. Drug. Deliv. Rev.* **1999**, *38*, 317-338.
2. Rui, Y.; Thompson, D. H. *Chem. Eur. J.* **1996**, *2*, 1505-1508.
3. Rui, Y.; Thompson, D. H. *J. Org. Chem.* **1994**, *59*, 5758-5762.
4. Mayer, L. D.; Hope, M. J.; Cullis, P. R. *Biochim. Biophys. Acta* **1986**, *858*, 161-168.
5. Thompson, D. H.; Gerasimov, O. V.; Wheeler, J. J.; Rui, Y.; Anderson, V. C. *Biochim. Biophys. Acta* **1996**, *1279*, 25-34.
6. Lee, T.-C. *Biochim. Biophys. Acta* **1998**, *1394*, 129-145.
7. Sugiura, T.; Waku, K., Eds. *Platelet Activating Factor and Related Lipid Mediators*; Plenum Press, 1987.
8. Fonteh, A. N.; Chilton, F. H. *J. Immunol.* **1992**, *148*, 1784-1791.
9. Snyder, F.; Lee, T.-C.; Blank, M. L. In *Advances in Lipobiology*; Gross, R. W., Ed.; Jai Press, 1997; Vol. 2, pp 261-286.
10. Glaser, P. E.; Gross, R. W. *Biochemistry* **1994**, *33*, 5805-5812.
11. Murphy, R. C. *Chem. Res. Toxicol.* **2001**, *14*, 463-472.
12. Touchstone, J. C.; Alvarez, J. G.; Levin, S. S.; Storey, B. T. *Lipids* **1985**, *20*, 869-875.
13. Gerasimov, O. V.; Schwan, A.; Thompson, D. H. *Biochim. Biophys. Acta* **1997**, *1324*, 200-214.
14. Rui, Y.; Wang, S.; Low, P. S.; Thompson, D. H. *J. Am. Chem. Soc.* **1998**, *120*, 11213-11218.
15. Wymer, N. J.; Gerasimov, O. V.; Thompson, D. H. *Bioconj. Chem.* **1998**, *9*, 305-308.
16. Shin, J.; Gerasimov, O. V.; Thompson, D. H. *J. Org. Chem.* **2002**, *67*, 6503-6508.
17. Shum, P.; Kim, J.-M.; Thompson, D. H. *Adv. Drug. Deliv. Rev.* **2001**, *53*, 273-284.
18. Lee, R. J.; Low, P. S. *J. Liposome Res.* **1997**, *7*, 455-466.
19. Qualls, M. M.; Thompson, D. H. *Int. J. Cancer* **2001**, *93*, 384-392.

Chapter 5

Development of Neutral Liposome Plasmid DNA Complexes for Gene Transfer: Non-Viral Gene Delivery Systems

Adarsh Iyengar and Seán M. Sullivan*

Department of Pharmaceutics, University of Florida, Gainesville, FL 32610
*Corresponding author: email: Sullivan@cop.ufl.edu

Plasmid based gene delivery systems have relied on the use of cationic amphiphiles to deliver genes to cells. The following chapter describes the development of a neutral liposome packaging system for plasmid DNA that yields high trapping efficiency (70%), liposomes diameter of 180 nm, has slow clearance rates from the blood stream compared to plasmid alone or when formulated with cationic amphiphiles, and can accommodate incorporation of targeting ligands with retention of particle size and no decrease in plasmid trapping efficiency.

Introduction

Synthetic membrane systems were initially developed to study the biophysical properties of membranes, such as plasma membranes, mitochondrial membranes, membranes of endocytic vacuoles, and the membranes of enveloped viruses. These studies led to the extension that model membrane systems could mimic the viral membrane system with regard to fusion of the plasma membrane or intracellular vacuole membrane, i.e., endosomes and lysosomes. One more manifestation was to use the model membrane system to deliver genes to cells. The first application for model membrane gene delivery used liposomes composed of phosphatidylethanolamine and phosphatidylserine. Addition of liposomes containing this lipid composition fused to the plasma membrane in the presence of calcium. *(1-6)* Plasmid DNA was then packaged into the liposomes and shown to yield gene expression. *(7-9)* During the course of these experiments, it was discovered that the predominant route of entry for these liposomes into the cells was through endocytosis. In order for the cells to be transfected, the DNA had to escape from the endocytic vacuoles. Hence, a new trigger for the release of the DNA was needed. Endosomes and lysosomes undergo acidification and this feature was pursued as a trigger for DNA release.

Phosphatidylethanolamine by itself will not form phospholipid bilayers. Instead it will form a hexagonal phase, which has been proposed to be the fusion intermediate in membrane fusion. *(10)* However, phosphatidylethanolamine can form stable bilayers when combined with other phospholipids or amphiphiles. Stabilization with an amphipile containing a weak acid for a head group, pK 5 to 6, can stabilize bilayer formation at neutral pH. Decreasing the pH, however, results in protonation of the weak acid and prevents bilayer stabilization, resulting in the formation of the hexagonal phase by the phosphatidylethanolamine. Hence, if this phase could be formed by the liposomes in the endocytic compartment, this should lead to membrane/membrane fusion and release of the liposome entrapped contents into the cytosol, very similar to the way some enveloped viruses infect cells. *(11)* Examples of molecules that have been used to stabilize the bilayer configuration with phosphatidylethanolamine are oleic acid, dioleolyl-succiniylglycerol, and palmitoylhomocysteine. *(12-14)* One example of this system used a pH-sensitive liposome formulation in combination with antibody targeting to cancer cells. The system was tested *in vivo* by growing the tumor cells in the peritoneal cavity and then injecting the pH-sensitive immunoliposomes intraperitoneally. The plasmid DNA encoded a reporter gene under an inducible promoter. Isolation of the cells from the peritoneum and stimulation with the inducing agent showed that the gene delivery was selective for the antibody and much greater expression was obtained with the pH-sensitive formulation. *(15)*

Because these liposomes were in a semistable state, they did not fare well in the blood stream in the presence of apoliproteins and serum proteins. Avenues were explored to stabilize the liposomes but these stabilizing agents often led to inhibition of the pH-sensitive fusion. As this line of research, stabilizing pH-sensitive liposomes to serum components, was proceeding a discovery was made that amphiphiles containing a cationic head group could not only bind to DNA but also facilitate cell uptake. The field of lipid-mediated gene delivery shifted away from pH-sensitive liposomes and focused on the development of cationic amphiphiles for gene delivery. *(16-18)* These amphiphiles had monocationic head groups, such as $-N(CH_3)_3$, or polycationic head groups, such as spermine $(NH_2-(CH_2)_3-NH-(CH_2)_4-NH-(CH_2)_3-NH_2)$. The other moiety that was modified was the hydrophobic domain. These domains were composed of diacyglycerols (ester linked acyl chains), diacyenylglycerols (ether linked acyl chains) and cholesterol. Cationic lipid-mediated gene delivery is an active area of research and there are clinical trials in progress to evaluate the therapeutic efficacy of these transfection complexes. These clinical trials are focused on local administration of the transfection complexes for the treatment of cancer. *(19)* The tumors are transfected with a cytokine expression plasmid that recruits T lymphocytes. Upon arrival, these T lymphocytes become stimulated to kill the tumor cells and in so doing, become programmed to kill other tumor cells. Although it is a great concept, demonstration of efficacy still remains to be clinically demonstrated.

Major limitations in locally administered cationic lipid/plasmid DNA complexes are (i) the number of cells that are transfected due to a small injection volume, (ii) the limited number of cells that come in contact with that injection volume, and (iii) of the cells that do come in contact, only a few are successfully transfected. Systemically administered transfection complexes can impact a much larger number of tissues and cells. This is a double-edged sword because the potential for adverse effects increases. This can be limited by administering the cationic transfection complexes through a catheter. One application has been used in the clinic where a DOTAP/DOPE liposome formulation was administered through a blood vessel following balloon angioplasty using a dispatch catheter. This catheter does not hamper the blood flow, and the transfection complexes are pushed out of ports into the vascular bed. Expression of vascular-derived growth factor (VEGF) showed increased blood vessel growth at the site of administration. The unique aspect about this study was that an adenovirus and a cationic lipid/plasmid DNA complex were compared in a human clinical trial and both showed similar results with regard to induction of new blood vessel growth. (20)

Administration of the cationic lipid/plasmid DNA complexes via catheterizaion restricts the distribution of the transfection complexes. This serves several functions, the first is that the therapeutic dose is reduced, and secondly, any adverse side effects due to the interaction of the gene delivery vehicle or expression of the gene in other organs or tissues are minimized. The cationic amphiphiles used to deliver plasmid DNA display a dose-dependent lack of tolerability in animal models. For example, in rodent animal models, liver sensitivity is observed. In larger animals, such as rabbits, pigs and dogs, lung sensitivity is observed in form of endothelial leak syndrome. It has also been observed that there is a burst in the release of secondary cytokines in animal models upon systemic administration of cationic lipid/ plasmid DNA transfection complexes. The induction is dose-related and appears to also be a function of the CpG content of the plasmid. A recent study has shown that reducing the amount of CpG repeats in the plasmid reduced the induction of secondary cytokine production and increased the longevity of gene expression. *(21)* There still remains the problem of the presence of cationic amphiphiles.

Cationic amphiphile can be eliminated by returning to the use of pH-sensitive liposomes or simple non-cationic lipids for delivery of DNA to cells. One problem not previously mentioned was the issue of trapping efficiency. To the academic researchers dealing with small-scale materials, this may not be as large of a concern. However, it is a concern for large-scale manufacture for both preclinical and clinical materials. Sonication or extrusion is used to form the liposomes. Sonication can shear the DNA and is not an option. Extrusion requires a high concentration of plasmid DNA that is difficult to achieve and can also result in shearing of the DNA upon repeated passes through the filter. There are currently two methods that yield high entrapment of plasmid DNA. The first is termed dehydration/rehydration liposomes (DRV). *(22,23)* The procedure involves the formation of small unilamellar liposomes ($d \leq 50nm$). The DNA is mixed with these liposomes and lyophilized. Hydration of the lyophilized cake yields liposomes with high DNA entrapments. One potential problem is the freezing and thawing of the plasmid DNA. This process can denature the plasmid, causing a loss in the degree of supercoiling. For cationic lipid-mediated transfection, this loss results in loss of gene expression compared to a more supercoiled plasmid DNA. Whether it makes a difference for neutral liposome-mediated transfection is unknown. This technology has been used for genetic vaccines in which the liposome-formulated plasmid is administered subcutaneously to generate an immune response. Surprisingly, unformulated DNA ("naked DNA") by itself can be used for the same purpose. *(24)*

A method was devised for obtaining high entrapment efficiency for neutral liposomes that does not require freezing and thawing of DNA, thus maintaining a high supercoil content, nor does it yield multilamellar membranes as observed for dehydration/rehydration liposomes. Unilamellar membranes may facilitate plasmid DNA escape from the liposomes both for lysosomal release and potential fusion with the plasma membrane. The process requires the combination of ethanol and divalent cations to trap DNA inside liposomes. The idea was initiated by results of plasmid DNA interactions with cells in the presence of divalent cations. *(25)* The study had shown that DNA could bind to cells as a function of Mg^{+2} concentration. These authors demonstrated in an earlier study that DNA could not absorb to neutral liposomes but cause invagination, yielding a liposome within a liposome with the DNA trapped inside the inner liposome. DNA absorption to the liposomes was dependent on the type of divalent cation and the cation concentration. Limitations of these findings toward the development of a gene delivery system were the low trapping efficiency and the release of the DNA upon cellular internalization, requiring the breakdown of two bilayers.

Materials and Methods

Trapping of plasmid DNA into neutral liposomes. Small unilamellar liposomes were prepared by sonication using 80mM lipid in 10mM Tris Buffer at pH 7.4. The liposomes were centrifuged at 12000 rpm to remove debris and sterile-filtered through 0.2 um polycarbonate-sterilizing membranes. Plasmid DNA was propagated in DH5α E.Coli under a kanamycin resistance selectable gene. A 2-column chromato-graphy system, comprised of an ion exchange column (TMAE) and a reverse chromatography column (Octylsepharose), were used to isolate the plasmid following alkaline lysis of the bacteria. *(26,27)* 250 μl of 80-μm liposomes were mixed with 0.1mg of plasmid DNA in 10 mM Tris at pH 7.4 to a final volume of 0.4 ml. 600 μl of absolute ethanol containing 8 mM calcium chloride was added. The addition was drop- wise over approximately 30 seconds with vortex mixing. The resulting aggregated complexes were dialyzed against 500 volumes of 10 mM Tris at pH 7.4 for 24 hours with two-times changes of buffer. For physiological experiments, neutral liposome complexes (NLCs) were dialyzed against 500 volumes of PBS over a 24-hours period.

Peptide synthesis and purification. Peptide synthesis was carried out by solid phase peptide synthesis on an Applied Biosystems Model 433A peptide synthesizer using *Fastmoc*[TM] chemistry. The amino acids were coupled to the amide MBHA resin using HBOt/ HBTU activation of the carboxyl groups and 30-minute coupling times. The dried peptide resins were then cleaved by stirring in a TFA/H_2O/ EDT/TIS (92.5:2.5:2.5:2.5% v/v) cleavage cocktail for two hours at room temperature. The resin was filtered off with a sintered glass funnel, and the peptide-containing extract was concentrated to a viscous consistency. The peptides were then precipitated with cold ether, and the precipitate was filtered off using a separate sintered glass funnel. After washing the precipitate with ether, the crude peptides were extracted with H_2O/acetonitrile solution (50/50% v/v) and lyophilized. The crude peptides were purified by preparative reversed phase HPLC using an H_2O/acetonitrile solvent system containing 0.1% TFA. The chromatographically pure fractions were pooled and lyophilized. The structure of the peptides was confirmed by mass spectrometry. Cyclization was carried out by dissolving the peptides in 10mM potassium ferricyanide at pH 8.5 to give a 0.2 mg peptide per ml solution. The solution was stirred for two hours at room temperature, and the completion of the cyclization was checked by HPLC analysis and Ellman's test. The pH of the solution was adjusted to 4 by dropwise addition of 5% acetic acid, and the ferricyanide was removed by treatment with 35 grams of damp AG1X-2 resin per liter of solution, or until the supernatant appeared clear and colorless. The resin was filtered off, and the peptide-containing supernatant was lyophilized. The peptide was again purified by preparative reverse phase HPLC using an H_2O/acetonitrile solvent system containing 0.1% TFA. Fractions containing pure peptides were pooled and lyophilized.

Peptide Conjugation to Succinyl DOPE. Succinyl DOPE was purchased from Avanti Polar Lipids (Alabaster, AL) as solutions in chloroform. The chloroform was evaporated to dryness, and the residue was re-dissolved in 5 ml of toluene. The solvent was again evaporated to dryness, and this toluene treatment was repeated four more times. The final residue was dried under vacuum overnight. The dried residue was re-dissolved in 0.5 ml of dichloromethane and diluted with 4 ml of DMF. Solid carbonyldiimide (CDI) was added at 10-molar excess, and the carboxyl group of succinyl DOPE was activated by stirring under nitrogen for one hour at room temperature. The peptide (2-molar excess over succinyl DOPE) was dissolved in 0.5 ml DMF and added to the activated succinyl DOPE. Ten ml of re-distilled triethylamine was added and coupling was allowed to proceed overnight under nitrogen at room temperature. The solvent was evaporated to dryness, and the residue was further dried overnight under vacuum. The dried residue was re-dissolved in about 10 ml of water, and the solution was adjusted to pH 7 using 1 N sodium hydroxide. The peptide-DOPE conjugates were then purified by reverse phase HPLC using a Vydac C4 column and a 5 mM ammonium phosphate, pH 7/acetonitrile solvent system. Fractions containing pure conjugates were pooled and then lyophilized. The structures of the conjugates were confirmed by mass spectrophotometry.

Cell adhesion and inhibition assay using HUVEC. A cell adhesion and inhibition assay was established as modified from Harbottle *et al.* to evaluate the binding affinity of the targeting peptides. *(28)* HUVEC (2×10^4 cells per tube) were preincubated with 3 RGD-based and 1 non-RGD based peptides (0.01 – 100 μM) at 37^0C for 30 minutes in suspension and transferred onto vitronectin coated 96-well microtiter Immulon-2 plates (Dynatech Laboratories Inc., Chantilly, VA). After 90 minutes of incubation at 37^0C, the percentage of live cells was measured at 450-nm absorbency by adding WST-1 proliferation reagent (Boehringer Mannheim, Indianapolis, IN) and incubating for 1-4 hours.

Preparation and Characterization of Targeted DOPC: CHOL Liposomes in Vitro. Lipids containing dioleoylphosphatidylcholine (DOPC) and cholesterol (CHOL, Avanti Polar Lipids, Inc., Alabaster, AL) at a 2:1 ratio, and various amounts of targeting ligands (0.1-0.2 molar ratio to DOPC) were mixed in chloroform. A trace amount of ^{3}H-cholesteryl hexadecyl ether (New England Nuclear, Boston, MA) was added to determine the specific activity of the liposomes. The mixture was dried by rotary evaporation to produce a film. The residual amount of chloroform was removed by drying under vacuum overnight. The lipid film was re-suspended in sterile PBS, and passed through an extruder (Lipex Biomembranes, Vancouver, Canada) using 50-nm pore size polycarbonate membranes to produce small unilamellar liposomes. HUVEC`s were grown in EBM-2 media supplemented with EGM-2 SINGLEQUOTS (BioWhittaker, Walkersville, MD) in a 37^0C incubator with 5% CO_2 in a humidified atmosphere. Cells were seeded at 5×10^4 per well into 24-well plates in triplicate and incubated overnight at 37^0C to reach 50-80% confluence. After the removal of growth media the following day, 0.25 ml of media containing ^{3}H-labeled liposomes (0.8 μmol/ml) were added to each well and incubated for one hour at 37^0C. To determine the binding specificity, some wells were pre-treated with 10-fold excess of free ligands in media for 10 minutes before the addition of liposomes. After the media was removed, cells were washed gently with PBS, trypsinized with 0.5 ml of 0.05% trypsin for 30 minutes, placed in

ScintiSafe plus 50% scintillation fluid (Fisher Scientific) and counted in a Beckman LS-6000SC counter.

Results and Discussion

Optimized conditions for the formation of stable NLCs were based on fixing the DNA and lipid concentrations and varying the ethanol and calcium concentrations simultaneously. The selection criteria were liposomes with a diameter of 200 nm or less and trapping efficiency. Twelve random concentrations were selected and trapping efficiency was determined using TO-PRO, a DNA binding fluorophore. The data were empirically fit to quadratic models of increasing complexity until a reasonable confidence limit ($\geq 95\%$) was obtained. (29) The purpose behind the design was to create a neutral liposome with encapsulated DNA that could then be targeted to specific cell types by attaching a ligand to the neutral liposome surface that bound to a unique receptor expressed on the cell surface. It was discovered that each new lipid composition required the ethanol and calcium concentrations to be optimized. Changing the lipid composition also resulted in different average diameters and different trapping efficiencies. For example, dioleoylphosphatidylcholine alone yielded 140-nm diameter liposomes with an average trapping efficiency of 67%, whereas incorporation of dioleoylphosphatidylethanolamine (DOPE) yielded a slightly larger average diameter of 160 nm with an average trapping efficiency of 75%. Incorporation of cholesterol into the lipid formulation increased the diameter to >200 nm and decreased the trapping efficiency to 37%. The purpose for incorporation of DOPE into the liposome formulation is threefold: (i) DOPE can facilitate fusion of membranes, (ii) cells have a receptor for phosphatidylethanolamine what may improve cell uptake, and (iii) DOPE provides a nucleophilic head group for liposome surface modification, such as PEG derivatization or ligand derivatization. The purpose for addition of cholesterol was to increase the integrity of the liposomal bilayer and prevent disruption due to interaction with serum components. However, the increase in size beyond 200 nm and the decrease in trapping efficiency made this approach unacceptable. As will be discussed later, this lipid component is not needed.

Extensive characterization was done on the DOPC and DOPC/DOPE liposomes to show that the plasmid DNA was not merely adsorbed to the surface of the liposome. This process included the use of TOPRO DNA binding in the absence and presence of detergent using NLCs in which the untrapped plasmid DNA was removed. Results showing no fluorescence in the absence of detergent indicated that all DNA was inside the NLC. Zeta potential measurements of the same NLCs revealed a net neutral surface charge, a further indication that the plasmid DNA was inside the liposomes.

Negative stain transmission electron microscopy confirmed the average particle size diameter to be 170 nm. In addition, no multilamellar morphology was observed for any of the preparations. To further support the existence of single bilayers, a fluorescent lipid, NBD-DOPE, was incorporated into the NLC at 0.1 mol%. Dithionite cannot diffuse across lipid bilayers and it quenches the NBD fluorescence. *(30)* The degree of fluorescence quenching in the absence and presence of detergent yielded a lamellarity of 1.22, indicative of unilamellar NLCs. For oligolamellar liposomes or multilamellar liposomes, this value would have increased to greater than one.

Before proceeding to *in vivo* biodistribution, both DOPC and DOPC/DOPE NLCs were characterized with regard to serum stability and acid pH stability. Results indicated that neither incubation in 90% fetal bovine serum or at pH 4 for one hour at $37^{\circ}C$ did increase the mean diameter, indicating that no aggregation of NLCs was induced, and no loss in entrapped plasmid DNA was observed.

The main purpose for the development of NLCs was to target the complexes to the tumor vasculature. Hence, biodistribution studies were conducted with DOPC NLCs. ^{3}H-cholesterylhexadecyl ether was incorporated into DOPC NLCs to monitor lipid distribution, and the plasmid was followed by quantitative PCR (qPCR). Tissues were harvested one hour and 18 hours after administration. Sixty percent of the lipid dose and 10% of the plasmid-administered dose were recovered at the 1-hour time point. The results indicated a 30% recovery of the injected dose in the blood stream, and less than 0.1% plasmid or lipid was found in the lungs. This is a dramatic change in plasmid biodistribution compared to cationic lipid/plasmid DNA complexes that are rapidly cleared from the blood stream ($t_{1/2} = 1$ minute) with about 14% accumulation in the lungs. *(31)* These results demonstrated that plasmid DNA could be formulated in neutral liposomes with high trapping efficiency and conservation of a particle size that can be endocytosed by cells. What remained is to demonstrate that the plasmid can be expressed upon entry to the cell.

No expression was observed from any of the tissues in the *in vivo* experiment. Transfection was further evaluated *in vitro* using endothelial cells for targeted gene expression and a luciferase expression plasmid to quantitate expression levels. The DOPC and DOPC/DOPE formulations were not taken up by HUVECs. An RGD peptide first described by Koivunen *et al.* was modified to remove one of the disulfide bonds. *(32)* The sequence was CDMRGDMFC. The removal of the internal disulfide bond increased the water solubility of the peptide, making it more easy to use in aqueous media but reducing the affinity for the $\alpha_V\beta_3$ integrin binding by an order of magnitude. The structures for the single and double disulfide peptides are shown below.

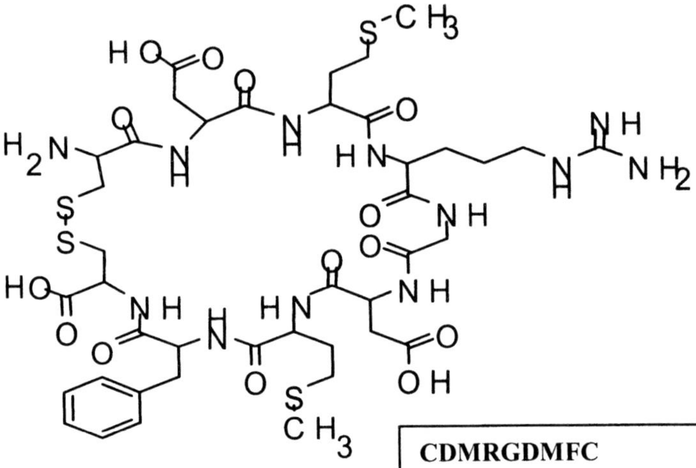

CDMRGDMFC

Single Disulfide Peptide

CDCRGDCFC

Double Disulfide Peptide

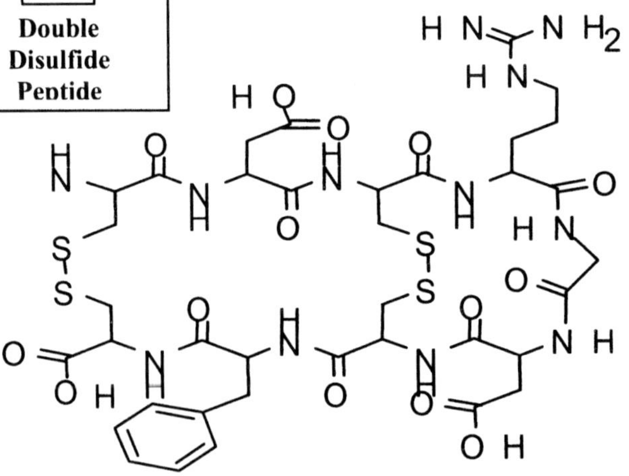

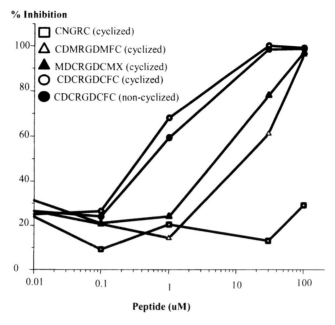

% Inhibition

□ CNGRC (cyclized)
△ CDMRGDMFC (cyclized)
▲ MDCRGDCMX (cyclized)
○ CDCRGDCFC (cyclized)
● CDCRGDCFC (non-cyclized)

Peptide (uM)

Figure 1. Percent inhibition of HUVEC attachment to vitronectin-coated plates as a function of peptide concentration. HUVECs were detached using PBS with 10mM EDTA at pH 7.4. 1 x 10⁵ cells were incubated in a 200-μl volume with each of the above peptides for 30 minutes at room temperature and then added to 96-well plates that had been treated with Vitronectin. After 2-hour incubation at 37°C, plates were washed and analyzed for the number of cells that adhered to the plate. Replacement of either the internal disulfide bond or the external disulfide bond with methionines decreased the ability of the peptide to inhibit cell attachment by an order of magnitude. There was also no difference between the cyclized and uncyclized peptide indicating that the cysteines may play another role in integrin binding. The CNGRC peptide does not bind to $\alpha_v\beta_3$ integrin and served as a negative control.

The peptide lacking the internal disulfide was covalently attached to succinimidyl-DOPE by an amide linkage converting the C-terminal carboxyl to an N-hydroxysuccinimidyl ester. Incorporation of the lipopeptide into ^{3}H-hexadecylcholesteryl labeled DOPC liposomes showed peptide-mediated binding to cells, and the binding could be inhibited with excess peptide. Furthermore, there was only a 3-fold reduction in binding affinity between the dual disulfide lipopeptide CDCRGDCFC-DOPE and the single disulfide lipopeptide CDMRGDMFC. These results are shown in Figure 2.

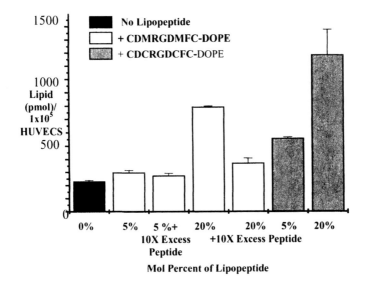

Figure 2. Lipopeptide-mediated binding of DOPC liposomes to HUVECs in vitro. 1 x 10^5 HUVECs were seeded in 24-well plates. 50 μM ^{3}H-cholesterylhexadecyl ether labeled DOPC liposomes containing varying mol percents of each lipopeptide were incubated in a 1-ml volume at 37°C for 1 hour. Cells were washed three times and removed from the plate with 1% Triton X-100, and cell associated radioactivity was measured. 10X excess peptide refers to addition of free peptide in 10-fold excess of the lipopeptide. Inhibition of CDCRGDCFC was not done due to limited solubility of the peptide.

The CDMRGDMFC-DOPE was incorporated into either the DOPC or DOPE/DOPC NLCs up to 20 mol% with little impact on particle size or trapping efficiency. Uptake studies with HUVECs yielded similar results to those obtained with the empty liposomes. NLCs were fluorescently labeled with 0.1 mol% of NBD-DOPE obtained from Avanti Polar Lipids. Fluorescent micrographs indicated that the lipopeptide-targeted NLCs were inside endosomes and lysosomes as evidenced by periplasmic accumulation of punctate fluorescence. However, luciferase expression in the HUVECs was barely above background. This would suggest that two rate-limiting steps needed to be overcome, escape from the endosomes and nuclear uptake of the released plasmid.

Current research is focused on formulating the NLCs to release the DNA from endosomes and lysosomes. This protocol can now be combined with the acidic pH-susceptible lipid formulations to facilitate

DNA transfection. Upon protonation of the carboxyl group, DOGS is no longer capable of stabilizing the bilayer and fusion occurs. Preliminary uptake studies show that this lipid is toxic to HUVECs and to human and rat brain tumor cells. Alternative pH-sensitive formulations are currently being tested with this system.

Conclusions

Overcoming the low trapping efficiencies initially experienced by liposome formulations make the NLCs a viable approach for gene therapy, especially since the potential toxic side effects of cationic lipids are eliminated. Secondly, the biodistribution results suggest that there may not be a need for derivatizing the surface with stealthing molecules to increase the circulation half-life. The ability to have the cells express the delivered gene is still a remaining problem. The employment of acidic pH-mediated release may address this problem, yielding a gene delivery system that more closely resembles a synthetic virus without the undesired side effects.

References

1. Papahadjopoulos, D.; Vail, W. J.; Pangborn, W. A.; Poste, G. *Biochim Biophys Acta.* **1976**, *448*, 265-283.
2. Newton, C.; Pangborn, W.; Nir, S.; Papahadjopoulos, D. *Biochim Biophys Acta.* **1978**, *506*, 281-287.
3. Portis, A.; Newton, C.; Pangborn, W.; Papahadjopoulos, D. *Biochemistry* **1979**, *18*, 780-790.
4. Wilschut, J.; Duzgunes, N.; Fraley, R.; Papahadjopoulos, D. *Biochemistry* **1980**, *19*, 6011-6021.
5. Duzgunes, N.; Nir, S.; Wilschut, J.; Bentz, J.; Newton, C.; Portis, A.; Papahadjopoulos, D. *J Membr Biol.* **1981**, *59*, 115-125.
6. Duzgunes, N.; Wilschut, J.; Fraley, R.; Papahadjopoulos, D. *Biochim Biophys Acta.* **1981**, *642*, 182-195.
7. Wilson, T.; Papahadjopoulos, D.; Taber, R. *Cell* **1979**, *17*, 77-84.
8. Fraley, R.; Subramani, S.; Berg, P.; Papahadjopoulos, D. *J Biol Chem.* **1980**, *255*, 10431-10435.
9. Fraley, R.; Straubinger, R.M.; Rule, G.; Springer, E.L.; Papahadjopoulos, D. *Biochemistry* **1981**, *20*, 6978-6987.
10. Hafez, I.M.; Cullis, P.R. *Adv Drug Deliv Rev.* **2001**, *47*, 139-148.
11. Schoch, C.; Blumenthal, R. *J Biol Chem.* **1993**, *268*, 9267-9274.

12. Duzgunes, N.; Straubinger, R.M.; Baldwin, P.A.; Friend, D.S.; Papahadjopoulos, D. *Biochemistry* **1985**, *24*, 3091-3098.

13. Collins, D.; Litzinger, D.C.; Huang, L. *Biochim Biophys Acta.* **1990**, *1025*, 234-242.

14. Connor, J.; Huang, L. *J Cell Biol.* **1985**, *101*, 582-589.

15. Huang, L.; Connor, J.; Wang, C.Y. *Methods Enzymol.* **1987**, *149*, 88-99.

16. Behr, J.P.; Demeneix, B.; Loeffler, J.P.; Perez-Mutul, J. *Proc Natl Acad Sci U S A.* **1989**, *86*, 6982-6986.

17. Felgner, P.L.; et al. *Proc Natl Acad Sci U S A.* **1987**, *84*, 7413-7417.

18. Gao, X.; Huang, L. *Biochem Biophys Res Commun.* **1991**, *179*, 280-285.

19. Kaushik, A. *Curr Opin Investig Drugs.* **2001**, *2*, 976-981.

20. Makinen, K.; Manninen, H.; Hedman, M.; Matsi, P.; Mussalo, H.; Alhava, E.; Yla-Herttuala, S. *Mol Ther.* **2002**, *6*, 127-133.

21. Yew, N.S.; Zhao, H.; Przybylska, M.; Wu, I.H.; Tousignant, J.D.; Scheule, R.K.; Cheng, S.H. *Mol Ther.* **2002**, *5*, 731-738.

22. Alino, S.F.; Garcia-Sanz, M.; Irruarrizaga, A.; Alfaro, J.; Hernandez, J. *J Microencapsul.* **1990**, *7*, 497-503.

23. Senior, J.; Gregoriadis, G. *Biochim Biophys Acta.* **1989**, *1003*, 58-62.

24. Wolff, J.A.; Malone, R.W.; Williams, P.; Chong, W.; Acsadi, G.; Jani, A.; Felgner, P.L. *Science* **1990**, *247*, 1465-1468.

25. Beliaev, N.D.; Budker, V.G.; Gorokhova, O.E.; Sokolov, A.V. *Mol Biol (Mosk).* **1988**, *22*, 1667-1672.

26. Anwer, K.; Bailey, A.; Sullivan, S.M. *Crit Rev Ther Drug Carrier Syst.* **2000**, *17*, 377-424.

27. Mahato, R.I. et al. *Hum Gene Ther.* **1998**, *9*, 2083-2099.

28. Hart, S.L.; Knight, A.M.; Harbottle, R.P.; Mistry, A.; Hunger, H.D.; Cutler, D.F.; Williamson, R.; Coutelle, C. *J Biol Chem.* **1994**, *269*, 12468-12474.

29. Steppan, D.; Werner, J.; Yeater R.P. Internet Publications, Gibsonia PA **1998**.

30. Gruber, H.; Schindler H. *Biochim Biophys Acta.* **1994**, *1189*, 212-224.

31. Anwer, K.; Kao, G.; Proctor, B.; Rolland, A.; Sullivan, S. *J Drug Target.* **2000**, *8*, 125-135.

32. Koivunen, E.; Wang, B.; Ruoslahti, E. *Biotechnology* (NY) **1995**, *13*, 265-270.

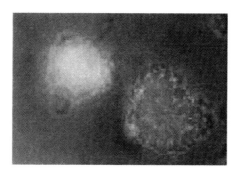

Figure 7. Gel-entrapped-proniosome-derived-niosomes (GEProDeN) stained with Sudan 4 dye. This is an exposure with dual illumination, including brightfield (green) illumination and epifluorescence (orange) illumination. This method shows that the locations of the niosomes and the entrapped dye are correlated.

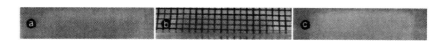

Figure 8. Eosin Yellowish-release from GEProDEN (a) and from hydrogel (b). A blank niosome-containing gel is shown in panel (c). The grid behind the samples is visible only in the sample which does not contain niosomes. These images were obtained after 6 hours.

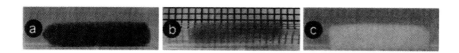

Figure 9. GEProDEN containing Sudan 4, a poorly soluble drug. The drug is only released in niosomes (a), not as free drug (b). As seen in panels (a) and (c), light scattering due to release of niosomes obscures the grid behind the sample.

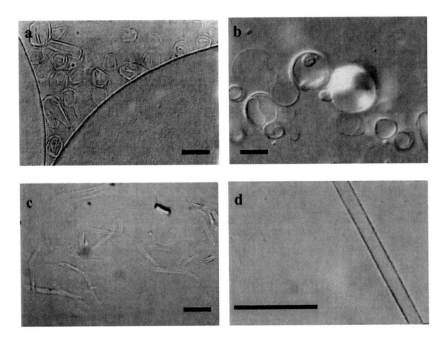

Figure 2. *Photomicrographs showing (a) multi-lamellar polyhedral niosomes in an aqueous channel, (b) spherical niosomes made from sorbitan monostearate, cholesterol and Solulan (45:45:10), (c) microtubules formed from polyhedral niosomes when extruded from capillaries smaller than their size, (d) a typical microtubule also produced by extrusion, (e) discomes produced by incubating surfactant I : Solulan C24 (50:50) (Cable, C. Ph.D. thesis, University of Strath-clyde, Glasgow, UK, 1990), (f) a hexadecane gel at room temperature containing surfactant tubular aggregates dispersed in organic medium (Reproduced with permission from Reference 2), and (g) toroidal vesicular structures in an isopropyl myristate formulation at the transition temperature between sol and gel phases. (Reproduced with permission from Reference 2) (Bars = 10 μm)*

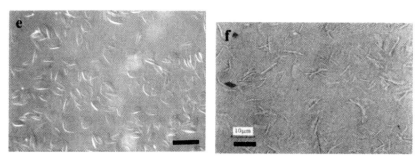

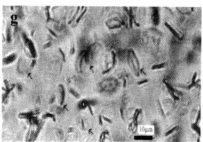

Figure 2. *Continued.*

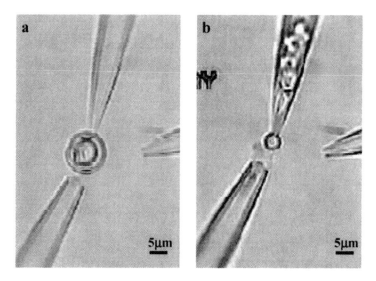

Figure 5.   Desquamation by micromanipulation of a Rhodamine B containing spherical liposome, leading to the release of the encapsulated dye.

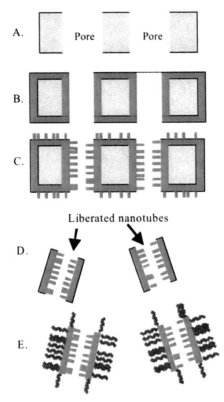

Figure 3. Schematic of Differential Inside/Outside Modification. Cross-section of Al2O3 template membrane showing two pores (A). Sol-gel synthesis of SiO$_2$ nanotubes (B). Silanization of inner nanotube surface (C). Removal of surface films and dissolution of alumina template (D). Secondary silanization on outer nanotube surface (E).

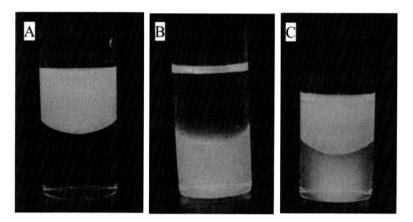

Figure 4. Fluorescently-modified nanotubes in biphasic cyclohexane (top)/ water (bottom) mix. Dansylamine inside/C18 outside nanotubes partition into cyclohexane phase (A). Quinineurathane inside/bare silica outside nanotubes partition into water phase (B). Mix of both types independently phase separates (C).

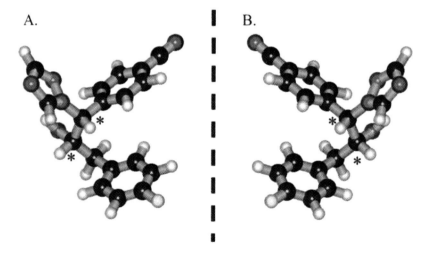

Figure 6. Three-dimensional structures of the RS-enantiomer (A) and SR-enantiomer (B) of FTB. (*) denotes the chiral centers. The geometry optimization was done by Ab Initio calculation with minimal basis set in HyperChem 6.03. The drug is in clinical trials by Hormos Medical, Turku, Finland. (Reprinted with permission from Lee et al. Science, 2002, 296, 2198. Copyright 2002 American Association for the Advancement of Science.)

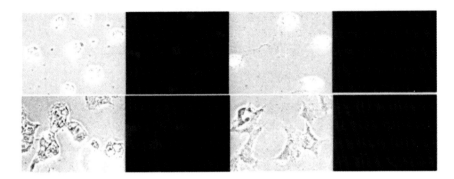

Figure 4. Binding of Rh-labeled PEG-PE micelles to EL4 cells (top panel) and to BT20 cells (bottom panel). Left half: bright field and fluorescent micro-scopy of 2C5-micelles; right half: bright field and fluorescent microscopy of plain micelles.

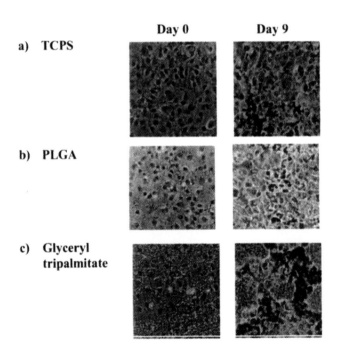

Figure 3. 3T3-L1 cells on a) TCPS, b) PLGA, and c) glyceryl tripalmitate. Day 0 immediately after cell seeding, day 9 after differentiation to adipocytes and red oil O-staining of intracellular lipid droplets.

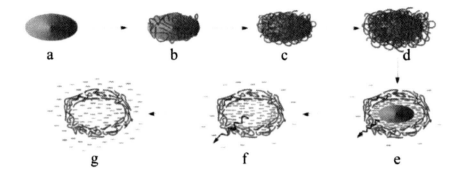

Figure 6. Scheme of the polyelectrolyte multilayer deposition process and subsequent core dissolution. The initial steps (a-d) involve stepwise shell formation on a fluorescein core. After the desired number of polyelectrolyte layers is deposited, the coated particles are exposed to pH 8 (e) and core dissolution with fluorescein penetration into the bulk is initiated, resulting in fully dissolved cores and empty capsules (f).

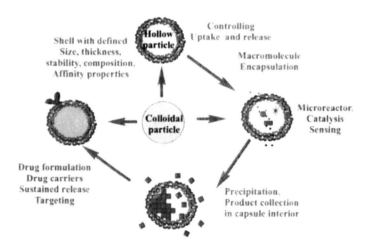

Figure 11. Comprehensive illustration of applications of the step-wise shell formation on colloidal particles.

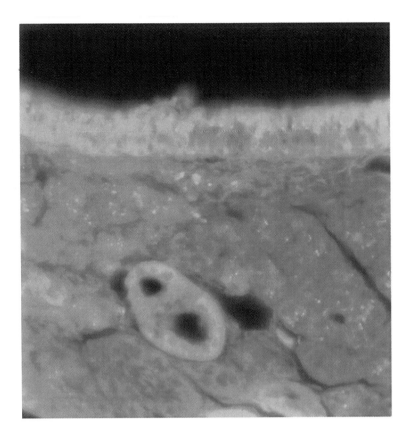

Figure 2. Fluorescent micrograph of a cross section of nasal mucosa from rat administered intranasaly with a suspension of PLA-PEG nanoparticles (mean size 1 μm). Fluorescent spots corresponding to the nanoparticles can be seen crossing the epithelium and reaching the submucosal space.

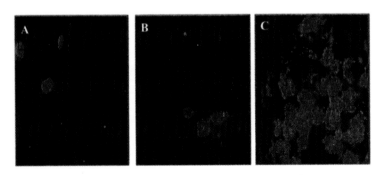

Figure 7. CLSM image of Caco-2 cell monolayers using propidium iodide as impermeable dead cell staining probe; (A) cells incubated with SPH polymer, (B) cells incubated with SPHC polymer, (C) cells treated with 0.1% SDS for 10 min.

Chapter 6

Does Shape Matter? Spherical, Polyhedral, and Tubular Vesicles

Alexander T. Florence[1,*], Behrooz Nasseri[1], and Parinya Arunothyanun[1,2]

[1]Centre for Drug Delivery Research, The School of Pharmacy, University of London, London WC1N 1AX, United Kingdom
[2]Current address: Government Pharmaceutical Organisation, Bangkok, Thailand
*Corresponding author: email: Alexander.Florence@ams1.ulsop.ac.uk

Surfactant and lipid vesicles can be produced in a variety of geometries, discoidal, polyhedral, toroidal and tubular. Here some properties of spherical and polyhedral non-ionic surfactant vesicles have been compared flow being one parameter. Shape is less important than membrane characteristics in controlling release of entrapped drug, but the flow properties of vesicular suspensions are, of course, markedly dependent on shape. The elasticity and flow behavior of such vesicular systems have been little studied but we postulate by analogy with erythrocytes that these are pertinent to the behavior of these potential drug delivery systems *in vivo*, an attribute not discussed in the literature.

Introduction

As most particulate drug delivery vectors are spherical, little attention has been paid to the influence of shape on the behavior of delivery systems. We have been interested for some time in non-ionic surfactant vesicle (niosome) design, and have as a result produced in aqueous media niosomes of a variety of shapes, namely discoidal, polyhedral, and tubular systems. *(1)* In non-aqueous solvents we have also observed spherical, tubular and toroidal inverse vesicles. *(2)* Other groups have found prolate vesicles and so-called non-axisymmetric "star-fish" vesicles. *(3,4)* As shape directly influences the flow properties of suspensions, the question of the effect of vesicle shape and properties on their rheological characteristics arises. Little work has been done on the rheology of liposomes or niosomes, yet one can postulate that the flow properties of spherical and aspherical vesicles in the capillary blood supply will be important. As Sackmann pointed out cell (and vesicle) membranes are "extremely soft with respect to bending and shearing but practically noncompressable with respect to lateral stretching", a construction which allows erythrocytes to travel "several hundred kilometers throughout our body" without loss of material. *(5)* The influence of deformability and hence shape on a range of blood cell behaviors has been discussed in detail. *(6)* Clear differences are seen in the rheology and properties of suspensions of spherical and polyhedral vesicles prepared from non-ionic surfactants and their behavior in capillaries in the laboratory. *(7)*

Results and Discussion

There are two different, but related, effects of vesicle flow: the effect of vesicle shape on flow properties and the effect of flow on the shape of elastic vesicles (or cells), the latter being discussed theoretically. *(8)* There are several instances in the use of vesicles in drug delivery technology where capillary flow is of relevance (i) in the fate of elastic vesicles in their transport through the skin *(9)*, (ii) in targeting, vectors arrival at target sites may be dictated not only by the diameter and surface characteristics of the carrier, but also by their elastic properties using the analogy of the fate of red cells *(6)*, and (iii) in the production of delivery systems by extrusion technologies. *(10-12)*

In this chapter we discuss issues surrounding the shape of niosomes and ask whether rheological characteristics matter *in vivo*. Based on *in vitro* data on the behavior of niosomes and liposomes under stress, we also consider the potential fate of vesicles in the capillary blood supply, with specific reference to vesicle damage or rupture and the consequent loss of entrapped solutes. Our proposition is that shape matters (i) because it affects flow and potential fate *in vivo*, through for example extravasation, and (ii) that as shape differences are determined by membrane composition there are secondary differences in the physical properties of vesicles of different shapes, including solute release and swelling, which must also be taken into account. In addition, the elasticity and visco-elasticity of vesicular systems may be important in their role as drug delivery vectors and may differentiate vesicles from inelastic solid nano- or microparticles.

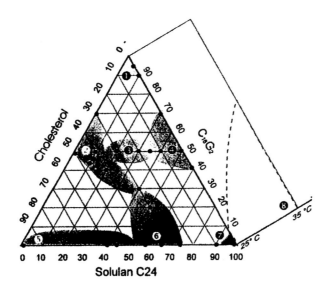

Figure 1. The $C_{16}G_2$-cholesterol-Solulan C24 ternary phase-diagram. Region 1, polyhedral vesicle (2-10 μm); region 2, spherical, helical and tubular vesicles (0.5-10 μm); region 3, discomes (10-30 μm), large vesicles (40 μm) and small spherical and helical vesicles (0.5-10 μm); region 4, discomes (12-60 μm) and possibly Solulan C24 micelles; region 5, cholesterol crystals; region 6, spherical vesicles (0.5-10 μm); region 7, a clear liquid (Solulan C24 micelles); region 8, mixed micelles formed at elevated room temperature. (Reproduced with permission from reference 13. Copyright 1997.)

Polyhedral systems are found in cholesterol-poor regions of the phase diagram, shown in Figure 1, for one of the typical systems we have studied, namely the three component mixture comprising cholesteryl-24-polyoxyethylene ether (Solulan C24), cholesterol and the non-ionic surfactant, $C_{16}G_2$, a hexadecyl diglyceryl ether. *(13)* Typical spherical and asymmetric systems from such mixtures are shown in Figure 2. Shape is determined by the properties of the bilayer membranes at given temperatures. Polyhedral vesicles, for example, convert reversibly to spherical systems above a critical temperature. Differences in shape not only affect the capillary flow, but they translate into differences in osmotic behavior, membrane diffusion characteristics, and elastic properties, all of which are important in determining behavior as delivery vectors *in vivo* unless other unknown and over-riding factors impinge. *(14)* The release of LHRH from polyhedral niosomes is greater than the release from their spherical equivalents, the behavior of both systems being highly dependant on the medium in which release was measured. *(15)*

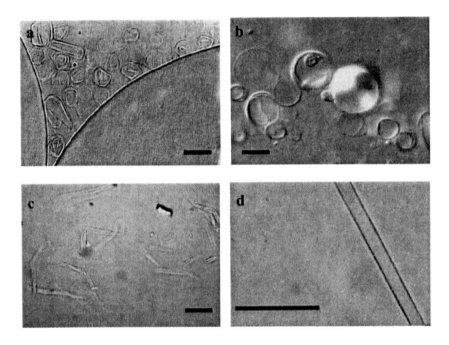

Figure 2. Photomicrographs showing (a) multi-lamellar polyhedral niosomes in an aqueous channel, (b) spherical niosomes made from sorbitan monostearate, cholesterol and Solulan (45:45:10), (c) microtubules formed from polyhedral niosomes when extruded from capillaries smaller than their size, (d) a typical microtubule also produced by extrusion, (e) discomes produced by incubating surfactant I : Solulan C24 (50:50) (Cable, C. Ph.D. thesis, University of Strathclyde, Glasgow, UK, 1990), (f) a hexadecane gel at room temperature containing surfactant tubular aggregates dispersed in organic medium (Reproduced with permission from Reference 2), and (g) toroidal vesicular structures in an isopropyl myristate formulation at the transition temperature between sol and gel phases. (Bars = 10 μm) (Reproduced with permission from reference 2. Copyright 1999 Elsevier Science.) (See page 2 of color insert.)

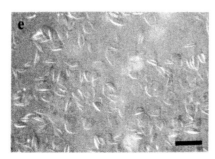
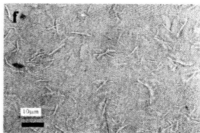

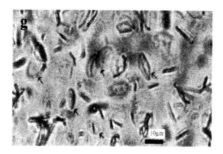

Figure 2. *Continued.* *(See page 3 of color insert.)*

Our studies on the flow properties of spherical and polyhedral vesicles in which estimates of surface hydration of non-ionic vesicle formulations were made, indicated clearly the higher viscosity of polyhedral systems (Figure 3). This work led us to consider the flow properties of vesicles in capillaries. Figure 4 shows the movement of an elastic spherical niosome and its deformation as the capillary thins. As shapes changes the contact area between the membrane and wall of the capillary increases, a phenomena which might well have some biological relevance. The behavior of a polyhedral vesicle is also shown. In narrow capillaries under pressure spherical vesicles, being visco-elastic, can survive intact. With polyhedral systems, as the capillary narrows and pressure is maintained, permanent shape changes occur. *(11,12)* Fusion of polyhedral niosomes under pressure in capillaries with diameters less than the diameter of the niosomes lead to the production of tubular systems up to 80 μm in length and approximately 1 μm in diameter. *(16)* Can such fusion occur *in vivo,* for example at a capillary bifurcation or during extravasation?

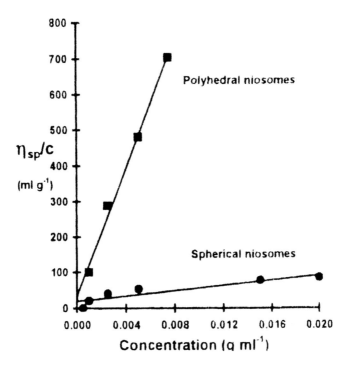

Figure 3. Plot of reduced specific viscosity (η_{rel} - 1)/C, versus concentration of lipid/surfactants at 25 °C for polyhedral niosome and spherical/tubular niosome suspensions, prepared from $C_{16}G_2$/cholesterol/Solulan C24 in the ratios 91:0:9 and 45:45:10. (Reproduced from reference 7. Copyright 1999 American Chemical Society.)

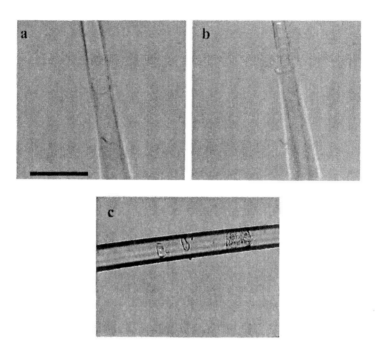

Figure 4. Flow of (a) a spherical vesicle in a capillary in which $r_{vesicle} = r_{capillary}$, (b) where $r_{vesicle} > r_{capillary}$ and deformation of the elastic system occurs, and (c) polyhedral vesicles where flow patterns clearly differ from those of spherical systems. (Bar = 10μm)

Much of the debate on whether the shape of vesicles matters is dependent on knowledge of the nature of the capillary blood supply and the forces exerted on and the damage done to vesicles as they move in capillaries. Earlier studies of doxorubicin remaining in and released from spherical niosomes after intravenous administration showed that around 60% of the drug remained within spherical niosomes eight hours after i.v. administration. *(17)* The extent to which this loss is due to normal diffusion or to the shear stress on the vesicles is not known. However, spherical vesicles can be stressed by micromanipulators and the outer bilayers removed, as shown in Figure 5, causing a rapid release of some of the encapsulated material (dye in this experiment). These might well be extreme forces but in experiments in which polyhedral vesicles were extruded through capillaries of decreasing diameter, from less than 1 μm to around 4 μm, the greater shear experienced by niosomes exiting through the narrower capillaries led to the greatest loss of entrapped carboxyfluorescein (Figure 6). The extent to which such assaults are commonplace *in vivo* is not known. The intrinsic release rates of spherical and polyhedral systems are ordinarily dependent on membrane properties. An additional complication in estimating what happens *in vivo* is that release from non-stressed systems is so different.

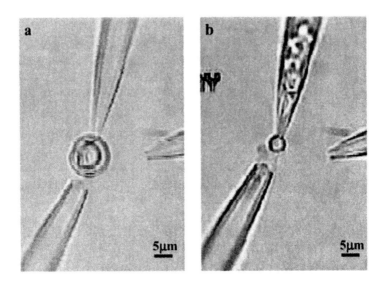

Figure 5. Desquamation by micromanipulation of a Rhodamine B containing spherical liposome, leading to the release of the encapsulated dye. (See page 3 of color insert.)

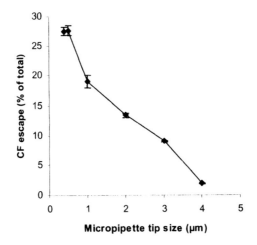

Figure 6. Initial (T=0) levels of entrapped CF release from polyhedral niosomes of size range 2–15 μm after extrusion via micropipette tips of reducing size.

Conclusions

This paper has simply posed the question "does the shape of vesicles matter?" and provides no concrete proof that *in vivo* it does. However we know that the closest relative of a lipid vesicle - a red blood cell – is influenced by its deformability, hence we maintain that shape matters. Shape differences are determined by membrane composition, hence there are differences in the physical properties of niosomes and other vesicles of various shapes, these sometimes leading to differences in the rate of release of contents and osmotic behavior. Elasticity is important in determining behavior in capillary beds and trafficking through cellular structures, but its true influence certainly requires more detailed investigation. Vesicle shapes are permanent only if the system has no elastic properties. Movement of intact vesicles across the skin and other semipermeable membranes is a function of their deformability. *(9)* Vesicles also show quite pronounced thermal fluctuations due to the "softness" of their membranes. *(18)* The presence of transition temperatures close to body temperature causes tubular structures to undergo shape transformation. It may be possible to take advantage of such shape changes to influence the movement of vesicles *in vivo*, for example after delivery to the eye or to intramuscular sites.

References

1. Uchegbu, I.F.; Florence, A.T. Non-ionic surfactant vesicles (Niosomes): Physical and Pharmaceutical Chemistry. *Adv. Coll. Inter. Sci.* **1995**, *58*, 1-55.
2. Murdan, S.; Gregoriadis, G.; Florence, A.T. Inverse toroidal vesicles: precursors of tubules in sorbitan monostearate organogels. *Int. J. Pharm.* **1999**, *183*, 47-49.
3. Döbereiner, H-G.; Evans, E.; Kraus, M.; Seifert, U.; Wortis, M. Mapping vesicle shapes into the phase diagram: A comparison of experiment and theory. *Phys. Rev. E.* **1997**, *55*, 4458-4474.
4. Wintz, W.; Döbereiner, H-G.; Seifert, U. Starfish vesicles. *Europhys. Lett.* **1996**, *33*, 403-408.
5. Sackmann, E. Membrane bending energy concept of vesicle- and cell-shapes and shape transitions. *FEBS Lett.* **1994**, *346*, 3-16.
6. Chien, S. Biophysical behavior of red cells in suspensions. In Surgenor, D.M. The Red Blood Cell. **1975**, *11*, New York: Academic Press.
7. Florence, A.T.; Arunothayanun, P.; Kiri, S.; Bernard, M-S.; Uchegbu, I.F. Some rheological properties of non-ionic surfactant vesicles and the determination of surface hydration. *J. Phys. Chem. B.* **1999**, *103*, 1995-2000.

8. Bruinsma, R. Rheology and shape transitions of vesicles under capillary flow. *Physica. A.* **1996**, *234*, 249-270.

9. Cevc, G,; Schätzlein, A,; Richardsen, H. Ultradeformable lipid vesicles can penetrate the skin and other semi-permeable barriers unfragmented. Evidence from double label CLSM experiments and direct size measurements. *Biochim. Biophys. Acta.* **2002**, *1564*, 21-20.

10. Hope, M.J.; Nayer, R.; Cullis, P. In *Liposome Technology*; Gregoriadis G., 2ⁿᵈ Ed.; CRC Press, Boca Raton. 1993.

11. Florence, A.T.; Nasseri, B. Microfabrication of lipidic structures. *Yakuzaigaku. J. Pharm. Sci. Tech.* **2001**, *61*, 8-9.

12. Arunothayanun, P.; Sooksawate, T.; Florence, A.T. Extrusion of niosomes from capillaries: approaches to a pulsed delivery device. *J. Control. Rel.* **1999**, *60*, 391-397.

13. Uchegbu, I.F.; Schätzlein, A.; Vanlerberghe, G.; Morgatini, N.; Florence, A.T. Polyhedral non-ionic surfactant vesicles. *J. Pharm. Pharmacol.* **1997**, *49*, 606-610.

14. Arunothayanun, P.; Uchegbu, I.F.; Florence, A.T. Osmotic behavior of polyhedral non-ionic surfactant vesicles (niosomes). *J. Pharm. Pharmacol.* **1999**, *51*, 651-657.

15. Arunothayanun, P.; Turton, J.A.; Uchegbu, I.F.; Florence, A.T. Preparation and *in vitro/in vivo* evaluation of luteinizing hormone releasing hormone (LHRH)-loaded polyhedral and spherical/tubular niosomes. *J. Pharm. Sci.* **1999**, *88*, 34-38.

16. Nasseri, B.; Florence, A.T. Microtubules formed by capillary extrusion and fusion of surfactant vesicles. *Int. J. Pharm.* **2003**, in press.

17. Uchegbu, I.F.; Double, J.A.; Turton, J.A.; Florence, A.T. Distribution, metabolism and tumoricidal activity of doxorubicin administered in sorbitan monostearate (Span 60) niosomes in the mouse. *Pharm. Res.* **1995**, *12*, 1019-1024.

18. Sackmann, E.; Duwe, H.P.; Engelhardt, H. Membrane bending elasticity and its role for shape fluctuations and shape transformations of cells and vesicles. *Faraday Discuss. Chem. Soc.* **1986**, *81*, 281-290.

Chapter 7

Lipid Microtubules as Sustained Delivery Vehicles for Proteins and Nucleic Acids

Nancy J. Meilander[1], Gerald M. Saidel[1],
and Ravi V. Bellamkonda[1,2,*]

[1]Department of Biomedical Engineering, Case Western Reserve University,
Wickenden 225, 10900 Euclid Avenue, Cleveland, OH 44106
[2]Current address: The Wallace H. Coulter Department of Biomedical
Engineering at Georgia Tech at Emory, Atlanta, GA 30332 (email:
ravi@bme.gatech.edu)

Lipid microtubule-based delivery systems are capable of the
sustained release of proteins and nucleic acids for biomedical
applications. The microtubules are hollow and open-ended
with an average diameter of 0.5 μm and an average length
ranging from 25-45 μm. They are non-inflammatory and can
be embedded into hydrogels for localization. Sustained
release of globular proteins can be attained in a manner
correlated to their size and loading concentration. A
mathematical model has been developed that can accurately
predict the release profiles. In addition, sustained release of
compacted plasmid DNA can be achieved using the lipid
microtubule delivery system. Released compacted DNA
retains its structure and bioactivity after release.

Introduction

Several polymeric delivery systems are available to release proteins and other bioactive compounds *(1-4)*, and a number of delivery systems are being investigated for the delivery of nucleic acids. *(5-12)* However, some polymeric delivery systems require organic solvents to dissolve the polymer and harsh physical forces such as homogenization and sonication to mix the immiscible phases during fabrication and loading. *(5-7,12-15)* Organic solvents can denature proteins, and residual solvents may affect the *in vivo* response. *(16)* In addition, forces from blending techniques and low pH from PLGA degradation may degrade proteins and DNA. *(7,8,17,18)* While fabrication techniques that avoid these hazardous conditions are under development, the microtubule delivery system can circumvent these issues by safely loading and releasing therapeutic agents without exposure to organic solvents or damaging forces. *(5,8,18)* The lipid microtubule-hydrogel delivery system we describe is injectable, versatile, and can be localized into specific areas *in vivo*.

Results and Discussion

Lipid Microtubules

Lipid microtubules, made from the diacetylenic lipid 1,2-bis(tricosa-10,12-diynoyl)-*sn*-glycero-3-phosphocholine (DC$_{8,9}$PC, Figure 1), were initially described by Yager and Schoen. *(19,20)* These microtubules are hollow and open-ended, with walls formed by one or more lipid bilayers. They form spontaneously during a controlled cooling process. The chiral interactions between lipid molecules cause the bilayer to twist and form a tubular structure. *(20, 21)* Since the chiral packing of the lipid molecules is very structured, the walls are highly ordered, and release of therapeutic agents from the lumen reservoir occurs via the two ends of each microtubule. *(22)* With a lumen diameter of approximately 0.5 μm and an average length of 25-45 μm (depending on the cooling rate), each microtubule has a high aspect ratio that allows for a large storage volume relative to the diameter. *(20,23)* They are stable in physiological solutions at 37°C for prolonged periods of time. *(24, 25)*

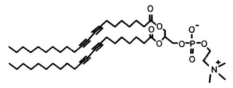

Figure 1. Chemical structure of DC$_{8,9}$PC.

Fabrication. The fabrication protocol for lipid microtubules has been previously described. *(26)* Briefly, lipid was dissolved in 70% ethanol (1 mg/ml) at 55°C and slowly cooled to 25°C. As the lipid passed through the phase transition temperature, the tubules self-assembled. The microtubules were dried in the presence of trehalose, a cryoprotectant, to preserve the tubular structures. Dry microtubules were loaded at room temperature by rehydration with an aqueous solution of the therapeutic agent (protein or DNA). Excess agent was removed by diluting the microtubules with saline solution, centrifuging (safe for proteins and DNA), and removing the supernatant. Throughout the loading process, the agent was never exposed to organic solvents or harmful external forces.

Characterization. Once self-assembled, the microtubules were characterized via light microscopy. Loaded microtubules were diluted, and an aliquot was placed on a glass slide and covered with a coverslip to create a single layer of microtubules (Figure 2). Using a MagnaFire digital camera (Optronics, Goleta CA) and Image Pro Express software (Media Cybernetics, Des Moines IA), microtubules were counted and lengths were measured. A typical microtubule batch yielded on the order of 10^8 tubules per mg lipid, and the average length ranged from 25-45 µm.

The loading efficiency can be defined as the ratio of the experimentally determined mass to the theoretically maximum mass of agent loaded in 1 mg of microtubules. The theoretically maximum mass was based on the assumption that the entire internal volume of the microtubules was filled with the agent at the same concentration as the loading solution. The internal volume was calculated using a diameter of 0.5 µm, the measured average length, and the measured yield. The actual mass of therapeutic agent in the tubules was determined by sonicating loaded microtubules to rupture the tubular structures and using a detection assay for the therapeutic agent. For globular proteins, the loading efficiency was 100%. *(26)*

Biocompatibility. To evaluate the *in vivo* response to microtubules, a rodent implantation model was utilized. Microtubules were injected subcutaneously in adult rats. On Day 10, skin flaps were removed, fixed, and evaluated. H&E staining revealed very few inflammatory cells for all implantation sites. The inflammatory and fibrotic reactions to the microtubule injections were not significantly different from the reactions to saline injections. *(26)* Lipid microtubules have been used for drug delivery applications both *in vitro* and *in vivo* without any deleterious effects. *In vitro* cell proliferation was not affected by co-incubation with microtubules, and PC12 cells were able to extend neurites in the presence of microtubules. *(24,26)* *In vivo*, lipid microtubules themselves did not affect angiogenesis in the chick chorioallantoic membrane assay, and no signs of inflammation were present when microtubules releasing nerve growth factor were incorporated into polymer channels for nerve regeneration (data not shown). *(27)* Thus, microtubules are a safe, non-inflammatory vehicle for delivering therapeutic agents *in vitro* and *in vivo*.

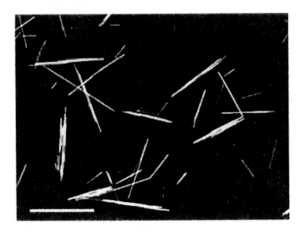

Figure 2. Light micrograph of lipid microtubules. Scale bar = 50 μm.

Hydrogel Carrier for Microtubules

Due to their small size, microtubules can be injected directly into a site of interest. However, their small size may also allow them to diffuse away from the injection site. To localize the lipid microtubules in a particular location, microtubules can be embedded in carriers including agarose hydrogel. Derived from red algae, agarose is a thermoreversible, biocompatible hydrogel consisting of alternating copolymers of 1,3-linked β-D-galactopyranose and 1,4-linked 3,6-anhydro-α-L-galactopyranose (Figure 3). Agarose is very porous and allows small molecules such as proteins and nucleic acids to diffuse through while the microtubules remain in the hydrogel. *(28)*

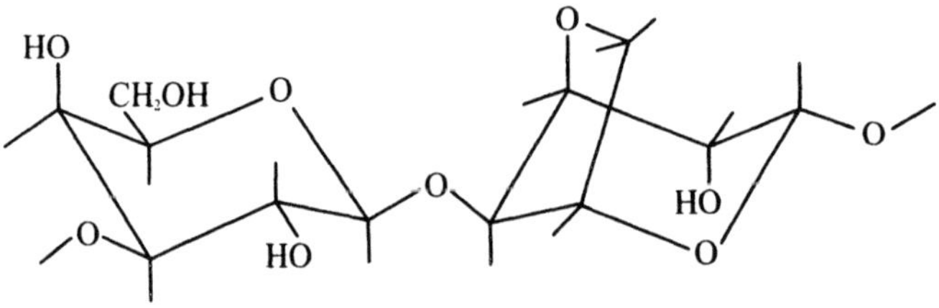

Figure 3. Repeat unit of agarose.

System Design Parameters. Both the carrier (hydrogel) and the micro-tubules can be modified to suit the application. Agarose concentration affects the porosity and the agent diffusivity within the hydrogel. Also, the gelling temperature can be changed by varying the extent of hydroxyethyl substitution on the agarose backbone. Since agarose is injectable in both the liquid and gelled states, some agarose formulations can be injected as a solution and will gel rapidly at 37°C. Microtubule length affects release characteristics, with longer microtubules releasing for a longer period of time. Increasing the tubule concentration in the hydrogel will allow for a greater amount of agent to be loaded. The agent concentration and size can also be varied to obtain the desired release profile. With these options, the microtubule-hydrogel delivery system is able to provide a variety of release profiles.

Sustained Release of Proteins

The sustained release properties of lipid microtubules have been demon-strated previously using proteins such as transforming growth factor-β, nerve growth factor, and cleaved high molecular weight kininogen. *(25-27)* We have characterized the microtubule-hydrogel delivery system by determining the release profiles of proteins *in vitro*. Globular proteins of varying molecular weights were released to determine the effects of molecular weight and protein concentration on the release profile. To predict the rate of release from our microtubule-hydrogel delivery system, a mathematical model based on the one-dimensional form of Fick's second law of diffusion was developed and compared to the experimental data.

Protein Release. To determine the effect of protein size on the release profile, microtubules were loaded with 0.45 mM solutions of three different test proteins: myoglobin (18 kDa), albumin (66 kDa), and thyroglobulin (660 kDa). *(26)* The microtubules were embedded in 1% (w/v) SeaPrep agarose hydrogel at a tubule concentration of 8.3 mg/ml. The release profiles demonstrated that size was inversely related to the release rate, with the smaller proteins releasing at a faster rate (Figure 4). When microtubules were loaded with 0.45, 1.51, and 2.26 mM albumin solutions, the mass of released protein increased with the loading concentration, but the percent of loaded protein released was unaffected by the loading concentration. *(26)*

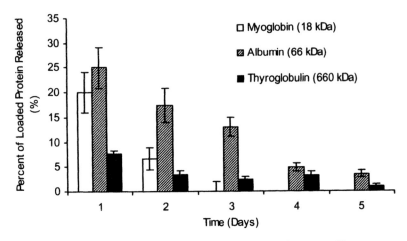

Figure 4. Effect of protein size on the release profile

Mathematical Model Development. A mathematical model, based on our *in vitro* experimental set-up, (Figure 5), was developed to predict the release profile from the microtubule-hydrogel delivery system. The basic assumption of the model is that the diffusivity of the protein within the gel is much smaller than the diffusivity in both the saline solution above the gel and the protein solution within the microtubules. Therefore, the rate limiting process is diffusion within the gel, and the microtubules act as reservoirs to provide a continuous supply of protein. The duration of this supply is dependent on the volume within the microtubules.

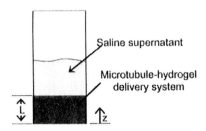

Figure 5. Schematic of protein release experiment.

The dynamic concentration distribution within the gel, as delivered by the microtubules, can be described by one-dimensional diffusion as

$$\frac{\partial C(z,t)}{\partial t} = D_e \frac{\partial^2 C(z,t)}{\partial z^2} \quad \text{with} \quad 0 < z < L,$$

where C is the protein concentration, z is the distance from the bottom of the gel, t is the time, D_e is the effective diffusivity of the protein in the microtubule-hydrogel, and L is the length of gel as shown in Figure 6.

The initial agent concentration (c_0) in the delivery system is assumed to be uniform, and the concentration gradient is zero at the bottom of the gel ($z = 0$) since no diffusion occurs there. Also, the saline solution has negligible protein, so the protein concentration at the top of the gel ($z = L$) is assumed to be zero. With these conditions and the above diffusion equation, the total mass, M, released from the system after time, T, was calculated as

$$M(T) = \frac{8c_0AL}{\pi^2} \sum_{n=1}^{\infty} \frac{(-1)^{n+1}}{(2n-1)^2} \left(\sin\frac{(2n-1)\pi}{2} \right) \exp\left(\frac{-(2n-1)^2 D_e \pi^2 T}{4L^2} - 1 \right),$$

where A is the cross-sectional area of the hydrogel.

Model Validity. The solution was computed using MATLAB (The Mathworks, Inc., Natick MA). Parameter values were based on the protein release experiments. Strong congruence was shown between the diffusion model and the experimental data obtained for three albumin loading concentrations (Figure 6). The release profiles for microtubules loaded with equivalent molar amounts (1.51 mM) of albumin and myoglobin were also compared to the model output. The theoretical release was consistent with the experimental release for both proteins (data not shown).

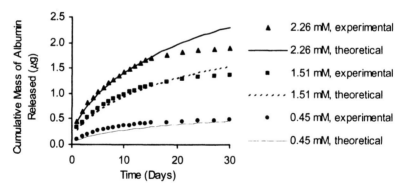

Figure 6. Congruence between mathematical model and experimental data for albumin release. The correlation (γ) is greater than 0.97 for each protein concentration.

Thus, the model correlates well with the experimental data. If the initial agent concentration, overall hydrogel dimensions, and effective diffusivity of the agent are known, the cumulative mass released at a given time can be calculated. Using this model, we can predict release profiles as well as theoretically analyze the effects of experimental parameters.

Sustained Release of Nucleic Acids

Non-viral gene therapy protocols are often limited by inefficient gene transfer and transient gene expression. Sustained release of non-viral DNA may improve the overall gene expression levels and extend the duration of expression. Lipid microtubules can provide the slow release of compacted plasmid DNA for at least 95 days. Released DNA was structurally similar to unreleased (freshly compacted) DNA and functionally able to transfect cells, though at a lower efficiency than freshly compacted DNA.

Compacted DNA Release. The reporter plasmid for these studies contained the luciferase gene controlled by the elongation factor-1α promoter and the CMV enhancer. The compaction conjugate consisted of a cationic peptide (N-terminal cysteine followed by 30 lysine residues with acetate as the negative counterion) covalently coupled to polyethylene glycol (10 kDa). The DNA was compacted by mixing the plasmid and compaction conjugate for a two-fold excess of positive charge and a final DNA concentration of 0.2 mg/ml. Once compacted, the DNA was sterilized using a 0.2 μm filter and centrifugally concentrated.

Dry microtubules were loaded by rehydration with compacted DNA solution (3 mg/ml DNA). Excess DNA was removed, and 5 mg loaded microtubules (containing 5.5 μg DNA per mg lipid) were mixed with SeaPlaque agarose for a final volume of 0.6 ml and a final concentration of 0.5% SeaPlaque. After gelation, saline supernatant was added to the samples, and they were incubated at 37°C. Periodically, the supernatant was removed and replaced with fresh saline. The mass of released DNA in the saline supernatant was quantified via UV-absorbance at 260 nm, and the release profile was generated (Figure 7). The released DNA was then evaluated for structural and functional integrity.

Structural Characterization of Released DNA. Structurally, released DNA was similar to freshly compacted DNA at all timepoints tested. Released DNA samples (Day 1, 20, and 50) were evaluated for structural integrity using sedimentation, electron microscopy, and serum stability. Since there was no significant difference between the timepoints tested, results are shown for DNA collected on Day 20 of release. In all characterization assays, freshly compacted DNA was the positive control.

A sedimentation assay, comparing the DNA UV-absorbance pre- and post-centrifugation, revealed that released DNA was non-aggregated. To evaluate DNA morphology, freshly compacted and released DNA were negatively stained with uranyl acetate and observed on a transmission electron microscope (JEOL USA, Inc., Peabody MA). The micrographs revealed similar long rods and toroids in the freshly compacted (Figure 8A) and the released (Figure 8B) DNA. Since compacted DNA has increased nuclease resistance compared to naked DNA, a serum stability assay was utilized to verify that released DNA retained this property. *(29)* Freshly compacted and released DNA samples were incubated for two hours with 75% mouse serum at 37°C, digested with trypsin to remove the compaction peptide, extracted with phenol-chloroform-isoamyl alcohol, and visualized using gel electrophoresis and ethidium bromide staining. Released DNA remained compacted and resistant to degradation by serum nucleases. Although no degradation was detected, the released plasmid DNA was converted from supercoiled to linear and nicked forms (data not shown).

Functional Characterization of Released DNA. To test the activity of the released DNA, bovine aortic smooth muscle cells (BASMC) were transfected with naked, freshly compacted, and released DNA (2 µg/ml) in reduced serum medium (OptiMEM, Invitrogen Corp., Carlsbad CA) with and without the cationic lipid transfection reagent Lipofectin (Invitrogen Corp.). DNA-Lipofectin complexes were formed according to the manufacturer's protocol. When the cells were 40-60% confluent, the growth medium (containing 10% serum) was replaced with OptiMEM containing the various forms of DNA, and the cells were incubated for 4 hours. At that time, the transfection medium was replaced with growth medium, and the cells were incubated for 20 hours. The cells were lysed 24 hours post-transfection, and luciferase activity was quantified using the luciferase assay reagent (Promega, Madison WI). The DC Bio-Rad protein assay was used to quantify total cellular protein (Bio-Rad Laboratories, Hercules CA), and luciferase activity was reported as relative light units per microgram of protein (RLU/µg protein).

Released DNA was capable of transfecting the BASMC (Figure 9). With Lipofectin, released DNA produced luciferase activity significantly above background but lower than naked DNA-Lipofectin complexes. Without Lipofectin, luciferase activity from released DNA was significantly higher than both the negative control and naked DNA. However, in all instances, activity from released DNA was lower than that from freshly compacted DNA. This may be due to the conversion of supercoiled DNA to nicked and linear DNA as revealed in the serum stability assay.

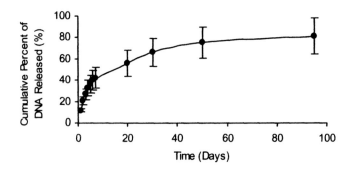

Figure 7. Cumulative release of compacted DNA from the microtubule-hydrogel delivery system.

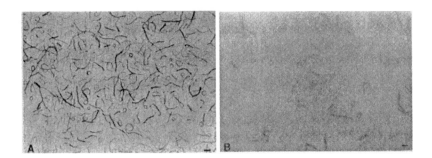

Figure 8. Electron micrographs of compacted DNA that is freshly compacted (unreleased) (A), and released from the microtubule-hydrogel delivery system on Days 7-20 (B). Scale bars = 100 nm.

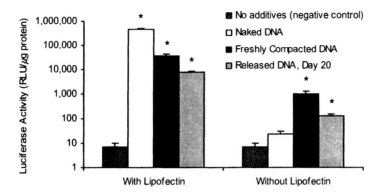

*Figure 9. Released DNA transfected BASMC with and without Lipofectin. (*P-value < 0.001 compared to negative control.)*

Conclusions

Lipid microtubules are a safe, predictable tool for delivering a variety of biological agents, including proteins and nucleic acids. The tubules are compatible with cells *in vitro* and do not invoke an inflammatory response *in vivo*. Since the microtubule delivery system is easily customized, its usefulness extends to applications that include therapeutic drug delivery, cancer treatment, tissue regeneration, and gene therapy.

Acknowledgements

The authors thank Osman Muhammad for the electron microscopy, the employees of Copernicus Therapeutics, Inc. (Cleveland, OH) for their advice and consultations, Matthew Shive, Ph.D. for assistance with the rodent implantation model, and Nicholas Ziats, Ph.D. for the biocompatibility evaluation. Funding was provided by the National Science Foundation (CAREER Award to RVB) and the Whitaker Foundation (fellowship to NJM).

References

1. Hatefi, A.; Amsden, B. Biodegradable injectable in situ forming drug delivery systems, *J. Control. Release* **2002**, *80*, 9-28.
2. Jain, R. A. The manufacturing techniques of various drug loaded biodegradable poly(lactide-co-glycolide) (PLGA) devices, *Biomater.* **2000**, *21*, 2475-2490.

3. Sinha, V. R.; Khosla, L. Bioabsorbable polymers for implantable therapeutic systems, *Drug Dev. Ind. Pharm.* **1998**, *24*, 1129-1138.

4. Kumar, M. N.; Kumar, N. Polymeric controlled drug-delivery systems: perspective issues and opportunities, *Drug Dev. Ind. Pharm.* **2001**, *27*, 1-30.

5. Ando, S.; Putnam, D.; Pack, D. W.; Langer, R. PLGA microspheres containing plasmid DNA: preservation of supercoiled DNA via cryopreparation and carbohydrate stabilization, *J. Pharm. Sci.* **1999**, *88*, 126-130.

6. Wang, D.; Robinson, D. R.; Kwon, G. S.; Samuel, J. Encapsulation of plasmid DNA in biodegradable poly(D, L-lactic-co- glycolic acid) microspheres as a novel approach for immunogene delivery, *J. Control. Release* **1999**, *57*, 9-18.

7. Walter, E.; Moelling, K.; Pavlovic, J.; Merkle, H. P. Microencapsulation of DNA using poly(DL-lactide-co-glycolide): stability issues and release characteristics, *J. Control. Release* **1999**, *61*, 361-374.

8. Hsu, Y. Y.; Hao, T.; Hedley, M. L. Comparison of process parameters for microencapsulation of plasmid DNA in poly(D,L-lactic-co-glycolic) acid microspheres, *J. Drug Target.* **1999**, *7*, 313-323.

9. Bonadio, J.; Smiley, E.; Patil, P.; Goldstein, S. Localized, direct plasmid gene delivery in vivo: prolonged therapy results in reproducible tissue regeneration, *Nat. Med.* **1999**, *5*, 753-759.

10. Ismail, F. A.; Napaporn, J.; Hughes, J. A.; Brazeau, G. A. In situ gel formulations for gene delivery: release and myotoxicity studies, *Pharm. Dev. Technol.* **2000**, *5*, 391-397.

11. Fukunaka, Y.; Iwanaga, K.; Morimoto, K.; Kakemi, M.; Tabata, Y. Controlled release of plasmid DNA from cationized gelatin hydrogels based on hydrogel degradation, *J. Control. Release* **2002**, *80*, 333-343.

12. Jong, Y. S.; Jacob, J. S.; Yip, K.-P.; Gardner, G.; Seitelman, E.; Whitney, M.; Montgomery, S.; Mathiowitz, E. Controlled release of plasmid DNA, *J. Control. Release* **1997**, *47*, 123-134.

13. Edelman, E. R.; Adams, D. H.; Karnovsky, M. J. Effect of controlled adventitial heparin delivery on smooth muscle cell proliferation following endothelial injury, *Proc. Natl. Acad. Sci. U.S.A.* **1990**, *87*, 3773-3777.

14. Cleek, R. L.; Rege, A. A.; Denner, L. A.; Eskin, S. G.; Mikos, A. G. Inhibition of smooth muscle cell growth in vitro by an antisense oligodeoxynucleotide released from poly(DL-lactic-co-glycolic acid) microparticles, *J. Biomed. Mater. Res.* **1997**, *35*, 525-530.

15. Wyatt, T. L.; Saltzman, W. M. Protein delivery from nondegradable polymer matrices, *Pharm. Biotechnol.* **1997**, *10*, 119-137.

16. Raghuvanshi, R. S.; Goyal, S.; Singh, O.; Panda, A. K. Stabilization of dichloromethane-induced protein denaturation during microencapsulation, *Pharm. Dev. Technol.* **1998**, *3*, 269-276.

17. Capan, Y.; Woo, B. H.; Gebrekidan, S.; Ahmed, S.; DeLuca, P. P. Preparation and characterization of poly (D,L-lactide-co-glycolide) microspheres for controlled release of poly(L-lysine) complexed plasmid DNA, *Pharm. Res.* **1999**, *16*, 509-513.

18. van de Weert, M.; Hennink, W. E.; Jiskoot, W. Protein instability in poly(lactic-co-glycolic acid) microparticles, *Pharm. Res.* **2000**, *17*, 1159-1167.

19. Yager, P.; Schoen, P. E. Formation of tubules by a polymerizable surfactant, *Mol. Cryst. Liq. Cryst.* **1984**, *106*, 371-381.

20. Schnur, J. M. Lipid tubules: A paradigm for molecularly engineered structures, *Science* **1993**, *262*, 1669-1676.

21. Spector, M. S.; Selinger, J. V.; Schnur, J. M. Thermodynamics of phospholipid tubules in alcohol/water solutions, *J. Am. Chem. Soc.* **1997**, *119*, 8533-8539.

22. Price, R.; Patchan, M. Controlled release from cylindrical microstructures, *J. Microencapsulation* **1991**, *8*, 301-306.

23. Thomas, B. N.; Safinya, C. R.; Plano, R. J.; Clark, N. A. Lipid tubule self-assemble: Length dependence on cooling rate through a first-order phase transition, *Science* **1995**, *267*, 1635-1638.

24. Rudolph, A. S.; Stilwell, G.; Cliff, R. O.; Kahn, B.; Spargo, B. J.; Rollwagen, F.; Monroy, R. L. Biocompatibility of lipid microcylinders: effect on cell growth and antigen presentation in culture, *Biomater.* **1992**, *13*, 1085-1092.

25. Spargo, B. J.; Cliff, R. O.; Rollwagen, F. M.; Rudolph, A. S. Controlled release of transforming growth factor-beta from lipid-based microcylinders, *J. Microencapsulation* **1995**, *12*, 247-254.

26. Meilander, N. J.; Yu, X.; Ziats, N. P.; Bellamkonda, R. V. Lipid-based microtubular drug delivery vehicles, *J. Control. Release* **2001**, *71*, 141-152.

27. Panchal, S. C.; Meilander, N. J.; Bellamkonda, R. V.; Ziats, N. P. Slow release of high molecular weight kininogen inhibits angiogenesis in vivo, *Soc. Biomater. 28th Ann. Mtg. Trans.* **2002**, *25*, 504.

28. Dillon, G. P.; Yu, X.; Sridharan, A.; Ranieri, J. P.; Bellamkonda, R. V. The influence of physical structure and charge on neurite extension in a 3D hydrogel scaffold, *J. Biomater. Sci. Polym. Ed.* **1998**, *9*, 1049-1069.

29. Kowalczyk, T. H.; Pasumarthy, M. K.; Gedeon, C.; Moen, R. C.; Cooper, M. J. Light scattering by compacted DNA predicts its serum stability, *Mol. Ther.* **2000**, *1*, S120.

Chapter 8

Template-Synthesized Bionanotubes for Separations and Biocatalysis

Sang Bok Lee[1], David T. Mitchell[1], Lacramioara Trofin[1],
Tarja K. Nevanen[2], Hans Söderlund[2], and Charles R. Martin[1,*]

[1]Department of Chemistry and Center for research at the Bio/Nano
Interface, University of Florida, Gainesville, FL 32611-7200
[2]VTT Biotechnology, P.O. Box 1500, FIN–02044 VTT, Espoo, Finland
*Corresponding author: email: crmartin@chem.ufl.edu

Synthetic bio-nanotubes were developed and used for
separations, including separation of enantiomers, and
biocatalysis. The nanotubes were templated from alumina
films that have cylindrical pores with monodisperse
nanoscopic diameters. A thin film of silica was chemically
synthesized within the pores of these films to create the
nanotubes. The nanotubes can be functionalized with a variety
of chemistries, including proteins, by using silanes. Further,
the inner and outer surfaces can be modified independently.
Nanotubes liberated from the alumina template can be used as
extractants or biocatalysts. Arrays of modified nanotubes left
in the alumina template can be used as facilitated transport
separation membranes.

Introduction

There is enormous current interest in using nanoparticles for biomedical applications including enzyme encapsulation, DNA transfection, biosensors, and drug delivery. *(1-3)* Typically, spherical nanoparticles are used for such applications because spherical particles are easy to make. Self-assembling lipid tubules have also been used in biomedical applications, although it is difficult to control tubule diameter or length and the lipid tubules must be coated with ceramic or metal to make them rugged enough for biomedical use. *(4-6)* We have pioneered a technology, called template synthesis, for preparing monodisperse nanotubes of nearly any size and composed of nearly any material, or combination of materials. *(7,8)* These nanotubes have a number of attributes that make them potential candidates for biomedical applications. First, nanotubes have inner voids that can be filled with species ranging in size from large proteins to small molecules. In addition, nanotubes have distinct inner and outer surfaces that can be differentially functionalized. This creates the possibility of tailoring the outer nanotube surface to satisfy a particular biochemical requirement (e.g., biocompatibility), while immobilizing a desired biochemical species to the inner surface. The ability to control the dimensions allows for tailoring tube size to fit the biomedical problem at hand. The nanotubes can be used either in the template, as an array to produce a separations membrane, or as a collection of liberated nanotubes for extractions or bio-catalysis. Finally, the ability to make these nanotubes out of nearly any material creates the possibility of making nanotubes with desired properties such as ruggedness or biodegradability. *(9)*

We have used template-synthesized silica nanotubes (Figure 1A) to demonstrate a number of these concepts. Silica nanotubes are ideal vehicles for such proof-of-concept experiments because they are easy to make, readily suspend in aqueous solution, and because silica surfaces can be derivatized with an enormous variety of chemical functional groups using simple silane chemistry with commercially available reagents. *(10)* The silica nanotubes were synthesized within the pores of nanopore alumina template membranes (Figure 1B) using a sol-gel method. Templates with pore diameters ranging from 20 to 200 nm were used for these studies.

Materials and Methods

Commercial Anopore alumina membranes used as templates were obtained from Whatman (Clifton, NJ). These were disks 47 mm in diameter with cylindrical pores of nominally 200 nm diameter. All other sizes of templates were grown in-house by anodic oxidation of high purity aluminium. *(11)* Unless otherwise noted, chemicals were reagent grade, obtained from commercial sources and were used as received. Water was 18 MOhm pure from a Barnstead Epure model D4641 system. UV-VIS spectra were obtained using a Hitachi U-

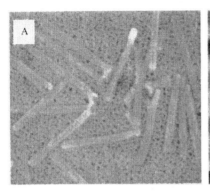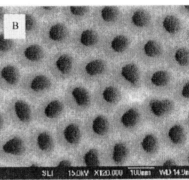

Figure 1. Silica nanotubes (60 nm diameter) produced by template synthesis in alumina template (A). Top view of alumina template membrane (B).

3501 spectrophotometer. Scanning electron microscopy (SEM) was performed using a Phillips 505 scanning electron microscope.

Template Synthesis. A sol-gel template process was used to prepare the nanotubes. *(12)* First, a sol-gel silica precursor was prepared by mixing absolute ethanol, tetraethylorthosilicate (TEOS, Aldrich, Figure 2A), and 1 M HCl (50:5:1 vol/vol). This solution was allowed to hydrolyze for 30 minutes. Alumina template membranes were then immersed into the sol-gel with sonication for 1 minute, after which they were air dried for 10 minutes at room temperature, and cured overnight at 150°C to complete the hydrolysis of the TEOS. The silica-coated membranes were polished on both surfaces with an aqueous aluminum oxide slurry of ~1um diameter particles. This removed the surface layers of SiO_2 that would otherwise bind the nanotubes together. To liberate the nanotubes, the membranes were immersed overnight in a 25% (wt/wt) solution of H_3PO_4 to dissolve the aluminum oxide template. The nanotubes were filtered from the acid solution and repeatedly rinsed with pH 7.0 buffer and water, then dried.

Silanization. Structures of all silanes used for surface modification are shown in Figure 2. C_{18} functionalized surfaces were prepared by immersing either the SiO_2-coated alumina membrane or freed nanotubes in a 5 vol% aqueous, 5 vol% octadecyltrimethoxysilane (Aldrich, Figure 2B) solution in ethanol, pH adjusted to 5.0 with acetate. *(13)* The deposition solution was stirred for 20 minutes before addition of the membrane to allow formation of siloxane oligomers. Silane deposition was usually done overnight to insure maximum coverage of the C_{18}. Following deposition, the membranes were rinsed with ethanol and dried for 20 minutes at 150°C to cure the silane layer. The silicon dioxide surface layers of the membrane were removed by mechanical polishing with a slurry of ~1 um alumina particles and the template alumina was dissolved with a 25% wt/wt solution of phosphoric acid. The nanotubes were filtered and rinsed, as above.

Modifications with N-triethoxysilylpropylquinineurethan (Gelest, Morris-ville, PA, Figure 2C), N-triethoxysilylpropyldansylamide, (Gelest, Figure 2D), 2-[methoxy(polyethyleneoxy)propyl]trimethoxysilane (Shearwater, Huntsville, AL, Figure 2E), were analogous. Each was deposited from an ethanolic solution containing 5% (wt/vol) of the silane. The deposition solution was also 5% in distilled water by volume and was adjusted to pH 5.0 with sodium acetate. In all cases the silane solution was allowed to polymerize 20 minutes before addition of the membrane. Silane deposition was accomplished by immersing the SiO_2-coated template into these solutions, followed by an ethanol rinse and heat fixing at 140°C for 20 minutes. Depositions were usually performed overnight to maximize coverage. The modified nanotubes were released from the template by dissolving with 25% H_3PO_4, filtered from the acid solution, and rinsed repeatedly with water.

Protein functionalized SiO_2 nanotubes were generally prepared from the unmodified nanotubes via an aldehyde terminated siloxane linker. (14) Unmodified nanotubes were stirred in a 5 vol% aqueous, 10 vol% triethoxy-silanebutyraldehyde (PSX1050, United Chemical Technologies, Figure 2F) solution in ethanol, pH adjusted to 5.0 with acetate. The aldehyde-modified nanotubes were filtered, rinsed with ethanol, and dried 24 hours in an oxygen free glove box. After drying, the nanotubes were incubated with a solution of protein in buffer (~1 mg protein/ml buffer). Incubation was at 4°C overnight. Aldehydes have been shown to react with pendant primary amines on proteins (lysine residues) to covalently link the proteins to the substrate. (15-17) This resulted in proteins being bound to both the interior and exterior of the nanotubes. The protein-modified nanotubes were filtered from the protein solution and extensively rinsed with buffer before use.

Liberated nanotubes with protein modification on the inside only were prepared using a three-step gluteraldehyde process. While still in the alumina template membrane, the nanotubes were silanized with an amino silane. The silica-coated alumina membrane was immersed for two hours in an ethanol solution containing 5 vol% 3-aminopropyltriethoxysilane and 5 vol% water. After rinsing with ethanol, the silane was cured by heating two hours at 80°C. The alumina template was then dissolved with aqueous 25% phosphoric acid and the nanotubes were filtered and extensively rinsed. The amino-modified interior surface was further modified with aldehyde by suspending the nanotubes in a 150 mM pH 7.4 phosphate buffer containing 2.5 vol% gluteraldehyde for five hours. The nanotubes were again filtered, rinsed with buffer, and suspended in protein solutions overnight at 4°C for protein attachment.

The a (R,S) and d (S,R) enantiomers of 4-[3-(4-fluorophenyl)-2-hydroxy-1-[1,2,4]triazol-1-yl-propyl]-benzonitrile and the Fab antibody fragment ENA11His were kindly provided by Dr. Hans Soderlund and coworkers at VTT Biotechnology, Finland. All extraction experiments were from pH 8.5 sodium phosphate buffer containing 5 vol% dimethylsulfoxide. Membrane separation experiments used membranes of aligned ENA11His-modified nanotubes in the alumina template. These were mounted between the two halves of a U-tube permeation cell. *(18-21)* A feed solution that was a racemic mixture of the RS and SR enantiomers (typically 0.1 mM in each enantiomer dissolved in pH 8.5 phosphate buffer that was 10 vol% in DMSO) was placed on one side of the membrane. The receiver solution on the other side of the membrane was the phosphate/DMSO buffer. The fluxes of the RS and SR enantiomers across the membrane were determined by periodically assaying for these enantiomers in the receiver solution. Separation and concentration determination of the enantiomers was done using a Shimadzu VP system High Performance Liquid Chromatograph (HPLC) under the following conditions: An Ultron ES-OVM column was used at 30 C with a running buffer of 20 mM ammonium phosphate adjusted to pH 5.0 containing 20 vol% methanol. The flow rate was 1.0 mL/min. Detection was at 230 nm and the detection limit was at a signal to noise level of 5. The injection loop had a volume of 20 µL.

Glucose oxidase was obtained from Sigma. The activity of glucose oxidase was assayed according to a modified literature procedure. *(22)* First a 50 mM, pH 5.1 acetate buffer was prepared containing 0.17 mM *o*-dianisidine and 1.72% (wt/vol) β–D-glucose. To 2.90 mL of this solution was added 0.10 mL of aqueous peroxidase solution at a concentration of 60 units/mL. Glucose oxidase-modified nanotubes were added to this mixture and shaken to disperse the nanotubes. Production of the oxidized *o*-dianisidine was monitored using visible spectroscopy at 500 nm.

Results and Discussion

Differential Inside/Outside Modification

One of the most interesting and useful features of the nanotube architecture compared to spherical nanoparticles is that the inside and outside surfaces are both easily accessible. We have developed the following simple procedure for applying different functional groups to the inner vs. outer surfaces of these nanotubes (see Figure 3 for schematic). While still embedded within the pores of the template membrane, the inner nanotube surfaces are reacted with the first silane. This silane cannot attach to the outer nanotube surfaces because the outer surfaces are in contact with the pore wall and are thus masked. The template is dissolved to liberate the nanotubes, which unmasks the outer nanotube surfaces. *(11)* The nanotubes are then exposed to a second silane to attach this silane to only the outer nanotube surfaces.

To prove this concept, a set of nanotubes was prepared with the green fluorescent silane N-(triethoxysilylpropyl)dansylamide attached to their inner surfaces, and the hydrophobic octadecyl trimethoxysilane (C_{18}) to their outer surfaces. These nanotubes were added to a vial containing water and the immiscible organic solvent cyclohexane, which were mixed and allowed to separate. Because these nanotubes are hydrophobic on their outer surfaces, they partition into the (upper) cyclohexane phase (Figure 4A). This may be contrasted to nanotubes that were labeled on their inner surfaces with the blue

A. Tetraethylorthosilicate

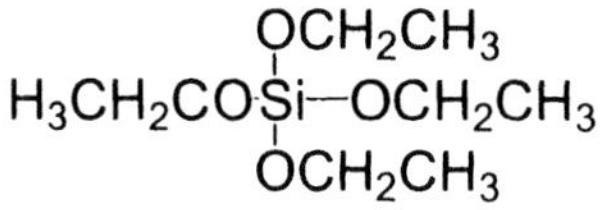

$$OCH_2CH_3$$
$$H_3CH_2CO\overset{|}{\underset{|}{Si}}-OCH_2CH_3$$
$$OCH_2CH_3$$

B. N-Octadecyltrimethoxysilane

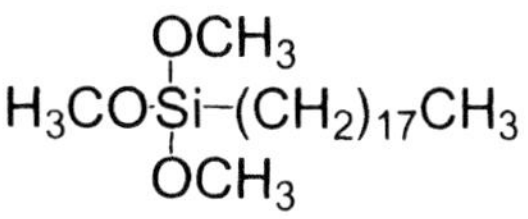

$$OCH_3$$
$$H_3CO\overset{|}{\underset{|}{Si}}-(CH_2)_{17}CH_3$$
$$OCH_3$$

C. N-Triethoxysilylpropylquinineurethan

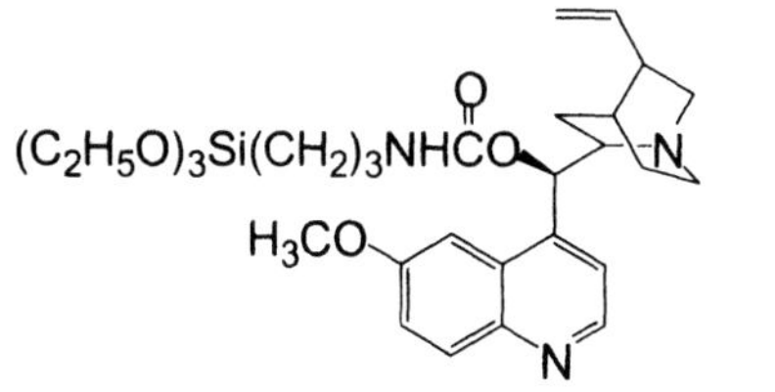

$(C_2H_5O)_3Si(CH_2)_3NHCO$

H_3CO

D. N-Triethoxysilylpropyldansylamide

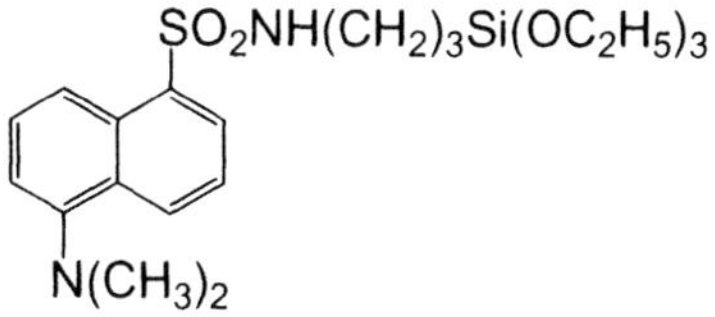

$SO_2NH(CH_2)_3Si(OC_2H_5)_3$

$N(CH_3)_2$

E. 2-[Methoxy(polyethyleneoxy)-
propyl]trimethoxysilane

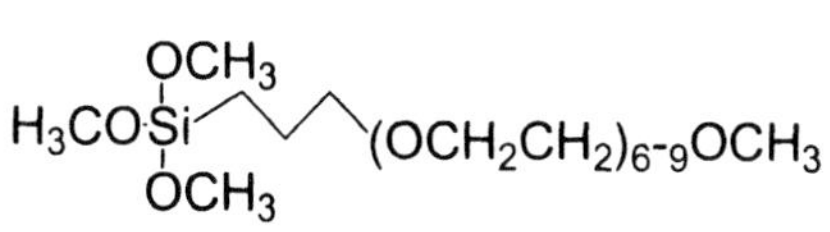

$$OCH_3$$
$$H_3CO\overset{|}{\underset{|}{Si}}\quad (OCH_2CH_2)_{6-9}OCH_3$$
$$OCH_3$$

F. 3-Triethoxysilanebutyraldehyde

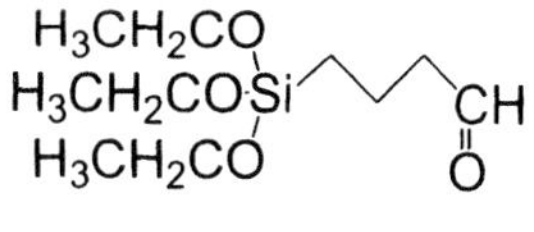

$$H_3CH_2CO$$
$$H_3CH_2CO\overset{|}{Si}\quad CH$$
$$H_3CH_2CO\quad\quad \overset{\|}{O}$$

Figure 2. Structures of silanes.

104

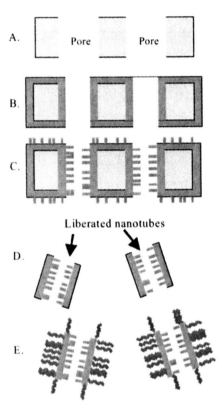

Figure 3. Schematic of Differential Inside/Outside Modification. Cross-section of Al2O3 template membrane showing two pores (A). Sol-gel synthesis of SiO₂ nanotubes (B). Silanization of inner nanotube surface (C). Removal of surface films and dissolution of alumina template (D). Secondary silanization on outer nanotube surface (E). (See page 4 of color insert.)

fluorescent silane triethoxysilylpropylquinineurethan, but were not labeled with silane on their outer surfaces. When the same experiment is done with these nanotubes, the quinineurethan fluorescence is seen only from the aqueous phase (Figure 4B). When both sets of nanotubes are added to the solvent mixture in the same vial, the tubes with the C_{18} outer surface chemistry go to the cyclohexane and the tubes with the silica outer surface chemistry go to the aqueous phase (Figure 4C).

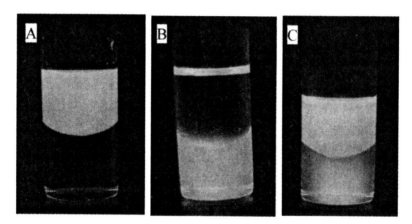

Figure 4. Fluorescently-modified nanotubes in biphasic cyclohexane (top)/ water (bottom) mix. Dansylamine inside/C18 outside nanotubes partition into cyclohexane phase (A). Quinineurathane inside/bare silica outside nanotubes partition into water phase (B). Mix of both types independently phase separates (C). (See page 5 of color insert.)

Extraction Experiments

One application for such differentially functionalized nanotubes is as smart nanophase extractors to remove specific molecules from solution. Nanotubes with hydrophilic chemistry on their outer surfaces and hydrophobic chemistry on their inner surfaces are ideal for extracting lipophilic molecules from aqueous solution. The hydrophobic molecule 7,8-benzoquinoline (BQ), which has an octanol/water partition coefficient of $10^{3.8}$ was used as a model compound for such nanophase solvent extraction experiments. *(23)* 5 mg of the silica-outer/C_{18}-inner nanotubes were suspended into 5 mL of 1.0×10^{-5} M aqueous BQ. The suspension was stirred for 5 minutes and filtered to remove the nanotubes. UV spectroscopy showed that 82% of the BQ was removed from the solution. When a second 5 mg batch of these nanotubes was added to the filtrate, >90% of the original amount of BQ was removed from the solution.

Control nanotubes that did not contain the hydrophobic C_{18} inner surface chemistry extracted less than 10% of the BQ (Figure 5).

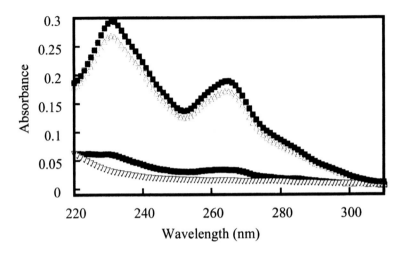

Figure 5. UV spectra of 7,8-benzoquinoline extracted with C18 modified silica nanotubes. (◆) Control solution (10^{-5} M benzoquinoline); (△) After extraction with SiO_2 tubules; (●) After extraction with C-18 SiO_2 tubules; (▽) After second extraction with C-18 SiO_2 tubules.

Nanotubes with C_{18} inside will in principle extract any lipophilic molecule. While this generic extraction ability might be useful for some applications, nanotubes that are molecule-specific would also be useful. We show here that antibody-functionalized nanotubes can provide the ultimate in extraction selectivity – the extraction of one enantiomer of a racemic pair. Enantiomeric separations are an area of rapidly increasing concern. Drugs that are produced as racemic mixtures normally contain only one enantiomer that is efficacious, and there is increasing pressure on the pharmaceutical industry to market enantiomerically pure drugs. *(24,25)* Nanotubes can be used for enantio-selective separations in two ways. First, liberated nanotubes can be used as selective extractants. Second, the nanotubes can be left in the template, and the resulting nanotube membrane can be used to selectively transport the desired enantiomer from the racemic mixture into a receiver solution on the other side of the membrane. Both methods require a molecular-recognition agent that is enantioselective.

Antibodies are perhaps the most specific of the molecular-recognition proteins. Antibodies developed by Dr. Hans Soderlund and coworkers have been shown to be selective in binding one enantiomer of the drug 4-[3-(4-

fluorophenyl)-2-hydroxy-1-[1,2,4]triazol-1-yl-propyl]-benzonitrile, FTB, an inhibitor of aromatase enzyme activity. This molecule has two chiral centers and thus four stereoisomers, RR, SS, SR, and RS (Figure 6). The antibody used selectively binds the RS relative to the SR enantiomer. Cloning, production, and purification of this RS enantiospecific Fab-fragment (termed ENA11His) have been reported previously. *(26)*

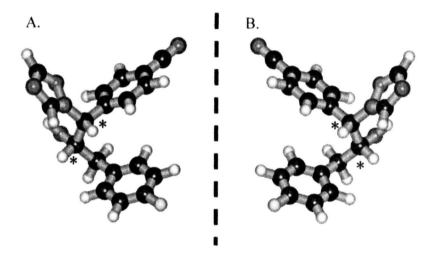

A.   B.

Figure 6. Three-dimensional structures of the RS-enantiomer (A) and SR-enantiomer (B) of FTB. (*) denotes the chiral centers. The geometry optimization was done by Ab Initio calculation with minimal basis set in HyperChem 6.03. The drug is in clinical trials by Hormos Medical, Turku, Finland. (Reprinted with permission from Lee et al. Science, 2002, 296, 2198. Copyright 2002 American Association for the Advancement of Science.) (See page 5 of color insert.)

ENA11His was immobilized to both the inner and outer surfaces of the silica nanotubes via an aldehyde silane linker as described in detail in Materials and Methods. *(27,28)* For extraction experiments, ENA11His-functionalized nanotubes that had been liberated from the alumina template were added to racemic mixtures of the SR and RS enantiomers of FTB. The tubes were then collected by filtration and the filtrate was assayed for the presence of the two enantiomers using a chiral HPLC method. The results of the extraction experiments are shown in Figure 7. Chromatogram A is from a solution that was 20 μM in both enantiomers, while chromatogram B was obtained for the same solution after exposure to the Fab-functionalized nanotubes. 75% of the RS enantiomer and none of the SR enantiomer was removed by the nanotubes. When the concentration of the racemic mixture was dropped to 10 μM, all of the

RS enantiomer was removed (chromatogram C). A set of control nanotubes was taken through the same fabrication procedure but without attachment of the aldehyde-silane coupling agent; these nanotubes did not extract measurable quantities of either enantiomer from the 20-μM solution.

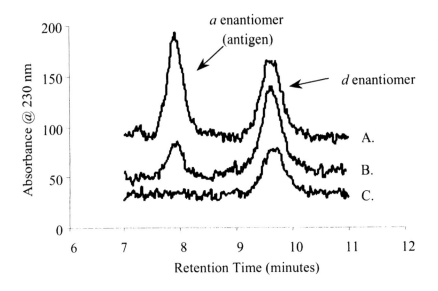

Figure 7. Chromatograms from enantioselective extractions: Racemic starting solution 20 μM in both a and d enantiomers (A); Same solution after extraction with 18 mg/mL ENA11His-modified nanotubes (B); Racemic 10 μM starting solution after extraction with 18 mg/mL ENA11His-modified nanotubes (C).

These experiments were done with the ENA11His immobilized to both the inner and outer surfaces of the nanotubes. We have also developed a chemistry that allows us to attach the protein to only the inner surfaces of liberated nanotubes. In this approach, the inner surfaces of the nanotubes were treated with aminopropyltrimethoxysilane while the tubes were still within the pores of the template membrane. The template membrane was then dissolved and the amino sites on the inner surfaces were coupled to free amino groups on the ENA11His using the well-known glutaraldehyde coupling reaction. *(23)* When 18 mg of these interior-only ENA11His-nanotubes were incubated with 1 mL of a 10 μM racemic mixture of the drug, 80% of the RS (and none of the SR) enantiomer was extracted. This amount corresponds to 0.44 nmol RS enantiomer per mg tubes, whereas almost double that amount, 0.80 nmol/mg, was extracted by the nanotubes with Fab on both their inner and outer surfaces.

For possible *in vivo* applications, biocompatibility is an important issue. It is well known that materials can be made biocompatible, as evidenced by decreased protein adsorption, by attaching poly(ethylene glycol) (PEG) chains to their surfaces. *(29,30)* We have used a PEG silane (MW ~5000, Shearwater), to improve the biocompatibility of the silica nanotubes. When 5 mg of unmodified silica nanotubes were incubated with 1 mg/mL IgG immunoproteins, more than half of the protein was removed from solution via adsorption to the nanotubes. In contrast, when an identical amount of PEG-modified nanotubes was incubated with this IgG solution, less than 3% of the protein was removed from the solution.

Enzyme Modified Nanotubes As Bioreactors

The above experiments show that proteins such as antibodies can be attached to the nanotubes and that after attachment the proteins are still functional and active. These proteins exhibit high binding specificities but stop short of catalyzing reactions. Enzymes, however, are by definition catalytic proteins. Enzyme-modified nanotubes may function as bioreactors, if the enzyme can be attached without denaturation.

Glucose oxidase, a robust and well-studied enzyme, was chosen as a model system. *(31)* The attachment of the enzyme to the nanotubes was carried out via an aldehyde silane bridge, as described in Materials and Methods. Assaying the protein for activity after attachment was necessary to determine if the protein structure survives the attachment process intact.

The activity of the attached glucose oxidase was determined using a modified literature assay. *(22)* The assay uses hydrogen peroxide, a by-product of the oxidation of glucose by glucose oxidase, to oxidize *o*-dianisidine. When reduced, *o*-dianisidine does not absorb in the visible region, while it shows a strong absorbance peak at 500 nm after oxidation. Thus, monitoring that wavelength with visible spectroscopy should show an increase in absorbance if the glucose oxidase is active. This increase should be linear over time as long as there are ample amounts of substrate and cofactors to continue the reaction.

Figure 8 shows this to be the case. For the first 100 seconds of this graph, the absorbance of the assay solution was monitored to show that no active enzyme was present. At ~100 seconds, the glucose oxidase modified nanotubes were added to the solution and the absorbance at 500 nm began increasing immediately. The increase in absorbance is linear as long as the nanotubes are left in the solution. By measuring the rate of product formation, the activity of the glucose oxidase on the nanotubes can be determined. This activity was found to be 0.5±0.2 units per mg nanotubes. One unit of glucose oxidase activity is the amount required to oxidize one µmol of glucose per minute.

110

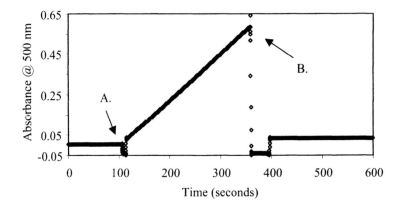

Figure 8. Activity assay of glucose oxidase-modified nanotubes. Enzyme-modified nanotubes added to the assay solution (A) and filtered from solution (B). Absorbance was at 500 nm.

Figure 8 also proves that the glucose oxidase is strongly bound to the nanotubes and does not leach off in appreciable amounts. This is shown by filtering the solution through 20 nm diameter alumina to remove the enzyme-modified nanotubes. Any leached or unbound glucose oxidase would be passed through the filter and would continue to catalyze oxidation of *o*-dianisidine, resulting in increasing absorbance. In Figure 8, the reaction mixture was filtered at 350 seconds. The absorbance after filtration drops to near zero because the oxidized o-dianisidine product forms micelles that are removed from solution by filtering. Absorbance at 500 nm was then monitored a further 200 seconds. No increase is seen during this period, verifying that the enzyme is strongly bound to the nanotubes via the aldehyde silane route.

Membrane Separations

As mentioned above, membranes composed of arrays of modified nanotubes embedded in the alumina template can also be used for separating enantiomers. Although there are other examples of antibody/particle systems used for enantio and other bioseparations, there appear to be no examples of antibodies in membrane-permeation enantioseparations. *(26,32,33)* This is perhaps because the binding constants for antibodies are often so large that the binding event is essentially irreversible. *(33-36)* Strong binding is undesirable because the membrane must ultimately release the target molecule so that it can be collected in the receiver solution. We show here that the binding affinity in synthetic nanotube membranes containing ENA11His enantioselective antibody fragments can be chemically tuned by adding dimethlysulfoxide (DMSO) to the racemic and receiver solutions. (8,37,38) These membranes effect chiral separations by selectively transporting the enantiomer that binds to the antibody relative to the enantiomer that has lower affinity for the antibody.

To create enantioselective membranes, nanopore alumina films as shown in Figure 1B were used as host membranes for template synthesis of silica nanotubes and immobilization of ENA11His enantioselective antibody fragments. (12,39,40) Films having pores with diameters of 20 and 35 nm were used for these studies. Deposition of the silica nanotubes and attachment of the antibody were as detailed in the experimental section. The ENA11His-containing membrane was mounted between two halves of a U-tube permeation cell. (18-21) A racemic feed solution of the RS and SR enantiomers (typically 0.1 mM in each enantiomer dissolved in pH 8.5 phosphate buffer that was 10% in DMSO) was placed on one side of the membrane. The permeate solution on the other side of the membrane was initially just the phosphate/DMSO buffer. Fluxes of each enantiomers across the membrane were determined by periodically assaying for these enantiomers in the permeate solution using a chiral HPLC method.

The slopes of straight-line plots of moles transported versus time (Figure 9) provide the fluxes of the RS and SR enantiomers across the anti-RS-containing nanotube membrane. The ratio of the RS flux to the SR flux is the transport selectivity coefficient, α. An average α value of 2.0 ± 0.2 was obtained for three identical membranes prepared from the 35-nm pore-diameter alumina, indicating that these membranes transport the RS enantiomer twice as fast as the SR enantiomer. The same α value was obtained after storage of the membrane for one week in the phosphate/DMSO buffer.

Because it is the RS enantiomer that specifically binds to the immobilized anti-RS, these data suggest that this Fab fragment is facilitating the transport of this enantiomer. (18,41-44) If this assumption is correct, theory predicts that the RS flux should initially increase linearly with feed concentration, and that the flux-vs.-feed-concentration curve should then flatten at higher concentrations. (18)

We investigated the effect of the concentration of the enantiomers in the racemic feed solution on the fluxes (Figure 10) and observed this Langmuiran-shaped curve for the RS enantiomer. The plot for the SR enantiomer is more linear, although some curvature is observed at the highest concentrations, which suggests that this enantiomer interacts weakly with the anti-RS. Facilitated transport theory also predicts that the highest selectivity coefficient should be obtained at the lowest feed concentration, and this result was also observed (inset Figure 10). A maximum selectivity coefficient of $\alpha = 2.6$ was obtained for this membrane.

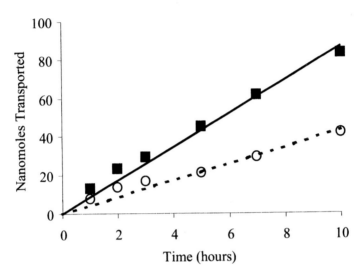

Figure 9. Plots of nanomoles of RS-enantiomer (solid line) and SR-enantiomer (dotted line) transported from the feed solution into the permeate solution vs. time through a silica-nanotube alumina membrane modified with Anti-RS Fab fragment. The membrane had 35 nm diameter pores. The feed solution was 0.1 mM in both the RS- and SR-enantiomers, dissolved in 10% DMSO-PBS buffer at pH 8.5. (Reprinted with permission from Lee et al. Science, 2002, 296, 2198. Copyright 2002 American Association for the Advancement of Science.)

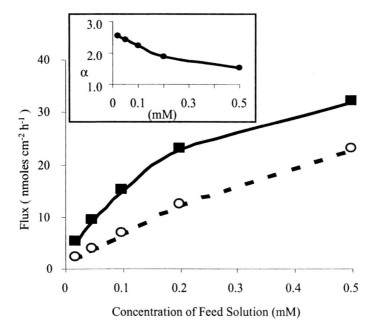

Figure 10. Plots of RS-enantiomer (solid line) and SR-enantiomer (dotted line) flux vs. concentration of the enantiomers in the feed solution for the membrane in Figure 9. The buffer in this case was 15% in DMSO. The inset shows the dependence of the selectivity coefficient α on the feed concentration. (Reprinted with permission from Lee et al. Science, 2002, 296, 2198. Copyright 2002 American Association for the Advancement of Science.)

Column chromatography experiments showed that the binding strength between the RS enantiomer and the anti-RS decreased with increasing DMSO content of the buffer. *(26,38)* If the facilitated transport mechanism is operative, these data would suggest that the RS flux would be highest at low DMSO contents and that the flux would decrease with increasing DMSO content. Furthermore, the RS flux should ultimately become equal to the SR flux because at high DMSO content neither enantiomer interacts appreciably with the anti-RS. *(26,38)* Figure 11 shows that all of these predictions are observed experimentally. The weak interaction of the SR enantiomer with anti-RS is also confirmed by these studies because the SR flux shows a slight decrease with increasing DMSO content. These studies also illustrate that there is an optimal DMSO content that maximizes the value of the selectivity coefficient (inset Figure 11).

114

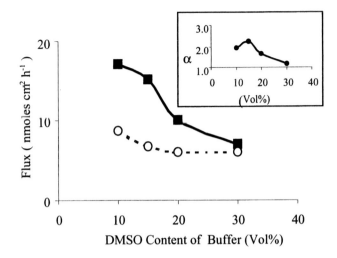

Figure 11. Plots of RS-enantiomer (solid line) and SR-enantiomer (dotted line) flux vs. DMSO content in the buffer solution for the membrane in Figure 2. The feed solution was 0.1 mM in each enantiomer. The inset shows the dependence of the selectivity coefficient α on the DMSO content of the buffer solution. (Reprinted with permission from Lee et al. Science, 2002, 296, 2198. Copyright 2002 American Association for the Advancement of Science.)

The selectivity in a facilitated-transport process can be increased by shutting down the non-facilitated (diffusional) transport of the unwanted chemical species. In porous membranes, this can be accomplished by decreasing the pore size in the membrane. *(18,45-47)* We explored this issue by measuring RS vs. SR flux in analogous membranes prepared with alumina films having 20 nm-diameter pores. The selectivity coefficient increased to $\alpha = 4.5$ for this smaller pore-diameter membrane. However, as would be expected, the fluxes for both enantiomers are lower in the smaller pore-diameter membrane (Figure 12).

Conclusions

We have shown that template synthesis can be used to produce highly monodisperse nanotubes of silica. These nanotubes can be modified with a variety of chemistries, including proteins, through silanization of the silica surface. Furthermore, the inside and outside surfaces can be modified independently. Nanotubes modified on the inside with C_{18} extract drugs from aqueous solution. Nanotubes can also be modified with enantioselective antibodies and used to extract one enantiomer from a racemic solution. Enzymes

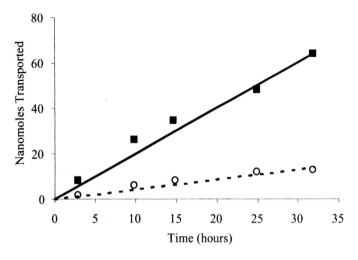

Figure 12. Plots as per Figure 9 but with 20-nm pore-diameter alumina membrane. The feed solution was 0.1 mM in each enantiomer / 15 % DMSO-PBS (pH 8.5). These alumina membranes were 35 μm thick with pore density of $2.3x10^{10}$ cm^{-2}. (Reprinted with permission from Lee et al. Science, 2002, 296, 2198. Copyright 2002 American Association for the Advancement of Science.)

can be covalently attached to the nanotubes, and are shown to be functional and active after attachment. Arrays of nanotubes left in the template can be modified with enantioselective antibodies to produce membranes that facilitate the transport of the antigen enantiomer.

Because in principle antibodies can be obtained that selectively bind to any desired molecule or enantiomer, the concepts presented here might provide a general approach for obtaining extractants or selectively-permeable membranes for a host of enantio- and bioseparations. However, throughput (i.e., flux) in a membrane-separations process is just as important as selectivity, and methods for enhancing flux across such membranes need to be developed. As per our prior work, this can be accomplished by augmenting diffusive flux with electroosmotic or pressure driven transport, and/or making an ultrathin film composite. *(8,29,48)*

In closing it is important to again emphasize that the template route can be used to prepare nanotubes of nearly any material. For example we have previously described a procedure for preparing nanotubes composed of the well-known biodegradable polymer poly(lactic acid). *(9)* Such biodegradable nano-tubes should prove useful for in vivo applications of biomedical nanotube technology.

116

Acknowledgements

This work was supported by the National Science Foundation, the Office of Naval Research, the UF Engineering Research Center for Particle Science and Technology, and the National Technology Agency, Finland. The FTB was kindly provided by Hormos Medical Ltd.

References

1. Chang, T.M.S.; Prakash, S.; *Mol. Biotech.* **2001**, *17*, 249.
2. Park, S.A.; Taton, T.A.; Mirkin, C.A. *Science* **2002**, *295*, 1503.
3. Langer, R. *Science* **2001**, *293*, 58.
4. Goldstein, A.S.; Gelb, M.H.; Yeager, P. .*J. Controlled Release* **2001**, *70*, 125.
5. Schnur, J.M.; Price, R.R.; Rudolph, A. *J. Controlled Release* **1994**, *28, 3*.
6. Spector, M.S.; Selinger, J.V.; Singh, A.; Rodriguez, J.M.; Price, R.R.; Schnur, J.M. *Langmuir* **1998**, *14*, 3493.
7. Martin, C.R. *Science* **1994**, *266*, 1961.
8. Miller, S.A.; Young, V.Y.; Martin, C.R. *J. Am. Chem. Soc.* **2001**, *123*, 12335.
9. Cepak, V.M.; Martin, C.R. *Chem. Mater.* **1999**, *11*, 1363.
10. Steinle, E.D.; Mitchell, D.T.; Wirtz, M.; Lee, S.B.; Young, V.Y.; Martin, C.R. *Anal. Chem.* **2002**, *74*, 2416.
11. Hornyak, G.L.; Patrissi, C.J.; Martin, C.R. *J. Phys. Chem. B* **1997**, *101*, 1548.
12. Lakshmi, B.B.; Patrissi, C.J.; Martin, C.R. *Chem. Mater.* **1997**, *9*, 2544.
13. Plueddemann, F.P. *Silane Coupling Agents;* Plenum: New York City, NY, 1982.
14. Bruning, C.; Grobe, J. *Chem. Comm.,* **1995**, 2323.
15. Franzelius, C.; Ackermann, I.; Angermaier, L.; Machbert, G. *J. Anal. Toxicology* **1998**, *22*, 359.
16. Stubbings, D.; Bubb, M.O.; Conradie, J.D. *Anal. Biochem.* **1993**, *210, 159*.
17. Yoshioka, N.; Mukai, Y. *J. Chromatog.* **1991**, *566, 361*.
18. Lakshmi, B.B.; Martin, C.R. *Nature* **1997**, *388, 758*.
19. Nishizawa, M.; Menon, V.P.; Martin, C.R. *Science* **1995**, *268, 700*.
20. Bayley, H.; Martin, C.R. *Chem. Rev.* **2000**, *100*, 2575.
21. Lee, S.B.; Martin, C.R. *Chem. Mater.* **2001**, *13*, 3236.
22. *Methods of Enzymatic Analysis;* Bergmeyer, J.; Grassl, M., Eds.: Verlag Chemie: Deerfield Beach, 1983; Vol. 2.
23. De Voogt, P.; Wegener, J.W.M.; Klamer, J.C.; van Zijl, G.; Grovers, H. *Biomed. Environ. Sci.* **1998**, *1*, 194.
24. Crosby, J. *Tetrahydron* **1991**, *47*, 4789.
25. Overdevest P.E.M. et al. In *Surfacant-Based Separations,* Scamehorn, J.F.; Harwell, J.H., Eds.; ACS: Washington, DC, 1999.

26. Nevanen, T.K.; Soderholm, L.; Kukkonen, K.; Suortti, T.; Teerinen, T.; Linder, M.; Soderlund, H.; Teeri, T.T. *J. Chromatog. A* **2001**, *925*, 89.
27. Kroger, D.; Liley, M.; Schiweck, W.; Skerra, A.; Vogel, H. *Biosensors Bioelectron.* **1999**, *14*, 155.
28. Huang S.-C.; Caldwell, K.D.; Lin, J.-N.; Wang, H.-K.; Herron, J.N. *Langmuir* **1996**, *12*, 4292.
29. Yu, S.; Lee, S.B.; Kang. M.; Martin, C.R. *Nanolett.* **2001**, *1*, 495.
30. Harris, J.M. *Poly(Ethylene Glycol) Chemistry: Biotechnical and Biomedical Applications;* Plenum: New York City, NY, 1992.
31. Martin, C.R.; Parthasarathy, R.V. *Adv. Mater.* **1995**, *7*, 487.
32. Kojima, K.; *Biochem. Biophys. Methods* **2001**, *49*, 241.
33. Chase, H.A. *Chem. Eng. Sci.* **1984**, *39*, 1099.
34. Harlow, E.; Lane, D. *Antibodies;* Cold Spring Harbor Lab: New York, 1988.
35. Hemminki, A.; Niemi, S.; Hautoniemi, L.; Soderlund, H.; Takkinen. K. *Immunotechnology* **1998**, *4*, 59.
36. Nachman, M. *J. Chromatogr.* **1992**, *597*, 167.
37. Jirage, K.B.; Hulteen, J.C.; Martin, C.R. *Science* **1997**, *278*, 655.
38. The effect of DMSO on the binding affinity for this antibody was demonstrated with column chromatography experiments. *(26)* Low DMSO-content buffers (2%) resulted in essentially irreversible binding of the hapten to the antibody, and high DMSO-content buffers (>30%) destroyed the antibody/hapten interaction.
39. Foss, C.A.J.; Hornyak, G.L.; Stockert, J.A.; Martin, C.R *J. Phys Chem.* **1994**, *98*, 2963.
40. Masuda, H.; Yamada, H.; Satoh, M.; Asoh, H.; Nako, M.; Tamura, T. *Appl. Phys. Lett.* **1997**, *71*, 2770.
41. Noble, R.D. *J.Membr. Sci.* **1992**, *75*, 121.
42. Westmark, P.R.; Gardiner, S.J.; Smith, B.D. *J. Am. Chem. Soc.* **1996**, *118*, 11093.
43. Park, Y.S.; Won, J.; Kang, Y.S. *Langmuir* **2000**, *16*, 9662.
44. Yang, J.; Huang, P. *Chem. Mater.* **2000**, *12*, 2693.
45. Javaid, A.; Hughey, M.P.; Varutbangkul, V.; Ford, D.M. *J. Membr. Sci.* **2001**, *187*, 141.
46. Hulteen, J.C.; Jirage, K.B.; Martin, C.R. *J. Am. Chem. Soc.* **1998**, *120*, 6603.
47. Lee, S.B.; Martin, C.R. *Anal. Chem.* **2001**, *73*, 768.
48. Liu, C.; Martin, C.R. *Nature* **1991**, *352*, 50.

Polymeric Micelles as Carriers in Drug and Gene Delivery

Chapter 9

Polymeric Micelles as Targetable Pharmaceutical Carriers

Vladimir P. Torchilin*, Anatoly N. Lukyanov, Zhonggao Gao, Junping Wang, and Tatyana S. Levchenko

Department of Pharmaceutical Sciences, Bouve College of Health Sciences, Northeastern University, Boston, MA 02115
*Corresponding author: email: vtorchil@lynx.dac.neu.edu

Micelles formed by Poly(ethylene glycol)/phospatidylethanol-amine (PEG-PE) conjugates are stable under physiological conditions, accumulate spontaneously in tumors via the enhanced permeability and retention (EPR) effect, and can be loaded with various anticancer agents. These micelles were modified with anticancer monoclonal 2C5 antibody to prepare targeted PEG-PE micelles able to recognize a broad variety of tumors. Modified micelles carry between 10 and 50 antibody molecules each. The micelle-bound antibody retains its specific activity. 2C5-targeted immunomicelles recognize tumors of different types *in vitro*, and show an enhanced efficiency of their tumor accumulation *in vivo*.

Introduction

Poly(ethylene glycol)/phospatidylethanolamine (PEG-PE) conjugates form very stable micelles in aqueous media. The protection provided by the PEG-based corona makes these micelles long-circulating, while the hydrophobic PE-core may be used as a cargo space for poorly soluble compounds, including anti-cancer drugs. *(1-4)*

Certain features of PEG-PE micelles such as their characteristic size, stability, and the longevity in circulation make them a very promising drug carrier for tumor delivery utilizing the enhanced permeability and retention (EPR) effect. The EPR effect is based on a spontaneous penetration of the particles into the tumor interstitium through enlarged fenestrations typical, in particular, for tumor vasculature. *(5-7)* Because of their small diameter, micelles may be a valuable alternative to other particulate delivery systems, such as liposomes and microparticles, for tumor delivery. It has been shown that in some cases particles with a diameter of 100 nm or larger do not penetrate tumor interstitium, apparently because of a small tumor vasculature cutoff size. *(8, 9)* The small size of 5-50 nm, therefore, makes the use of micelles advantageous in the case of such tumors. *(10, 11)*

Similar to other particulate delivery systems, the drug delivery potential of PEG-PE micelles can be greatly enhanced by attaching targeting ligands, such as antibodies, to their surface. *(12, 13)* In an attempt to develop a drug delivery system that would recognize a broad variety of tumors, we have used a nucleosome-specific antibody, 2C5, which can recognize tumors via tumor cell surface-bound nucleosomes, to prepare targeted PEG-PE immunomicelles. *(14, 15)* We report here the results of the preparation and characterization of 2C5 targeted immunomicelles, and their ability to recognize tumors of different types *in vitro* and *in vivo*.

Materials and Methods

PEG-PE with a PEG residue of 2000 Da, and phosphatidylethanolamine lissamine rhodamine B (Rh-PE) were purchased from Avanti Polar Lipids, Inc., (Alabaster, AL) and were used without further purification. ^{111}In with specific radioactivity of 395 Ci/mg of In equivalent was purchased from Perkin Elmer Life Sciences, Inc. (Boston, MA) and was used within 5 days upon arrival. Distilled and deionized water was used in all experiments. Diethylene triamine pentaacetic acid-phosphatidylethanolamine conjugate (DTPA-PE) and p-nitro-phenylcarbonyl-PEG-dipalmitoyl phosphatidylethanolamine (pNP-PEG-PE) were synthesized according to published procedures. *(4,16)*

Monoclonal 2C5 antibody was produced using a 2C5E3 hybridoma cell line (American Type Culture Collection, Manasas, VA). Cells were cultivated in RPMI 1640 cell culture medium supplemented with 10% fetal calf serum, streptomycin/penicillin, Na-pyruvate, and β-mercaptoethanol. After a substantial level of antibody had been detected in the cell-cultivating medium using ELISA (5-6 days after inoculation), cells were removed by centrifugation at 2000xg for 15 minutes. The supernatant was concentrated 10-fold by ultrafiltration using Amicon filters with a cutoff size of 100 kDa (Millipore Corp., Bedford, MA). The protein was precipitated by addition of $(NH_4)_2SO_4$ to the final concentration of 47% and centrifuged at 14,000xg for 60 min. Precipitated protein was dissolved in 0.01 M Tris, pH 8.6, and dialyzed against a 1000-fold excess of the same buffer. 2C5 antibody was purified using ion-exchange chromatography on DEAE-Toyopearl 650M and subjected to affinity chromato-graphy on Protein-G Sepharose.

The micelles were formed by extensive 5-15 min vortexing of PEG-PE at a polymer concentration of 5 mM in 10 mM HEPES buffered saline at pH 7.4 (HBS).

To prepare 2C5-modified micelles, PEG–PE was supplemented with 2 mol% of pNP-PEG-PE, and the micelles were formed in 5 mM Na-citrate buffered saline at pH 5.0. To 0.5 ml of the micellar solution obtained, an equal volume of 12 mM solution of 2C5 antibody in 40 mM Tris-buffered saline, pH 9.0, was added. In some cases, the protein was labeled with fluorescein (1-3 residues per protein molecule) using carboxyfluorescein succinimidyl (Molecular Probes, Inc., Eugene, OR). The mixture was incubated for 3 hours at room temperature and dialyzed against a 5000-fold excess of HBS, using cellulose ester membranes with a cutoff size of 300,000 Da (Spectrum Medical Industries, Inc., Rancho Dominguez, CA). The amount of micelle-bound 2C5 was quantified following the fluorescence of fluorescein probe at the exitation wavelength of 490 nm and emission wavelength of 520 nm ($F_{490/520}$).

Size and size distributions of micelles were determined by dynamic light scattering using a N4 plus MD Coulter Submicron Particle Size Analyzer (Coulter Corporation, Miami, FL).

The immunological activity of micelle-attached 2C5 was estimated by standard ELISA. ELISA plates were coated with 50 µl of 1 µg/ml nucleosomes (water soluble fraction of calf thymus nucleohistone, Worthington Biochemical Corp., Lakewood, NJ) and incubated overnight at 4°C. To the plates coated with nucleosomes, 50 µl of 2C5 immunomicelles at 20 µg/ml of PEG-PE were added and incubated for 4 hours at room temperature. The plates were washed 3 times with HBS and coated with horseradish peroxidase-anti mouse IgG conjugate (ICN biomedical, Inc., Aurora, OH), diluted according to the manufacturer recommendation. The conjugate was removed after 3 hours incubation at room temperature, and the plates were washed 3 times with HBS. Bound peroxidase was quantified by degradation of its substrate, diaminobenzidine supplied as a ready for use solution (Neogen, Lexington, KY). The intensity of color developed was analyzed by an ELISA reader, Labsystems Multiscan MCC/340 (Labsystems and Life Sciences International, LTD, UK).

Murine Lewis lung carcinoma (LLC) and EL4 T lymphoma cells as well as human mammary adenocarcinoma BT20 cells were purchased from American Type Culture Collection. The cells were propagated under ATCC recommended conditions.

The immunomicelles-cell interaction was studied using micelles containing 0.5 mol % of Rh-PE. EL4 cells were grown in suspension to the density of about $2x10^4$ cells/ml and transferred to Hank's solution by centrifugation at 700xg for 10 minutes. The cells were washed twice by centrifugation under the same conditions and resuspended in Hank's buffer at about $1x10^5$ cells/ml density. Rh-PE-labeled antibody-free micelles or immunomicelles were added to the suspension of EL4 cell at the PEG_{2000}-PE concentration of $4.2x10^{-4}$ M. Following, the cells were incubated for 1 hour at 37°C under 5% CO_2, washed trice with Hank's solution, concentrated to the density of $1x10^6$ cells/ml by centrifugation, and mounted individually on fresh glass slides using a fluorescence-free Trevigen™ mounting medium (Trevigen, Gaithersburg, MD). Mounted slides were studied with a Nikon Eclipse E400 microscope under bright light, or under epi-fluorescence using a Rh/TRITC filter.

BT-20 cells were grown on cover slips placed into 6-well tissue culture plates. After the cells reached a confluence of 60 to 70%, the plates were washed twice with Hank's solution. Rhodamine-labeled 2C5 immunomicelles containing micelles dispersed in Hank's buffer at a PEG_{2000}-PE concentration of $4.2x10^{-4}$ M were added to the washed cells, and the cells were incubated for 1 hour at 37°C under 5% CO_2. After incubation, the cover slips were washed twice with Hank's buffer, mounted, and studied for the presence of Rh fluorescence as described above for EL4 cells.

For animal experiments, the micelles were radiolabeled with ^{111}In via an amphiphilic chelating agent, DTPA-PE, added to their composition. The study was performed in female C57B1/6J mice. The mice were inoculated subcutaneously into the left rear flanks with 20,000 LLC cells dispersed in 100 µl of HBS. After the tumor diameters reached ca. 0.5-1 cm (1-2 weeks post inoculation), the mice were injected with 100 ml of 0.5 mM ^{111}In-labeled micellar formulations via the tail vein. At 0.5-2 hours post injection, the mice were sacrificed by cervical dislocation. Blood, tumors, and samples of muscle were extracted and analyzed for the presence of micelle-associated ^{111}In radioactivity.

Results and Discussion

PEG-PE conjugates form very stable, long-circulating micelles that selectively accumulate in tumors via the EPR effect. *(1,2,4)* Table I summarizes the data on PEG-PE micelles loaded with anticancer agents from earlier publications as well as some new formulations. As Table I indicates, PEG-PE micelles can be loaded with various anticancer agents. In most cases, drug-loaded micelles have a size very close to that of the blank ("empty") particles, indicating that drug-loaded micelles, similar to blank particles, should be able to penetrate leaky vasculature typical for tumors and deliver their load via passive targeting (EPR effect).

Table I. PEG-PE micelles loaded with anticancer agents

Micelle Composition*	Drug load (drug/carrier)	Size (nm)	Publication
PEG_{750}-PE	N/A	7-15 nm	*(4)*
	Chlorine e6 trimethyl ester to 32 wt %	5-20 nm	N/A
	Vitamin K3 to 50 wt %	2-5 nm	N/A
PEG_{2000}-PE	N/A	7-20 nm	*(3,4)*
	Chlorine e6 trimethyl ester to 30 wt %	7-20 nm	*(3)*
	Tamoxifen to 25 wt %	7-20 nm	N/A
	Taxol to 1.5 wt %	7-20 nm	*(3)*
	Vitamin K3 to 30 wt %	10-20 nm	N/A
ePC/PEG_{2000}-PE, 4/1 mol	N/A	20-60 nm	N/A
	Taxol to wt 4%	20-60 nm	N/A
PEG_{5000}-PE	N/A	10-35 nm	*(3,4)*
	Dequalinium to 3 wt %	10-40 nm	*(2)*
	Tamoxifen to 20 wt %	10-40 nm	*(3)*
	Taxol to wt 1%	13-40 nm	*(3)*
	Vitamin K3 to 30 wt %	7-40 nm	N/A

* - ePC – egg phosphatidylcholine; the number associated with PEG shows its molecular weight.

PEG-PE micelles were modified with monoclonal 2C5 antibodies, known to recognize the surface of various tumor cells but not normal cells, to further improve their drug targeting potential. *(14)* The use of this antibody as a drug carrier targeting ligand would allow preparation of drug delivery systems able to recognize tumors of various types. 2C5-targeted PEG-PE immunomicelles were prepared utilizing a new coupling reagent, pNP-PEG-PE, earlier developed by us for attaching specific amino group-containing ligands to normal and long-circulating liposomes. *(16,17)* The amphiphilic reagent pNP-PEG-PE is capable of inserting into the hydrophobic phase of liposomes and micelles with its lipid part, and of covalent attaching to primary NH_2-groups of protein and peptides with its p-nitrophenol-activated PEG terminus. A typical result of bound 2C5 quantification obtained using a fluorescein labeled protein is shown in Figure 1. *(18)* Under the experimental conditions used, 30% of added 2C5 was attached to the micelles. This amount corresponds to between 10 and 50 protein molecules bound to a single micelle. Protein binding to control micelles lacking pNP-PEG-PE was negligibly small.

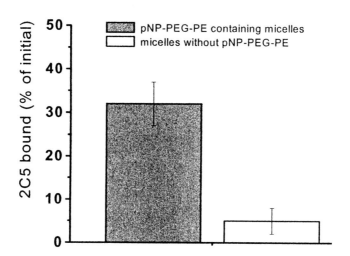

Figure 1. Binding of 2C5 antibodies to PEG-PE micelles.

One of the advantages of micelles over alternative particulate drug carriers is their relatively small size. This small size allows micelles to penetrate the interstitium of tumor cells with small vasculature cutoff size, which are non-accessible for other drug carriers with larger particle diameters. *(8, 9)* The data shown in Figure 2 demonstrate that modification of micelles with 2C5 mono-clonal antibodies has a very small effect on the micelle size, indicating that 2C5

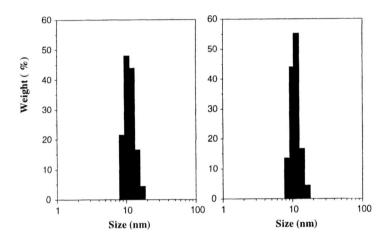

Figure 2. Size distribution of PEG-PE micelles before (left) and after modification with 2C5 antibody (right).

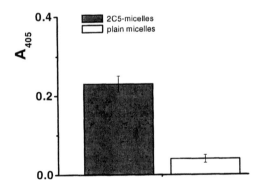

Figure 3. Binding of PEG-PE micelles to a monolayer of nucleosomes.

targeted PEG-PE immunomicelles will be capable of delivering drugs to tumors with a low vasculature cutoff size.

The preservation of specific activity of micelle-bound antibody is crucial for drug targeting. The data shown in Figure 3 indicate that the 2C5 antibody attached to PEG-PE micelles via pNP-PEG-PE retains its affinity. *(18)* 2C5-immunomicelles bind to a 2C5-specific nucleosomes, whereas control micelles, prepared by the same method but lacking pNP-PEG-PE, show only very minor binding, comparable to the background signal typical for this method.

The use of 2C5 antibody as a targeting ligand allows for the preparation of drug delivery systems with specificity against tumors of various types (Figure 4). Binding of 2C5-immunomicelles to cancer cells was observed for two totally different cell lines, murine EL4 T lymphoma and human mammary adenocarcinoma BT20. Incubation of the same cell lines with micelles lacking antibodies resulted in virtually no micelle-to-cell binding.

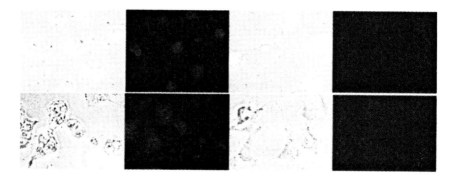

Figure 4. Binding of Rh-labeled PEG-PE micelles to EL4 cells (top panel) and to BT20 cells (bottom panel). Left half: bright field and fluorescent micro-scopy of 2C5-micelles; right half: bright field and fluorescent microscopy of plain micelles. (See page 6 of color insert.)

The accumulation of plain and 2C5-targeted PEG-PE micelles in sub-cutaneous LLC tumors in mice is shown in Figure 5. At all time points studied, both plain and 2C5-targeted formulations demonstrated a much higher accu-mulation in the tumor cells compared to non-targeted muscle tissue. The enhanced accumulation of plain micelles in the tumor can be explained by the EPR effect, whereas improved accumulation of 2C5-targeted micelles clearly indicates that immunomicelles are capable of specific recognition and binding to tumor cells. This observation allows to assume that micelles targeted with 2C5 will be capable of delivering their load not only to tumors with a mature vasculature but also to tumors at earlier stages of their growth, and to meta-stases. This ability is not expected for plain micelles.

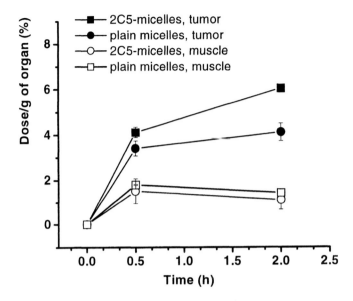

Figure 5. Accumulation of PEG-PE micelles in subcutaneous LLC tumor in mice.

Conclusions

Antibodies, such as the 2C5 monoclonal antibody, can be covalently attached to PEG-PE micelles utilizing the amphiphilic modifying agent, pNP-PEG-PE, with preservation of the antibody's specific activity. 2C5-targeted PEG-PE micelles specifically bind to tumor cells of various types *in vitro*, and demonstrate an enhanced accumulation in tumors *in vivo*.

Acknowledgements

This work was supported by NIH grant 5R01 GM60200-03 to Vladimir P. Torchilin.

References

1. Trubetskoy, V.S.; Gazelle, G.S.; Wolf, G.L.; Torchilin, V.P. *J. Drug Target.* **1997**, *4*, 381-388.
2. Weissig, V.; Lizano, C.; Torchilin, V.P. *J. Liposome Res.* **1998**, *8*, 391-400.

3. Gao, Z.; Lukyanov, A.N.; Singhal, A.; Torchilin, V.P. *Nano Letters* **2002**, *2*, 979-982.

4. Lukyanov, A.N.; Gao, Z.; Mazzola, L.; Torchilin, V.P. *Pharm. Res.* **2002**, *19*, 1424-1429.

5. Gabizon, A.A. *Adv. Drug Deliv. Rev.* **1995**, *16*, 285-294.

6. Maeda, H.; Wu, J.; Sawa, T.; Matsumura, Y.; Hori, K. *J. Control. Release* **2000**, *65*, 271-284.

7. Maeda, H. *Adv. Enzyme Regul.* **2001**, *41*, 189-207.

8. Parr, M.J.; Masin, D.; Cullis, P.R.; Bally, M.B. *J. Pharmacol. Exp. Ther.* **1997**, *280*, 1319-1327.

9. Weissig, V.; Whiteman, K.R.; Torchilin, V.P. *Pharm. Res.* **1998**, *15*, 1552-1556.

10. Jain, R.K. *Cancer Metastasis Rev.* **1987**, *6*, 559-593.

11. Jain, R.K. *Cancer Metastasis Rev.* **1990**, *9*, 253-66.

12. Torchilin, V.P. *Eur. J. Pharm. Sci.* **2000**, *11 (Suppl. 2)*, S81-91.

13. Torchilin, V.P. *J. Control. Release* **2001**, *73*, 137-172.

14. Iakoubov, L.Z.; Torchilin, V.P. *Oncol. Res.* **1997**, *9*, 439-446.

15. Iakoubov, L.Z.; Torchilin, V.P. *Cancer Detect. Prev.* **1998**, *22*, 470-475.

16. Torchilin, V.P.; Levchenko, T.S.; Lukyanov, A.N.; Khaw, B.A.; Klibanov, A.L.; Rammohan, R.; Samokhin, G.P.; Whiteman, K.R. *Biochim. Biophys. Acta* **2001**, *1511*, 397-411.

17. Torchilin, V.P.; Rammohan, R.; Weissig, V.; Levchenko, T.S. *Proc. Natl. Acad. Sci. USA* **2001**, *98*, 8786-8791.

18. Torchilin, V.P.; Lukyanov, A.N.; Gao, Z.; Mazzola, L. *Polym. Prepr.* **2002**, *43*, 677-678.

Chapter 10

Pluronic Block Copolymers as Novel Therapeutics in Drug Delivery

Alexander V. Kabanov[1,*], Elena V. Batrakova[1], and Valery Yu. Alakhov[2]

[1]College of Pharmacy, Department of Pharmaceutical Sciences, 986025 Nebraska Medical Center, Omaha, NE 68198–6025
[2]Supratek Pharma Inc., 531 Boulevard des Prairies, Building 18, Laval, Quebec H7B 1B7, Canada
*Corresponding author: email: akabanov@unmc.edu

Pluronic® block copolymers are found to be an efficient drug delivery system with multiple effects. The incorporation of drugs into the core of Pluronic® micelles results in increased solubility, metabolic stability, and circulation time for the drug. This review will focus on two aspects of Pluronic® block copolymers in drug delivery applications, the interactions of single molecular chains of Pluronic® copolymers ("unimers") with multidrug resistant cancer cells, resulting in sensitization of these cells with respect to various anticancer agents, and the inhibition of drug efflux transporters in both the blood brain barrier and the small intestine by unimers, which provides for the enhanced transport of selected drugs to the brain and increases oral bioavailability.

Introduction

The development of efficient drug delivery systems has attracted tremendous attention during the last two decades, driven by the recognition that a drug molecule must overcome enormous barriers before it reaches its target site within the body. In addition, delivery systems can address and correct problems related to the physical characteristic of a drug, including solubility and stability. Consequently, the technologies currently under development for drug delivery and drug targeting systems will have a tremendous impact on the improvement of novel drug therapies.

A major subset of existing drug delivery systems, those based on synthetic polymers, have attracted significant attention, as they appear particularly promising. *(1)* This has lead to the emergence of a new field called *"polymer therapeutics"*. Generally polymer therapeutics refers to any polymer that is used as a component of a drug product for the purpose of eliciting or modifying drug action. This includes polymers, which are inherently biologically active, polymer-drug conjugates, polymeric micelles, nanoparticles and polymer-coated liposomes. There are several fundamental properties of polymers useful in solving drug delivery problems. First, polymers are large molecules that can be designed to be intrinsically multifunctional and thus can be combined either covalently or non-covalently with drugs to overcome multiple problems such as solubility, stability, and permeability. Second, polymers can be combined with various targeting vectors to direct drugs to specific sites in the body. Third, polymers are ideal for the design of environmental stimulus-responsive materials allowing for controlled and sustained release of the drug at the site of action. Finally, polymers can have biological activity of their own and are capable of interacting with and modifying the activity of various endogenous drug transport systems within the body, thus affecting drug delivery.

One important and promising example of novel polymer therapeutics that benefit from each of the above properties are polymeric micelles formed by amphiphilic block copolymers. Polymeric micelles have been evaluated in multiple pharmaceutical applications as drug and gene delivery systems, as well as in diagnostic imaging as carriers for various contrasting agents. *(2-11)* The use of Pluronic® block copolymers in experimental medicine and pharmaceutical sciences has a long history. A number of excellent reviews are published that contain detailed discussions of many aspects of Pluronic®-based formulations, particularly, those using gels, w/o and o/w emulsions, nanoparticles coated by the block copolymer, and solid polymer blends. *(4,12-20)* These systems are formed either in the condensed state or with a high concentration of lipophilic components. The current review focuses on the relatively dilute isotropic solutions of block copolymers in aqueous media. These solutions exist in the form of either a molecular dispersion or as micelles of block copolymers. The core-shell architecture of the micelles is essential for their utility in drug delivery. The core is a water-incompatible compartment that is segregated from the aqueous exterior by the hydrophilic chains of the shell, thereby forming, within the core, a "cargo" for the incorporation of various therapeutic or diagnostic reagents. As a result, polymeric micelles can be used as efficient carriers for compounds, which alone exhibit poor solubility, undesired pharmacokinetics, and low stability in a physiological environment. Furthermore, Pluronic® block copolymers are capable of enhancing the performance of drugs by acting as biological response-modifying agents, which act directly upon the target cells. This review will focus on two aspects of Pluronic® block copolymers, the interaction with multidrug resistant cancer cells resulting in sensitization of these cells with respect to various anticancer agents, and the inhibition of drug efflux transporters in both the blood brain barrier (BBB) and in the small intestine resulting in enhanced transport of select drugs to the brain and increased oral bioavailability.

Results and Discussion

Pluronic® Block Copolymers: Structure and Solution Behavior

Pluronic® block copolymers (also known under their non-proprietary name "poloxamers") consist of ethylene oxide (EO) and propylene oxide (PO) blocks arranged in a basic A-B-A structure: EO_x-PO_y-EO_x. This arrangement results in an amphiphilic copolymer, in which the number of hydrophilic EO_x and hydrophobic PO_y units can be altered. The structure formula of Pluronic® block copolymers is shown below. Copolymers with various x and y values are characterized by distinct hydrophilic-lipophilic balances (HLB).

$$HO-\left[CH_2\text{-}CH_2\text{-}O\right]_x \left[\underset{\underset{CH_3}{|}}{CH_2\text{-}CH\text{-}O}\right]_y \left[CH_2\text{-}CH_2\text{-}O\right]_x-H$$

$$\text{EO} \qquad\qquad \text{PO} \qquad\qquad \text{EO}$$

A defining property of amphiphilic block copolymers is the ability of individual block copolymer molecules, termed "unimers", to self-assemble into micelles in aqueous solutions. The unimers form molecular solutions in water at block copolymer concentrations below the critical micelle concentration (CMC), while at concentrations above the CMC unimer molecules aggregate to form micelles. The micelles can be spherical, rod-like, or lamellar, depending on the length of the EO and PO blocks, concentration of the block copolymers, and the temperature. (21) All these types of micelles have a hydrophobic core formed by

PO chains and a hydrophilic shell formed by EO chains. Typically, Pluronic[®] copolymers used for drug delivery have a CMC ranging from 1 μM to 1 mM (ca. 5 x 10[-3] to 1 %wt.) at body temperature (37°C). The CMC is of paramount signifcance to drug delivery applications using block copolymers. *(22,23)* First, the CMC determines the stability of micelles against possible dilution of the drug delivery system in body fluids. *(7,23)* Second, the CMC determines the maximal achievable concentration of Pluronic[®] unimers, to which cells will be exposed, thereby defining the biological response-modifying effects, which Pluronic[®] itself will exert on these cells. *(24)*

The second most important feature from the drug delivery standpoint is the size of the micelles, which strongly affects blood circulation times and bioavailability of these particles. *(4,16,25-28)* The preferred size range for many pharmaceutical applications is from ca. 10 to 100 nm. Pluronic[®] block copolymer micelles are clearly within this preferred range. These particles demonstrate the most prolonged blood circulation times and are small enough to penetrate even very small capillaries in body tissues, offering an effective distribution in certain tissues. *(4,16,27)* Furthermore, particles smaller than 100 nm can be encapsulated by endocytic vesicles, allowing uptake into target cells via endocytosis. *(29)* Particles with diameters larger than 200 nm are frequently sequestered by the spleen as a result of mechanical filtration, followed by removal through the cells of the phagocyte system *(4,26)*, while particles with diameters of less than 5-10 nm are rapidly removed through extravasation and renal clearance. *(25)*

Micelle formation is critically dependent upon the temperature. This is a result of the successive dehydration of PO and EO chains upon temperature increase. *(30)* Below room temperature both types of blocks within a Pluronic[®] molecule are hydrated and relatively soluble in water. When the temperature increases, the PO block dehydrates and becomes insoluble, resulting in the formation of micelles. This temperature is referred to as the critical micelle temperature (CMT), which for most Pluronic[®] copolymers ranges from ca. 25 to 40 °C, i.e., is below or near body temperature. Consideration of the temperature dependence of micelle formation in drug delivery is important. In particular, one must be aware that micelles can disintegrate and release solubilized drug if they are stored below room temperature. Although the micelle disintegration is reversible and micelles can reassemble when the temperature is increased, the solubilized drug can precipitate and may be difficult to resolubilize as a consequence of kinetics factors.

Pluronic[®] micelles and unimers play very important roles in drug formulations. Micelles are used as carriers for various drugs, resulting in increased solubility, metabolic stability, and circulation time for the drugs. *(2-9)* By attaching a peptide or other biospecific molecule that can promote site-specific drug delivery to the surface of the EO corona, a micelle can be targeted to a specific site in the body. *(31,32)* Pluronic[®] unimers also have an important bio-logical role in drug delivery. It has been discovered that Pluronic[®] unimers exhibit biological response-modifying activities in certain drug formulations. *(22,33-35)* The following section considers pharmaceutical and biochemical aspects of Pluronic[®] drug delivery systems containing micelles and unimers.

Pharmacokinetics and Biodistribution of Block Copolymer Formulations

There are few reports on the subject of pharmacokinetics and tissue distribution of block copolymers in the body. One of such studies compared the biodistribution of various Pluronic[®] copolymers having various ratios of the lengths of the EO and PO segments. *(36)* This study determined the areas under the curves (AUC) for blood, liver, and spleen, as well as the tissue distribution coefficients ($P_{organ/blood}$) for both liver and spleen. As shown in Table I, the tissue distribution coefficients increase in the following Pluronic[®] order: F68 < F108 < P85 < L61. This suggests that the retention of the block copolymer in the organs increases with the length of the hydrophobic PO block or as the HLB decreases. The studies show that the block copolymer concentrations in the plasma remain quite high for several hours following administration. *(36)* These concentrations are in the same range as the established CMCs for the studied Pluronics[®], suggesting that micelles might be present in the circulation.

Table I. Pharmacokinetic and tissue distribution parameters of Pluronic[®] block copolymers after i.v. administration in mice. (36)

Tissue	F68 EO_{76}-PO_{29}-EO_{76}		F108 EO_{133}-PO_{50}-EO_{133}	
	AUC	$P_{org/blood}$[a]	AUC	$P_{org/blood}$[a]
Blood	0.111	-	0.026	-
Liver	0.225	2.03	0.079	3.03
Spleen	0.066	0.59	0.032	1.23

Tissue	F85 EO_{26}-PO_{40}-EO_{26}		L61* EO_2-PO_{30}-EO_2	
	AUC	$P_{org/blood}$[a]	AUC	$P_{org/blood}$[a]
Blood	2.180	-	0.044	-
Liver	7.365	3.38	0.215	4.93
Spleen	4.240	1.94	0.118	2.68

[a] The tissue distribution coefficient $P_{org/blood}$ is defined as the ratio of *AUC* in organ to *AUC* in blood.

An important factor for the biodistribution of micelles is their stability in biological systems. The stability of block copolymer micelles can be considered in terms of the equilibrium behavior ("*thermodynamic stability*") and dynamic behavior ("*kinetic stability*"). *(7)* The CMC and the partition coefficient are the major thermodynamic constants determining the stability of the micellar carrier and the drug release in equilibrium conditions (Figure 1). The dilution of micelles in body fluids results in a decrease in the portion of the micelle-incorporated drug. Furthermore, if the system is diluted below the CMC, the micelles are completely disintegrated and the drug is completely released in the external media. As mentioned earlier, the CMC values observed for Pluronic® block copolymers are in the range from ca. 5 x 10^{-3} to 1 %wt. In terms of micelle stability, this range can be characterized as "from moderately stable to relatively unstable micelles".

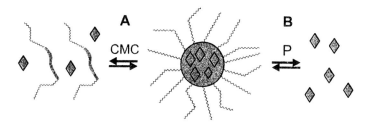

Figure 1. Mechanisms of drug release from the micelle: (A) disintegration of the micelles below CMC; (B) release of the drug as a result of partitioning.

However, this instability can be compensated by the high kinetic stability of block copolymer micelles, which is due to slow relaxation processes of the copolymers, resulting in a slow dissociation of the micelles after dilution to concentrations below the CMC. Micelles that are formed by block copolymers containing a hydrophobic block with a glass transition temperature exceeding 37°C are particularly stable in this respect. *(38,39)* The molecular motion of the chains in the core of such micelles is "frozen" and, thus, the block copolymer molecules are strongly physically attached to each other. *(9)* The drug release rates in such systems are also low due to slow diffusion of the solute through the core. Block copolymers of this type offer high blood circulation times combined with the slow release of the free drug in the body.

It is important to recognize that an increase in the circulation time through a stable drug-carrier complex will not necessarily improve the therapeutic index of the drug. Indeed, too strong of an attachment of the drug to the micelle carrier decreases drug release, which may result in lower concentrations of the drug in the body. There must be some optimum ratio between the effective incorporation of the drug in the carrier that increases stability and circulation time of the drug, and the effective release of the drug from the carrier within the critical site of action. Once this optimum is achieved, the therapeutic index is maximal.

The potential strength of the block copolymer approach in therapeutics is that the critical physicochemical parameters can be adjusted in a very broad range within a single homologous block copolymer set in order to maximize the therapeutics index for given drug delivery situation. This possibility has been illustrated using Pluronic® block copolymers. For these copolymers a relationship between partition coefficient P of a hydrophobic probe, pyrene, and CMC has been evaluated. (37) The experimental curve underlying this relationship is presented in Figure 2. As is seen in this figure, the CMC and P values are varied by over two orders of magnitude, when the block copolymer structure is changed. The copolymers at the upper left corner of this graph have the lowest CMC and highest P, characterized by the highest stability and strongest retention of the solute. In contrast, the copolymers at the lower left corner, having the highest CMC and lowest P, are readily disintegrating and releasing drug upon dilution. By varying the molecular parameters of the copolymers one can adjust the block copolymer-based formulation to achieve desired characteristics of the micelle stability and drug release.

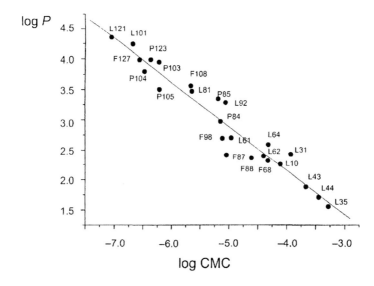

Figure 2. Relationship between the partitioning coefficients of pyrene and CMC in Pluronic® block copolymer systems. (Reproduced from reference 37. Copyright 2000 American Chemical Society.)

At present little is known about the effects of Pluronic® block copolymers on pharmacokinetics and biodistribution of drugs in the body. In one study the pharmacokinetics and tissue distribution of doxorubicin formulated with mixed micelles of Pluronic® L61 and F127 (termed "SP1049C", Supratek Pharma Inc., Montreal, Canada) in normal and tumor bearing animals has been examined. *(34)* Table II presents *AUC* data obtained from this study for plasma and various tissues. A comparison between a conventional doxorubicin formulation and the SP1049C formulation revealed little affect of the block copolymers on the pharmacokinetic profiles of the drug in liver, kidney, heart, and lung of both normal and tumor-bearing mice. However, at the same time the brain *AUCs* were increased 2.9- and 1.7-times in normal and tumor-bearing mice, respectively. This increase in the brain accumulation of doxorubicin may be related to the inhibition of the drug efflux systems, such as P-glycoprotein (Pgp), expressed in the blood brain barrier, by Pluronic®. A substantial, 1.7-time increase in the accumulation of doxorubicin in solid tumor was also observed with the SP1049C formulation compared to a conventional formulation. *(34)* An increased drug delivery to the tumor is important in view of the fact that Pluronic®-based compositions of doxorubicin have been shown to be substantially more effective *in vivo* in treating various solid tumors, compared to the free drug. *(34,40)*

Table II. The plasma pharmacokinetic parameters of free doxorubicin (DOX) and doxorubicin in SP1049C formulation in normal and tumor-bearing mice. (34)

Animal/ Formulation	AUC [μg x h/g]						
	Plasma	Brain	Heart	Kidney	Liver	Lung	Tumor
Normal mice							
DOX	7.1	9.0	111.5	271.5	147.1	307.5	-
DOX/SP1049C	14.6	26.0	139.8	312.1	192.3	282.2	-
Tumor-bearing mice							
DOX	7.1	5.6	156.2	263.7	154.2	207.5	30.1
DOX/SP1049C	8.5	9.2	177.2	270.9	173.5	268.2	50.8

Pluronic® Formulations for Treatment of Drug Resistant Tumors

Tumors with the multidrug resistant (MDR) phenotype are among some of the most difficult types to treat. MDR cells overexpress efflux proteins belonging to a superfamily of ATP binding cassette (ABC), such as P-glycoprotein (Pgp) and multidrug resistance-associated proteins (MRP) that pump drugs out of a cell. *(41,42)* Furthermore, several other proteins (i.e., glutathione S-transferase, metallothionein, thioredoxin, topoisomerase I, II, O^6-alkylguanine-DNA alkyltransferase etc.) are believed to contribute to the resistant phenotype as well. *(41)* This combination of several independent mechanisms of drug resistance complicates chemotherapy and reinforces the need for the development of novel drugs and drug formulations effective against drug resistant cancers. Alakhov *et al.* demonstrated that Pluronic® block copolymers sensitize resistant cells, resulting in an increase in the cytotoxic activity of the drug by two to three orders of magnitude. *(33,43,44)* By addition of P85 or L61, the cytotoxic effects of doxorubicin in multidrug resistant lines significantly surpassed those observed in sensitive lines. Similar effects of Pluronic® block copolymers have also been reported *in vivo. (34,40)* In these studies, mice bearing drug sensitive and drug resistant tumors were treated with doxorubicin alone and doxorubicin in Pluronic® compositions. The tumor panel included i.p. murine leukemias (P388, P388-Dox), s.c. murine myelomas (Sp2/0, Sp2/0-Dnr), i.v. and s.c. Lewis lung carcinoma (3LL-M27), s.c. human breast carcinomas (MCF-7, MCF-7ADR), and human head and neck carcinoma (KBv). *(34)* Using the National Cancer Institute criteria for tumor inhibition and increased lifespan, Pluronic®-formulated doxorubicin has met the efficiency criteria in all models (9 of 9), while doxorubicin alone was effective only in selected tumors (2 of 9). *(34)* Together these studies indicate improved treatment of drug resistant cancers with Pluronic® block copolymers.

The Pluronic® block copolymer related enhanced cytotoxicity in drug resistant cancer cells appears to be related to the effects of the copolymer on the Pgp drug efflux transport system. Defects in the intracellular accumulation of doxorubicin in resistant cancer cells expressing Pgp can be overcome by treatment with Pluronic®, while no alteration in drug uptake in the presence of Pluronic® was observed with non-Pgp expressing parental cancer cells, providing additional support for the specific effects of the copolymer on Pgp transport system in MDR cells. *(24,44)* This conclusion has been reinforced by recent studies, demonstrating that Pluronic® block copolymers (L61, P85) have pronounced effects, increasing accumulation and permeability of various Pgp-dependent drugs in mdr1-transfected cells that overexpress Pgp. *(35,45)* Additional support for the Pgp mediated mechanism of Pluronic® in Pgp expressing cells is that the block copolymer has no or little effect on the accumulation of non-Pgp dependent compounds in both resistant and parental cells. *(35,46)* Therefore, the increased absorption of the Pgp substrates in Pgp expressing cells is attributable to the effects of the block copolymer on the Pgp efflux system, rather than to nonspecific alterations in membrane permeability of the substrates.

However, recent studies suggest that the effects of Pluronic® block copolymers might go beyond the inhibition of the Pgp efflux pump only. Studies using the human pancreatic adenocarcinoma cell line, Panc-1, that expresses the MRP efflux pump, suggested that P85 inhibits efflux and increases cellular accumulation of the MRP-dependent probe, fluorescein, in these cells. *(47)* A more recent study reported that L61 partially inhibited MRP2-mediated transport of vinblastine in transfected canine kidney cells that stably express MRP2. *(45)* However, the potency of this inhibitor with respect to MRP2 in these cells was substantially lower than its potency with respect to the Pgp in the MDR1-transfected cells that express Pgp. Thus, the evaluation of the effects of Pluronic® block copolymers on MRP is far from completion.

Another impediment to treatment, which is present in MDR cells, involves the sequestration of drugs within cytoplasmic vesicles, followed by extrusion of the drug from the cell. *(48-52)* Drug sequestration in MDR cells is achieved through the maintenance of abnormally elevated pH gradients across organelle membranes by the activity of H^+-ATPase, an ATP-dependent pump. *(53)* Recent studies examined effects of Pluronic® block copolymers on intracellular localization of doxorubicin in the MDR cancer cell line, MCF-7/ADR. *(44)* In these cells, free doxorubicin is sequestered in cytoplasmic vesicles, which might further diminish the amount of the drug available for interaction with the nucleus. *(52)* Following incubation of the cells with doxorubicin and Pluronic®, the drug was released from the vesicles and accumulated, primarily, in the nucleus. *(44)* Overall, these studies suggest that Pluronic® copolymers affect several important mechanisms of drug resistance in cancer cells.

Various drug resistance mechanisms, including drug transport and detoxification systems, require consumption of energy to sustain their function in MDR cells. Hence, mechanistic studies have focused on the effects of Pluronic® block copolymers on metabolism and energy conservation in drug resistant cells. *(54,55)* These studies were based on earlier reports indicating that Pluronic® block copolymers can affect mitochondria function in non-MDR cells. There could be multiple reasons for the inhibitory activity of these compounds in mitochondria. Likely components contributing to the antimetabolic effects of nonionic detergents include their ability to serve as K^+ ionophores *(58,59)*, and to uncouple oxidative phosphorylation. *(60,61)* It is also possible that these detergents directly inhibit the NADH dehydrogenase complex by interacting with the hydrophobic sites of this complex in the mitochondria membrane. *(61,62)* Using lipophilic spin probes, Rapoport *et al.* have shown that two Pluronic® copolymers, P85 and P105, reduce the activity of the electron transport chains in mitochondria as assessed by the rates of bioreduction of these probes in HL-60 cancer cells. *(63)* These findings indicate that Pluronic® block copolymers could be transported inside the cells and reach mitochondria. This transport, in fact, was directly shown for selected Pluronics® (i.e., P85) labeled with fluorescent tags to examine their transport and localization inside cells. *(22,32)*

Slepnev *et al.* were first to demonstrate that following a two-hour exposure of Jurkat T-cell lymphoma cells to a Pluronic® block copolymer, P85, intracellular levels of ATP were depleted. *(64)* This treatment did not induce permeabilization of the cellular membrane since no leakage of intracellular ATP in the external media was observed. Therefore, ATP depletion was likely to be a result of inhibition of cellular metabolism rather than due to a loss of ATP in the environment. Another groundbreaking observation, in the context of the drug resistance phenomena, were the studies that compared the effects of the P85 on ATP levels in several cell types that either express Pgp and MRP, or do not express Pgp and MRP. *(54-57)* Exposure of both resistant and sensitive cells to P85 resulted in energy depletion, which was reversed when the block copolymer was removed. However, the resistant cells were much more responsive to P85, exhibiting profound decreases in ATP levels at substantially lower concentrations of the block copolymer compared to the sensitive cells. The effective concentrations of P85 that induced a 50% decrease in ATP levels in the cells (EC_{50}), as determined from the dose-response curves are presented in Table III. This table also presents the relative responsiveness of the Pgp and MRP overexpressing cells compared to the non-Pgp and non-MRP overexpressing cells. These data suggest that the responsiveness of the cells to P85 correlated with expression of Pgp and MRP. Based on the results of these studies, the appearance of the MDR phenotype is one factor that renders cellular metabolism responsive to treatment with Pluronics®.

Table III. Effects of P85 on ATP levels in Pgp and MRP overexpressing cells and cells that do not overexpress Pgp or MRP. The cells were exposed to P85 for 120 min prior to determining the intracellular ATP levels. (56)

Cells	Pgp or MRP overexpression	Initial ATP levels [nmol/mg protein][a]	EC_{50} [%]	Relative responsiveness to P85[b]
MCF-7	No	30 ± 1.5	2.25	-
MCF-7/ADR	Pgp, MRP	300 ± 20	0.009	250[c]
KB	No	1 ± 0.01	0.675	-
KBy	Pgp	4 ± 0.1	0.036	19[c]
C2C12	No	15 ± 1.4	4.5	-
HUVEC	No	40 ± 4.9	0.0675	-
Caco-2	Pgp, MRP	5.5 ± 0.4	0.00067	6670[d]
BBMEC	Pgp, MRP	1.6 ± 0.04	0.018	250[d]
LLC-PK1	No	61 ± 6.9	0.45	-
LLC-MDR1	Pgp	79 ± 1.7	0.0045	100[e]
MDCK-wt	No	1.7 ± 0.1	0.02	-
MDCK-MRP1	Pgp, MRP	6.7 ± 0.02	0.00003	670[f]
MDCK-MRP2	Pgp, MRP	3.9 ± 0.05	0.0004	50[f]
COR-L23	No	4.0 ± 0.35	10	-
COR-L23/R	MRP	4.0 ± 0.2	0.1	100[g]

[a]Mean ± SEM (n=4). [b]Calculated as the ratio of EC_{50} of non-Pgp non-MRP cells to EC_{50} of corresponding Pgp expressing cells. [c]Compared to MCF-7 cells. [d]Compared to C2C12 cells. [e]Compared to LLC-PK1 cells. [f]Compared to MDCK-wt cells. [g]Compared to COR-L23 cells.

Pluronic® block copolymers are known to induce drastic changes in the microviscosity of cell membranes as assessed using a hydrophobic membrane probe, 1,6-diphenyl-1,3,5-hexatriene (DPH). *(65,66)* These changes can be attributed to the alterations in the structure of the lipid bilayers as a result of adsorption of the block copolymer molecules on the membranes. Interestingly, it appears that Pluronic® block copolymers have different effects with respect to the membranes of some normal and cancer cells. The treatment with the same doses of P85 or L61 increased microviscosity ("fluidized") of the membranes of cancerous cells, while, in contrast, decreased the microviscosity ("solidified") of membranes of the normal blood cells. *(65)* Membrane fluidization by various agents including nonionic surfactants, such as Tween 20, Nonidet P-40 and Triton X-100, is known to contribute to inhibition of Pgp efflux function. *(67)* MDR modulation by membrane fluidizers occurs by abolishment of Pgp ATPase activity that results in the loss of Pgp-mediated drug efflux. *(67)* Furthermore, recent studies demonstrated that P85 inhibits Pgp ATPase activity, and that inhibition of this activity is observed with the same doses of the block copolymer as those that inhibit Pgp efflux in Pgp expressing cells. *(55,66)* Therefore, it is likely that these Pluronic® block copolymers have a "double-punch" effect in Pgp expressing cells: through ATP depletion and membrane fluidization, which both have a combined result of potent inhibition of Pgp. *(55,66)* Both factors are critical for the exhibition of the effect of P85 on Pgp efflux system in Pgp expressing cells. The interrelationship between membrane fluidization and energy depletion components of the Pluronic® affect can be better understood in view of the current picture of the Pgp structure, describing Pgp as a two-domain protein with ATP-binding sites in each domain. *(68)* Proper interaction of these two ATP-binding sites is crucial for the proper functioning of Pgp. It was suggested that binding of ATP in one domain causes a conformational change in the Pgp molecule necessary for the hydrolysis of ATP and translocation of the substrate. *(69)* Therefore, the structural perturbations in the lipid membranes induced by the block copolymer may decrease the affinity of ATP to its binding site and interfere with the ATPase activity. This means that higher concentrations of intracellular ATP would be required for normal functioning of Pgp, i.e., drug efflux system would become more vulnerable to decreases in intracellular ATP. It is possible that different drug transporters have different energy requirements in MDR cells and/or different sensitivity to changes in membrane microviscosity. As a result, the potency of Pluronic® block copolymers with respect to modulation of these drug transport mechanisms may also vary.

As is the case with any chemosensitizer, the effects of Pluronic® block copolymers in MDR cells exhibit significant dose-dependent behavior. However, due to the ability of the block copolymers to self-assemble into micelles and to solubilize hydrophobic drugs, the dose dependencies observed with these compounds are drastically different compared to the dose dependencies of many other Pgp modulators. Studies evaluating the dose response to various Pluronic®

block copolymers in MDR cells have demonstrated that increases in accumulation of the Pgp probe rhodamine 123, and potentiation of doxorubicin activity by Pluronic® in MDR cancer cells occur at block copolymer concentrations below the CMC. *(24)* This means that both effects are due to the block copolymer single chains, i.e., the unimers. As a result, the accumulation and cytotoxicity of drugs in MDR cells increase with increasing concentrations of Pluronic® until the CMC is reached and unimer concentration levels off because, above the CMC, block copolymer added in the system is consumed for the micelle formation. Under these conditions, the drug accumulation and cytotoxicity in MDR cells, first, level off and then decrease. *(24)* Therefore, the CMC provides the "cut-off point" for the maximal drug accumulation in MDR cells. The decreases in drug absorption in the cells above the CMC are very similar to those reported previously for other nonionic detergents that are MDR modulators, such as Cremophor EL. *(70,71)* The inhibition of cell transport in the presence of micelles is attributed to incorporation of the drug into the micelles, resulting in a decrease in the amount of the free probe available for diffusion through the cell membrane into cells.

The molecular composition of the block copolymer affects both the inhibition of the Pgp efflux system as well as the hypersensitization effects of Pluronic® in MDR cells. For example, studies of rhodamine 123 accumulation in resistant KBv cells in the presence of block copolymers differing in the lengths of EO and PO chains suggested that more hydrophobic block copolymers (having lower HLB) are more active than more hydrophilic block copolymers (having higher HLB). *(24)* Second, cytotoxicity studies using doxorubicin suggested that the potency of Pluronic® unimers in sensitization of the MDR cells increased with the increase in the copolymer hydrophobicity.

Summarizing the discussion above it appears that the effects of Pluronic® on Pgp are at least in part induced by alterations in the structure of the cell membranes by the block copolymers. Such interactions with the membranes involve incorporation of the hydrophobic PO chains of the block copolymer in the lipid bilayers. In contrast, hydrophilic EO chains do not interact with lipid membranes and are used to prevent binding of other polymers with the membranes. *(72)* At the same time, hydrophobic block copolymers are better transported inside the cells and/or are more potent inhibitors of metabolic processes than the hydrophilic copolymers. Furthermore, in the energy depletion studies, exposure of the MDR cells to a hydrophilic copolymer, such as F108, did not induce such a drastic decrease in intracellular ATP levels as those observed following exposure of the cells to the more hydrophobic copolymers P85 and L61. *(55,72)* Therefore, combined differences in membrane interactions, cellular transport, and energy depletion activity may contribute to the observed dependence of the potency of block copolymers on their structure in MDR cells.

To evaluate how efficacious these block copolymers are in inhibiting Pgp, the absorption of rhodamine 123 was examined in Pgp expressing cells. *(24)* A dose response curve for rhodamine 123 accumulation was obtained for each block copolymer as discussed in the previous section. Next, the maximal accumulation levels ("R123 enhancement factors") observed with the most effective doses of each Pluronic® were plotted as a function of the length of the hydrophobic PO block (y). This operation yielded a bell shaped dependency of the net efficacy of Pluronic® copolymers in inducing rhodamine 123 accumulation in cells (Figure 3). As is seen in the figure, the most efficacious block copolymers are those with intermediate lengths of the hydrophobic block ranging from 30 to 60 PO repeating units, while the block copolymers with shorter or longer PO blocks are less efficient. Furthermore, the resistance reversion indexes determined in the doxorubicin cytotoxicity study in KBv cells followed exactly the same pattern as the drug accumulation data shown in Figure 3. *(24)*

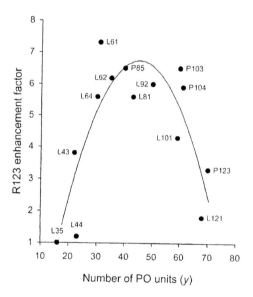

Figure 3. Optimization of Pluronic® block copolymer composition in MDR cells. The entire set of hydrophilic copolymers with HLB varying from 20 to 29 had no or little effect on drug transport and is not presented in this figure. Only the copolymers with HLB less than 20 exhibiting varying degrees of activity in MDR cells are presented. (Reproduced with permission from reference 24. Copyright 1999.)

This behavior was explained by the interplay of both hydrophobic-hydrophilic properties of Pluronic® molecules and their self-assembly behavior in aqueous solutions. The copolymers with long PO segments and short EO segments are the most potent. However, they also have much lower solubility and CMC, which limits the effective concentration of the unimers in the solution. On the other hand, the unimers with short PO segments a have high CMC and their concentration in solution can be very high. However, the potency of these unimers is low. As a result, the optimal net efficacy is observed with Pluronic® copolymers having intermediate lengths of PO chains and a relatively short EO segments, such as P85 and L61. The unimers of these copolymers are sufficiently potent and relatively high concentration of unimers can be reached in solution.

Pluronic® Effects on Brain and Oral Bioavalability of Drugs

There is an increasing interest in the role of Pgp and MRP in the tissue distribution of therapeutic agents based on reports that these transporters are expressed in 'normal' cells in the body, including brain microvessel endothelial cells (BMVEC), intestinal epithelial cells, and hepatocytes. For example, immunohistochemical and functional studies indicate that Pgp is expressed on the luminal (apical) plasma membrane of BMVEC that form the blood brain barrier (BBB). [72,73] Less is known regarding the role of the MRP drug efflux transport system in the BBB. There are several isoforms of MRP that appear to be expressed in the BBB, including MRP1, MRP4, MRP5, and MRP6. [74] In contrast to Pgp, which transports lipophilic and cationic compounds, MRP transports anionic compounds and/or glucuronide and glutathione conjugates. [75,76] Several studies indicate the presence of outwardly directed efflux transport systems for organic anions in the BBB. [77-79]

To date, there are two studies that indicate Pluronic® can enhance the brain penetration of selected drugs *in vivo*. In the first study, Kabanov *et al.* demonstrated increased delivery of the neuroleptic drug, haloperidol, to the brain in mice with the use of insulin or antibody conjugated Pluronic® micelles. [31,32] In addition, haloperidol delivery to the brain was also increased in the presence of P85. In the second study, Batrakova *et al.* examined the brain accumulation of digoxin in wild type mice, mdr1a knockout mice, and wild type mice treated with P85. [35] As expected, the brain accumulation of digoxin was significantly higher in the mdr 1a/b (-/-) knockout mice, due to the absence of Pgp efflux transport of digoxin at the BBB. [35] The kinetic profiles of radiolabeled digoxin in the plasma and the brain of wild type mice suggested that P85 prolonged the residence time and concentrations of Pluronic® in the brain. The relative contribution of Pgp inhibition to this central nervous system (CNS) delivery enhancement was evaluated by comparing P85 treated wild type female FBV mice with non-treated Pgp-deficient mice. These experiments demonstrated that delivery to the CNS of a prototypical Pgp substrate could be significantly enhanced by co-administration of Pluronic®.

Attachment of a specific ligand to the drug carrier enables binding of the carrier to the cell surface, entrapment of the carrier into endosomes, and trafficking of the carrier inside the cell. For example, the corona-forming EO chains in block copolymer micelles can be modified to incorporate ligand moieties and redirect these micelles along endocytic pathways. Receptor-mediated transport using Pluronic® micelles as the drug carrier has been reported recently. (32) This study revealed that P85 micelles, containing a fluorescent dye, are taken up into cells via an endocytosis mechanism. The absorption was drastically increased when a protein molecule, enterotoxin B, capable of binding with a cell receptor, was covalently linked to the surface of a micelle. Excess of free enterotoxin B effectively inhibited the uptake of the micelles with the enterotoxin B modified corona, suggesting specific interactions of the micelles with the cells through the receptor. A similar approach was recently used to evaluate the effects of the conjugation of specific ligands with Pluronic® micelles on drug processing and permeability in BMVEC. (22) To target receptor-mediated endocytosis in the BMVEC, P85 micelles were conjugated to insulin. The transport of the probe was significantly increased in the presence of the insulin vector compared to the transport of the probe in insulin-free micelles or in micelles with the same concentration of free insulin. Furthermore, the competitive inhibition of transport of insulin-vectorized micelles with an excess of free insulin was demonstrated. This study suggested that conjugation of insulin to Pluronic® micelles resulted in a shift from a vesicular transport of the micelle through simple endocytosis to a receptor-mediated endocytosis. In addition, by modifying the micelles with a ligand, the cellular processing could be altered to favor transcytosis as the major pathway and recycling to the lumenal side as the minor transport pathway, which results in enhancement in the flux of the drug across in the BBB. These studies provide a foundation for future development of a therapeutic method for enhancing the brain penetration of drugs using Pluronic® block copolymer technology.

There is an increasing body of evidence that outwardly directed drug efflux systems hinder oral bioavailability of selected drugs. Intestinal epithelial cells are known to express a functionally active Pgp as well as various isoforms of MRP, including MRP2, MRP3 and, to a lesser extent, MRP1 and MRP5. (80) In this respect it is believed that by inhibiting the function of these drug efflux systems it is possible to increase efficiency of delivery of these drugs through the oral route. The potential effectiveness of inhibition of the Pgp efflux system in enhancing oral bioavailability has been studied recently by examining the effects of nonionic detergents on peptide permeability in monolayers of the human colon epithelium cell line, Caco-2. (70,71) In these studies, the permeability of Caco-2 monolayers to selected peptides was significantly enhanced by nonionic surfactants, Polysorbate 80 and Cremophor EL. Consequently, *in vitro* studies examined the effects of Pluronic® block copolymers on drug absorption and permeability in Caco-2 monolayers. *(22,46)* The unimers of Pluronic® block copolymers inhibited the Pgp efflux system in Caco-2 monolayers, resulting in a significant enhancement of absorption and permeability of the probe. Table IV presents the apparent permeability coefficients (P_{app}) of various compounds in Caco-2 monolayers in the AP to BL direction. *(78)* As is seen from the data, P85 increases permeability in the monolayers with respect to a broad panel of drug and probe molecules, suggesting that it can be useful for increasing oral bioavailability of these compounds. Furthermore, recent reports have demonstrated increased oral uptake of two drugs, amikacin and tobramicin, which could be Pgp substrates, following oral administration to mice in the presence of poloxamer CRL-1605. *(81,82)* Taken together these studies provide substantial evidence that Pluronic® block copolymers can be useful in increasing oral absorption of select drugs by inhibiting drug efflux systems in intestinal epithelial cells.

Table IV. Effects of P85 on the permeability of various solutes in Caco-2 mono-layers in AP to BL direction. (78).

Solute	Drug transporter	$P_{app} \times 10^6$ [cm/s]		Effect
		Assay buffer	P85	
Mannitol	none	0.2 ± 0.004	0.2 ± 0.004	insignificant
Valproic acid	unknown	10.4 ± 0.5	14.3 ± 0.5	1.4
Loperamide	unknown	1.6 ± 0.1	3.3 ± 0.2	2.1
Doxorubicin	Pgp, MRP	14.5 ± 1.2	35.2 ± 0.7	2.4
Methotrexate[a]	MRP	3.9 ± 0.2	10.1 ± 0.3	2.6
Etoposide	Pgp, MRP	4.0 ± 0.6	10.6 ± 0.8	2.7
Rhodamine 123	Pgp	0.7 ± 0.1	2.3 ± 0.5	3.3
Fluorescein	MRP	3.8 ± 0.4	13.9 ± 0.5	3.7
Vinblastine[a]	Pgp, MRP	3.1 ± 0.4	13.3 ± 0.3	4.3
Ritonavir[a]	Pgp	3.3 ± 0.3	14.4 ± 0.4	4.4
Ziduvidin	MRP	2.9 ± 0.1	14.5 ± 0.4	5.0
Taxol	Pgp	0.36 ± 0.01	4.7 ± 0.4	13.1

[a] Additional data, not reported in Ref. *(78)*.

Conclusions

Pluronic® block copolymers are among the most potent drug delivery systems with a broad spectrum of biological response-modifying activities. Pluronic® unimers self-assemble into micelles, which incorporate drug molecules and transport them within the body. The unimers themselves sensitize multidrug resistant cells with respect to various anticancer agents, and inhibit drug efflux transporters in both the blood brain barrier (BBB) and the small intestine. This inhibition results in enhanced transport of selected drugs to the brain and increased oral bioavailability. These properties warrant further investigations regarding the use of Pluronic® formulations as novel promising drug delivery systems.

References

1. Langer, R. Drug delivery and targeting, Nature **1998**, *392,* 5-10.
2. Yokoyama, M. Block copolymers as drug carriers, *Crit. Rev. Ther. Drug Carrier Syst.* **1992**, *9,* 213-248.
3. Kwon, G.S., Kataoka, K. Block copolymer micelles as long-circulating drug vehicles, *Adv. Drug Deliv. Rev.* **1995**, *16*, 295-309.
4. Stolnik, S., Illum, L., Davis, S.S. Long circulating microparticulate drug carriers, *Adv. Drug. Deliv. Rev.* **1995**, *16,* 195-214.
5. Kabanov, A.V., Alakhov, V.Y. Block copolyrner micelles (microcontainers for drug targeting), In *Polymeric Materials Encyclopedia;* Salamone, J.C., Ed.; CRC Press: Boca Raton, New York, London, Tokyo, 1996; Vol. 1, pp 757-760.
6. Cammas, S., Kataoka, K. Site specific drug carriers: Polymeric micelles as high potential vehicles for biologically active molecules, In *NATO ASI Series;* Webber, S.E., Ed.; Ser. E, Kluwer Academic Publisher, 1996; Vol. 327, pp 83-113.
7. Alakhov, V.Y., Kabanov, A.V. Block copolymeric biotransport carriers as versatile vehicles for drug delivery, *Exp. Op. Invest. Drugs* **1998**, *7*, 1453-1473.
8. Kwon, G.S., Okano, T. Soluble self-assembled block copolymers for drug delivery, *Pharm. Res.* **1999**, *16,* 597-600.
9. Allen, C., Maysinger, D., Eisenberg, A. Nano-engineering block copolymer aggregates for drug delivery, *Coll. Surfaces, B: Biointerfaces* **1999**, *16,* 3-27.
10. Kataoka, K., Kabanov, A. *Polymeric Micelles in Biology and Pharmaceutics,* Special Issue: Colloids and Surfaces, B: Biointerfaces, Elsevier: Amsterdam, Lausanne, New York, Oxford, Shannon, Tokyo, 1999.
11. Kabanov, A.V., Alakhov, V.Y. Pluronic block copolymers in drug delivery: From K micellar nanocontainers to biological response modifiers, *Crit. Rev. Ther. Drug Carrier* Syst. **2002**, *19,* 1-73.
12. Schmolka, I.R. A review of block polymer surfactants, *J. Am. Oil Chem. Soc.* **1977**, *54,* 110-116.
13. Geyer, R.P. Perfluorochemicals as oxygen transport vehicles, *Biomater. Artif Cells Artif. Organs* **1988**, *16,* 31-49.
14. Allison, A.C., Byars, N.E. Adjuvant formulations and their mode of action, *Semin. Immunol.* **1990**, *2,* 369-374.

15. Schmolka, I.R. Physical basis for poloxamer interactions, *Ann. NY Acad. Sci.* **1994**, *720*, 92-97.
16. Hawley, A.E., Davis, S.S., Illum, L. Targeting of colloids to lymph nodes: influence of lymphatic physiology and colloidal characteristics, *Adv. Drug. Deliv. Rev.* **1995**, *17*, 129-148.
17. Newman, M.J., Actor, J.K., Balusubramanian, M., Jagannath, C. Use of nonionic block copolymers in vaccines and therapeutics, *Crit. Rev. Ther. Drug Carrier* Syst. **1998**, *15*, 89-142.
18. Malmsten, M. Block copolymers in pharmaceutics, In: *Amphiphilic block copolymers: Self assembly and applications;* Alexandridis, P., Lindman, B., Eds.; Elsevier: Amsterdam, Lausanne, New York, Oxford, Shannon, Singapore, Tokyo, 2000; pp 319-346.
19. Moghimi, S.M., Hunter, A.C. Poloxamers and poloxamines in nanoparticle engineering and experimental medicine, *Trends Biotechnol.* **2000**, *18*, 412-420.
20. Anderson, B.C., Pandit, N.K., Mallapragada, S.K. Understanding drug release from poly(ethylene oxide)-b-poly(propylene oxide)-b-poly(ethylene oxide) gels, *J. Contr. Rel.* **2001**, *70*, 157-167.
21. Nagarajan, R. Solubilization of hydrocarbons and resulting aggregate shape transitions in aqueous solutions of Pluronic (PEO-PPO-PEO) block copolymers, *Coll. Surfaces, B: Biointerfaces* **1999**, *16*, 55-72.
22. Batrakova, E.V., Han, H.Y., Miller, D.W., Kabanov, A.V. Effects of pluronic P85 unimers and micelles on drug permeability in polarized BBMEC and Caco-2 cells, *Pharm. Res.* **1998**, *15*, 1525-1532.
23. Kabanov, A.V., Nazarova, I.R., Astafieva, I.V., Batrakova, E.V., Alakhov, V.Y., Yaroslavov, A.A., Kabanov, V.A. Micelle formation and solubilization of fluorescent probes in poly(oxyethylene-b-oxypropylene-b-oxyethylene) solutions, *Macromol.* **1995**, *28*, 2303-2314.
24. Batrakova, E.V., Lee, S., Li, S., Venne, A., Alakhov, V., Kabanov, A. Fundamental relationships between the composition of pluronic block copolymers and their hypersensitization effect in MDR cancer cells, *Pharm. Res.* **1999**, *16*, 1373-1379.
25. Torchilin, V.P. *In vitro* and *in vivo* availability of liposomes, In: *Self-assembling complexes for gene delivery: From laboratory to clinical trial;* Kabanov, A.V., Felgner, P.L., Seymour, L.W., Eds.; John Wiley: Chichester, New York, Weinheim, Brisbane, Singapore, Toronto, 1998; pp 277-293.
26. Schiffelers, R.M., Bakker-Woudenberg, I.A., Snijders, S.V., Storm, G. Localization of sterically stabilized liposomes in Klebsiella pneumoniae-infected rat lung tissue: Influence of liposome characteristics, Biochim. Biophys. Acta **1999**, *1421*, 329-339.
27. Ishida, O., Maruyama, K., Sasaki, K., Iwatsuru, M. Size-dependent extravasation and interstitial localization of polyethyleneglycol liposomes in solid tumor-bearing mice, *Int. J. Pharm.* 1999, 190, 49-56.

28. Kong, G., Braun, R.D., Dewhirst, M.W. Hyperthermia enables tumor-specific nanoparticle delivery: Effect of particle size, *Cancer Res.* **2000**, *60,* 4440-4445.

29. Ogawara, K., Yoshida, M., Furumoto, K., Takakura, Y., Hashida, M., Higaki, K., Kimura, T. Uptake by hepatocytes and biliary excretion of intravenously administered polystyrene microspheres in rats, *J. Drug Target.* **1999**, *7,* 213-221.

30. Alexandridis, P., Nivaggioli, T., Hatton, T.A. Temperature effects on structural properties of Pluronic P104 and F108 PEO-PPO-PEO block copolymer solutions, *Langmuir* **1995**, *11,* 1468-1476.

31. Kabanov, A.V. *et al.* The neuroleptic activity of haloperidol increases after its solubilization in surfactant micelles. Micelles as microcontainers for drug targeting, *FEBS Lett.* **1989**, *258,* 343-345.

32. Kabanov, A.V., Slepnev, V.I., Kuznetsova, L.E., Batrakova, E.V., Alakhov, V.Y., Melik-Nubarov, N.S., Sveshnikov, P.G., Kabanov, V.A. Pluronic micelles as a tool for low-molecular compound vector delivery into a cell: effect of Staphylococcus aureus enterotoxin B on cell loading with micelle incorporated fluorescent dye, *Biochem. Int.* **1992**, *26,* 1035-1042.

33. Alakhov, V.Y., Moskaleva, E.Y., Batrakova, E.V., Kabanov, A.V. Hyper-sensitization of multidrug resistant human ovarian carcinoma cells by pluronic P85 block copolymer, *Bioconjug. Chem.* **1996**, *7,* 209-2 16.

34. Alakhov, V., Klinski, E., Li, S., Pietrzynski, G., Venne, A., Batrakova, E., Bronitch, T., Kabanov, A.V. Block copolymer-based formulation of doxorubicin. From cell screen to clinical trials, *Coll. Surf, B: Biointerfaces* **1999**, *16,* 113-134.

35. Batrakova, E.V., Miller, D.W., Li, S., Alakhov, V.Y., Kabanov, A.V., Elmquist, W.F. Pluronic P85 enhances the delivery of digoxin to the brain: *In vitro* and *in vivo* studies, *J. Pharmacol. Exp. Ther.* **2001**, *296,* 551-557.

36. Kabanov, A.V., Alakhov, V.Y. Micelles of amphilphilic block copolymers as vehicles for drug delivery, In: *Amphiphilic Block Copolymers: Self-Assembly and Applications;* Alexandridis, P., Lindman, B., Eds.; Elsevier: Amsterdam, Lausanne, New York, Oxford, Shannon, Singapore, Tokyo, 2000; pp 347-376.

37. Kozlov, M.Y., Melik-Nubarov, N.S., Batrakova, E.V., Kabanov, A.V. Relationship between pluronic block copolymer structure, critical micellization concentration and partitioning coefficients of low molecular mass solutes, *Macromol.* **2000**, *33,* 3305-3313.

38. Yokoyama, M., Sugiyama, T., Okano, T., Sakurai, Y., Naito, M., Kataoka, K. Analysis of micelle formation of an adriamycin-conjugated polyethylene glycol-poly(aspartic acid) block copolymer by gel permeation chromatography, *Pharm. Res.* **1993**, *10,* 895-899.

39. Kwon, G.S., Natio, M., Yokoyama, M., Okano, T., Sakurai, Y., Kataoka, K. Physical entrapment of adriamycin in AB block copolymer micelles, *Pharm. Res.* **1995**, *12,* 192-195.

150

40. Batrakova, E.V. *et al.* Anthracycline antibiotics non-covalently incorporated into the block copolymer micelles: *in vivo* evaluation of anti-cancer activity, *Br. J. Cancer* **1996**, *74*, 1545-1552.
41. Naito, S., Yokomizo, A., Koga, H. Mechanisms of drug resistance in chemotherapy for urogenital carcinoma, *Int. J. Urol.* **1999**, *6*, 427-439.
42. Kuwano, M., Toh, S., Uchiumi, T., Takano, H., Kohno, K., Wada, M. Multidrug resistance-associated protein subfamily transporters and drug resistance, *Anticancer Drug Des.* **1999**, *14*, 123-131.
43. Page, M., Alakhov, V.Y. Elimination of P-gp-mediated multidrug resistance by solubilization in Pluronic rnicelles, In: *Proc. Ann. Meet. Am. Assoc. Cancer Res.,* Vol. 33, 1992, p A3302.
44. Venne, A., Li, S., Mandeville, R., Kabanov, A., Alakhov, V. Hypersensitizing effect of pluronic L61 on cytotoxic activity, transport, and subcellular distribution of doxorubicin in multiple drug-resistant cells, *Cancer Res.* **1996**, *56*, 3626-3629.
45. Evers, R., Kool, M., Smith, A.J., van Deemter, L., de Haas, M., Borst, P. Inhibitory effect of the reversal agents V-104, GF120918 and Pluronic L61 on MDR1 Pgp-, MRP1- and MRP2-mediated transport, *Br. J. Cancer* **2000**, *83*, 366-374.
46. Batrakova, E.V., Han, H.Y., Alakhov, V., Miller, D.W., Kabanov, A.V. Effects of pluronic block copolymers on drug absorption in Caco-2 cell monolayers, *Pharm. Res.* **1998**, *15*, 850-855.
47. Miller, D.W., Batrakova, E.V., Kabanov, A.V. Inhibition of multidrug resistance-associated protein (MRP) functional activity with pluronic block copolymers, *Pharm. Res.* **1999**, *16*, 396-401.
48. Breuninger, L.M., Paul, S., Gaughan, K., Miki, T., Chan, A., Aaronson, S.A., Kruh, G.D. Expression of multidrug resistance-associated protein in NIH/3T3 cells confers multidrug resistance associated with increased drug efflux and altered intracellular drug distribution, *Cancer Res.* **1995**, *55*, 5342-5347.
49. Nooter, K., Stoter, G. Molecular mechanisms of multidrug resistance in cancer chemotherapy, *Pathol. Res. Pract.* **1996**, *192*, 768-780.
50. Cleary, I., Doherty, G., Moran, E., Clynes, M. The multidrug-resistant human lung tumour cell line, DLKP-A10, expresses novel drug accumulation and sequestration systems, *Biochem. Pharmacol.* **1997**, *53*, 1493-1502.
51. Shapiro, A.B., Fox, K., Lee, P., Yang, Y.D., Ling, V. Functional intracellular P-glycoprotein, *Int. J. Cancer* **1998**, *76*, 857-864.
52. Altan, N., Chen, Y., Schindler, M., Simon, S.M. Defective acidification in human breast tumor cells and implications for chemotherapy, *J. Exp. Med.* **1998**, *187*, 1583-1598.
53. Benderra, Z., Morjani, H., Trussardi, A., Manfait, M. Role of the vacuolar H+-ATPase in daunorubicin distribution in etoposide-resistant MCF7 cells overexpressing the multidrug-resistance associated protein, *Int. J. Oncol.* **1998**, *12*, 711-715.

54. Batrakova, E.V., Li, S., Alakhov, V.Y., Kabanov, A.V. Selective energy depletion and sensitization of multiple drug resistant cancer cells by Pluronic block copolymers., *Polym. Prepr.* **2000**, *41*, 1639-1640.

55. Batrakova, E.V., Li, S., Elmquist, W.F., Miller, D.W., Alakhov, V.Y., Kabanov, A.V. Mechanism of sensitization of MDR cancer cells by Pluronic block copolymers: selective energy depletion, *Br. J. Cancer* **2001**, *85*, 1987-1997.

56. Batrakova, E.V., Li, S., Alakhov, V.Yu., Elmquist, W.F., Miller, D.W., Kabanov, A.V. Sensitization of cells overexpressing multidrug resistant protein by Pluronic P85, *Pharm. Res.* **2003**, *10*, 1581-1590.

57. Kabanov A.V., Batrakova, E.V., Alakhov, V.Y. An essential relationship between ATP depletion and chemosensitizing activity of Pluronic® block copolymers, *J. Contr. Rel.* **2003**, *91(1-2)*, 75-83.

58. Van Zutphen, H., Merola, A.J., Brierley, G.P., Cornwell, D.G. The interaction of nonionic detergents with lipid bilayer membranes, *Arch. Biochem. Biophys.* **1972**, *152*, 755-766.

59. Atkinson, T.P., Smith, T.F., Hunter, R.L. Histamine release from human basophils by synthetic block co-polymers composed of polyoxyethylene and polyoxypropylene and synergy with immunologic and non-immunologic stimuli, *J. Immunol.* **1988**, *141*, 1307-1310.

60. Brierley, G.P., Jurkowitz, M., Merola, A.J., Scott, K.M. Ion transport by heart mitochondria. XXV. Activation of energy-linked K + uptake by non-ionic detergents, *Arch. Biochem. Biophys.* **1972**, *152*, 744-754.

61. Brustovetskii, N.N., Dedukhova, V.N., Egorova, M.V., Mokhova, E.N., Skulachev, V.P. Uncoupling of oxidative phosphorylation by fatty acids and detergents suppressed by ATP/ADP antiporter inhibitors, *Biochemistry (Mosc.)* **1991**, *56*, 1042-1048.

62. Kirillova, G.P., Mokhova, E.N., Dedukhova, V.I., Tarakanova, A.N., Ivanova, V.P., Efremova, N.V., Topchieva, I.N. The influence of pluronics and their conjugates with proteins on the rate of oxygen consumption by liver mitochondria and thymus lymphocytes, *Biotechnol. Appl. Biochem.* **1993**, *18*, 329-339.

63. Rapoport, N., Marin, A.P., Timoshin, A.A. Effect of a polymeric surfactant on electron transport in HL-60 cells, *Arch. Biochem. Biophys.* **2000**, *384*, 100-108.

64. Slepnev, V.I., Kuznetsova, L.E., Gubin, A.N., Batrakova, E.V., Alakhov, V., Kabanov, A.V. Micelles of poly(oxyethylene)-poly(oxypropylene) block copolymer (pluronic) as a tool for low-molecular compound delivery into a cell: Phosphorylation of intracellular proteins with micelle incorporated [gamma-^{32}P]ATP, *Biochem. Int.* **1992**, *26*, 587-595.

65. Melik-Nubarov, N.S., Pomaz, O.O., Dorodnych, T., Badun, G.A., Ksenofontov, A.L., Schemchukova, O.B., Arzhakov, S.A. Interaction of tumor and normal blood cells with ethylene oxide and propylene oxide block copolymers, *FEBS Lett.* **1999**, *446*, 194-198.

66. Batrakova, E.V., Li, S., Vinogradov, S.V., Alakhov, V.Y., Miller, D.W., Kabanov, A.V. Mechanism of pluronic effect on p-glycoprotein efflux system in blood brain barrier: contributions of energy depletion and membrane fluidization., *J. Pharmacol. Exp. Ther.* **2001**, *299*, 483-493.

67. Regev, R., Assaraf, Y.G., Eytan, G.D. Membrane fluidization by ether, other anesthetics, and certain agents abolishes P-glycoprotein ATPase activity and modulates efflux from multidrug-resistant cells, *Eur. J. Biochem.* **1999**, *259*, 18-24.

68. Ambudkar, S.V., Dey, S., Hrycyna, C.A., Ramachandra, M., Pastan, I., Gottesman, M.M. Biochemical, cellular, and pharmacological aspects of the multidrug transporter, *Ann. Rev. Pharmacol. Toxicol.* **1999**, *39*, 361-398.

69. Ramachandra, M., Ambudkar, S.V., Chen, D., Hrycyna, C.A., Dey, S. Human P-glycoprotein exhibits reduced affinity for substrates during a catalytic transition state, *Biochem.* **1998**, *37*, 5010-5019.

70. Nerurkar, M.M., Burton, P.S., Borchardt, R.T. The use of surfactants to enhance the permeability of peptides through Caco-2 cells by inhibition of an apically polarized efflux system, *Pharm. Res.* **1996**, *13*, 528-534.

71. Nerurkar, M.M., Ho, N.F., Burton, P.S., Vidmar, T.J., Borchardt, R.T. Mechanistic roles of neutral surfactants on concurrent polarized and passive membrane transport of a model peptide in Caco-2 cells, *J. Pharm. Sci.* **1997**, *86*, 813-821.

72. Batrakova, E.V., Li, S., Alakhov, V.Y., Miller, D.W., Kabanov, A.V. Optimal structure requirements for Pluronic block copolymers in modifying P-glycoprotein drug efflux transporter activity in BBMEC, *J. Pharm. Exp. Ther.* **2003**, *304 (2)*, 845-854.

73. Cordon-Cardo, C., O'Brien, J.P., Casals, D., Rittman-Grauer, L., Biedler, J.L., Melamed, M.R., Bertino, J.R. Multidrug-resistance gene (P-glycoprotein) is expressed by endothelial cells at blood-brain barrier sites, *Proc. Natl. Acad. Sci. USA* **1989**, *86*, 695-698.

74. Zhang, Y., Han, H., Elmquist, W.F., Miller, D.W. Expression of various multidrug resistance-associated protein (MRP) homologues in brain microvessel endothelial cells, *Brain Res.* **2000**, *876*, 148-153.

75. Hollo, Z., Homolya, L., Hegedus, T., Sarkadi, B. Transport properties of the multidrug resistance-associated protein (MRP) in human tumour cells, *FEBS Lett.* **1996**, *383*, 99-104.

76. Jedlitschky, G., Leier, I., Buchholz, U., Barnouin, K., Kurz, G., Keppler, D. Transport of glutathione, glucuronate, and sulfate conjugates by the MRP gene-encoded conjugate export pump, *Cancer Res.* **1996**, *56*, 988-994.

77. Adkison, K.D., Artru, A.A., Powers, K.M., Shen, D.D. Contribution of probenecid-sensitive anion transport processes at the brain capillary endothelium and choroid plexus to the efficient efflux of valproic acid from the central nervous system, *J. Pharmacol. Exp. Ther.* **1994**, *268*, 797-805.

78. Batrakova, E.V., Li, S., Miller, D.W., Kabanov, A.V. Pluronic P85 increases permeability of a broad spectrum of drugs in polarized BBMEC and Caco-2 cell monolayers, *Pharm. Res.* **1999**, *16*, 1366-1372.

79. Slepnev, V.P., DeCamilli, P. Endocytosis: An Overview, In: *Self-Assembling Complexes for Gene Delivery: From Laboratory to Clinical Trial;* Kabanov, A.V., Felgner, P.L., Seymour, L.W., Eds.; John Wiley: Chichester, New York, Weinheim, Brisbane, Singapore, Toronto, 1998; p 71.

80. Hirohashi, T., Suzuki, H., Chu, X.Y., Tamai, I., Tsuji, A., Sugiyama, Y. Function and expression of multidrug resistance-associated protein family in human colon adenocarcinoma cells (Caco-2), *J. Pharmacol. Exp. Ther.* **2000,** *292,* 265-270.

81. Banerjee, S.K., Jagannath, C., Hunter, R.L., Dasgupta, A. Bioavailability of tobramycin after oral delivery in FVB mice using CRL- 1605 copolymer, an inhibitor of P-glycoprotein, *Life Sci.* **2000,** *67,* 2011-2016.

82. Jagannath, C., Wells, A., Mshvildadze, M., Olsen, M., Sepulveda, E., Emanuele, M., Hunter, R.L., Jr., Dasgupta, A. Significantly improved oral uptake of amikacin in FVB mice in the presence of CRL-1605 copolymer, *Life Sci.* **1999,** *64,* 1733-1738.

Chapter 11

Clinically Available Endosomolytic Agent for Gene Delivery

K. Itaka[1], K. Miyata[1], A. Harada[1], H. Kawaguchi[2], K. Nakamura[2], and K. Kataoka[1,*]

[1]Department of Materials Science and Engineering, Graduate School of Engineering, The University of Tokyo, 7–3–1 Hongo, Bunkyo-ku, Tokyo 113–8656, Japan
[2]Department of Orthopaedic Surgery, Faculty of Medicine, The University of Tokyo, 7–3–1 Hongo, Bunkyo-ku, Tokyo 113–8655, Japan
*Corresponding author: email: kataoka@bmw.t.u-tokyo.ac.jp

The ability of hydroxychloroquine, a chloroquine derivative, to improve the gene transfection efficiency of a carrier system based on non-viral delivery was investigated. Hydroxychloroquine gave enhanced gene expression and low cytotoxicity in an *in vitro* transfection study. In particular, prolonged incubation for 24 hours with 100 μM hydroxychloroquine significantly enhanced the expression using a polyion complex (PIC) micelle system with excellent stability in serum-containing medium. Therefore, appropriate endosomolytic agents should be useful for *in vivo* gene delivery using non-viral delivery systems, with the FDA-approved hydroxychloroquine as one of the most promising candidates for this purpose.

Introduction

Chloroquine has widely been used for the enhancement of DNA/polycation complex based gene transfer. *(1-3)* Chloroquine was originally discovered as an anti-malaria drug, and its anti-inflammatory effects are well known. The mechanism of increasing the transfection efficiency assumes that choloroquine is a weak base, and that its consequent endosomotropism contributes to its activity by interfering with lysosomal degradation and enhancing the release of DNA into the cytoplasm. *(4)* Chloroquine, however, shows cytotoxicity and there still remain some difficulties with its application in clinical gene therapy.

One of the chloroquine derivatives, hydroxychloroquine, in which one of the N-ethyl substituents of chloroquine is ß-hydroxylated, is considered to be as effective as the parent molecule but with lower toxicity. *(5)* In fact, hydroxy-chloroquine is a FDA-approved drug, and high doses have been clinically used for the treatment of rheumatoid arthritis and lupus erythematosus. *(6-8)* In this study, we evaluate the ability of hydroxychloroquine to enhance transfection efficiency and discuss its feasibility as a clinically available endosomolytic agent.

Materials and Methods

Chemicals. Poly(L-lysine) with a degree of polymerization of 80, and poly (ethylene glycol-L-lysine) block copolymer (PEG-PLL; PEG Mw 12,000 g/mol; 71 PLL segments) were synthesized as reported previously. *(9)* The LipofectAMINE™ reagent and fetal bovine serum (FBS) were purchased from GIBCO BRL. Chloroquine and hydroxychloroquine were purchased from Sigma and Acros Organics, respectively.

Plasmid DNA. pGL3-Luc (Promega) was used in all experiments. This plasmid was amplified in competent DH5α Escherichia coli and purified using EndoFree™ Plasmid Maxi or Mega Kits (QIAGEN). The DNA concentration was determined by its UV absorbance measured at 260 nm.

Formation of DNA-loaded complex particles. PEG-PLL block copolymer and pDNA were separately dissolved in 10 mM of Tris-HCl buffer at pH 7.4. Polyion complex (PIC) micelles were formed by mixing both solutions at various charge ratios, based on the residual molar amount of the lysine unit to nucleotide. The poly(L-lysine)/DNA complex (Plys-polyplex) was similarly prepared by mixing the poly(L-lysine) and pDNA solutions. The polycationic lipid/DNA complex (lipoplex) was prepared by mixing the pDNA solution and LipofectAMINE™ reagent following the manufacturer's protocol. In all cases, the final DNA concentration was adjusted to 30 µg/ml.

Transfection. 293T cells were seeded in 24-well culture plates. After 24-hours incubation in the culture medium (Dulbecco's modified eagle medium; Sigma), the cells were rinsed, and 250 µl medium containing chloroquine or hydroxychloroquine was added to each well. 25 µl of the DNA-loaded complex solution was then applied to each well. For the transfection efficiency study (Figure 1), the cells were incubated for 4 hours. For the prolonged incubation study (Figure 3), the transfection time was varied from 3 to 24 hours. After removal of the transfection medium, the cells were further incubated in fresh culture medium. At 48 hours after the initial application of the DNA-loaded complexes, the luciferase gene expression was measured. Throughout this procedure, 10% FBS was included in the culture medium.

Cytotoxicity Assay. The cytotoxicity of chloroquine and hydroxy-chloroquine was evaluated by an MTT assay (Cell Counting Kit: Dojindo). 293T cells were plated into 96-well tissue culture plates. The medium was removed 24 hours later, and 100 µl DMEM (with 10% FBS) containing chloro-quine or hydroxychloroquine (10-100 µM) was added to each well. After several hours of incubation, the viability of the cells in each well was measured following the manufacturer's protocol. To compare the cytotoxicity between the two agents, the distribution of values was first analyzed in each group using the F-test. Between groups with normal distributions, the parametrical analysis using the Student's t-test (StatView-J 4.5; Stat View, Berkeley) was performed.

Results and Discussion

The presence of hydroxychloroquine in the transfection medium enhanced the gene expression of Plys-polyplex and PIC micelles (Figure 1). The results were concentration-dependent up to 100 µM, and almost equivalent to those found for chloroquine, indicating that hydroxychloroquine can be used under similar conditions as chloroquine. However, gene expression decreased for concentrations greater than 150 µM due to cytotoxicity. This observation is in accordance with reports showing 100 µM chloroquine as the optimum condition for *in vitro* transfection. *(1-3)* Conversely, both agents acted negatively on the transfection by lipoplex, presumably caused not only by the severe cytotoxicity in the co-presence of both lipoplex and the endosomolytic agent, but also the differences in the intracellular routing between lipoplex and complexes based on cationic polymers.

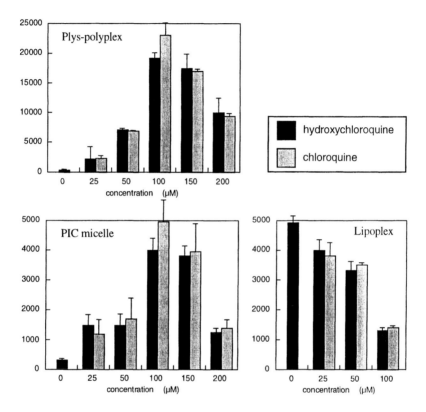

Figure 1. Transfection efficiency to 293T cells by Plys-polyplex, PIC micelles, and lipoplex in the presence of chloroquine or hydroxychloroquine (10-200 μM) in the culture medium. (n = 4; ± S.E.).

Cytotoxicity may be one of the most serious problems for the clinical application of endosomolytic agents. Indeed, we have observed that 100 μM chloroquine caused a serious cytotoxocity for most types of cells, especially in

158

culture media without serum. However, the viability considerably improved in media containing 10% serum. Figure 2 represents the viability of 293T cells in the presence of chloroquine or hydroxychloroquine in serum-containing medium. The cells could survive and proliferate even in 100 µM concentration for 24 hours. Similar results were obtained for other kinds of cell lines, although the degree of toxicity varied among these lines. It should be noted that the cytotoxicity of hydroxychloroquine was lower than that of chloroquine. For example, the number of live cells after 8 hours (p = 0.002) and 24 hours (p < 0.001) of incubation was significantly higher in the presence of 100 µM hydroxychloroquine than in the presence of 100 µM chloroquine.

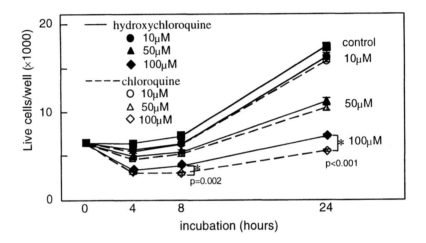

Figure 2. Viability of 293T cells in the presence of chloroquine or hydroxy-chloroquine (10-100 µM) in the culture medium. (n = 8; ± S.E.).

The effect of prolonged incubation was investigated next. The gene expression showed a remarkable increase with longer incubation in the co-presence of DNA-loaded complexes and 100 µM of hydroxychloroquine (Figure 3). This phenomenon was not observed in the absence of hydroxychloroquine (data not shown). Interestingly, the time-dependent increase in gene expression was more obvious for PIC micelles compared to Plys-polyplex, resulting in higher gene expression of the former after 24-hour incubation. This unique gene expression profile of PIC micelles may be explained by their excellent stability in the serum-containing medium as well as their appreciably lower cytotoxicity compared to Plys-polyplex. *(10,11)*

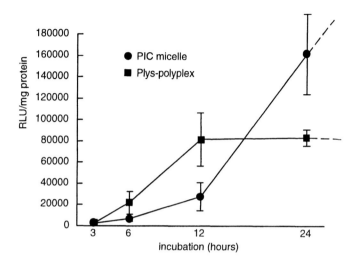

Figure 3. Transfection efficiency by prolonged incubation in the transfection medium (Plys-polyplex, PIC micelles) with 100 μM hydroxychloroquine. (n = 4; ± S.E.).

As reported in the literature, the steady-state blood concentration of hydroxychloroquine in patients with rheumatoid arthritis (daily dosis 400 mg) was 870.3 ± 329.3 ng/ml, equivalent to 2 μM. *(12)* Thus, if a somewhat higher concentration of hydroxychloroquine is permissible locally and temporarily, these conditions will effectively work for increasing the transfection efficiency. Moreover, DNA-loaded complexes and endosomolytic agents should not necessarily be used simultaneously, rather could be used separately or in a different way of administration. Although the conditions between *in vitro* and *in vivo* studies are quite different, and the ability of hydroxychloroquine to increase the transfection efficiency *in vivo* is not known, the results of this study indicate that the administration of hydroxychloroquine via a suitable method may be worth considering for clinical gene therapy with non-viral delivery systems.

Conclusions

The enhanced gene expression found for Plys-polyplex and PIC micelles with hydroxychloroquine present in the transfection medium, and the comparatively low cytotoxicity of hydroxychloroquine suggest that clinically available endosomolytic agents may improve effective *in vivo* gene delivery when used in combination with an appropriate delivery system possessing a considerable tolerability and low toxicity under physiological conditions, such as PIC micelles.

Acknowledgments

This work was financially supported by Grants-in-Aid for Scientific Research (No. 11167210 to K.K and No. 12877221 to H.K.) and Special Coordination Funds for Promoting Science and Technology from the Ministry of Education, Culture, Sports, Science and Technology of Japan as well as by the Core Research Program for Evolutional Science and Technology (CREST) from the Japan Science and Technology Corporation (JST).

References

1. Luthman, H.; Magnusson, G. *Nucleic Acids Res.* **1983**, *11*, 1295-308.
2. Erbacher, P.; Roche, A.C.; Monsigny, M.; Midoux, P. *Exp Cell Res.* **1996**, *225*, 186-94.
3. Wolfert, M.A.; Seymour, L.W. *Gene Ther.* **1998**, *5*, 409-14.
4. Wagner, E. *J. Control. Release* **1998**, *53*, 155-8.
5. *The Pharmacological Basis of Therapeutics, 10th edition* Hardman, J.G.; Limbird, L.E.; Gilman, A.G., Eds.; McGraw-Hill: Columbus, OH, 2001; pp 1077-1080.
6. Hamilton, E.B.; Scott, J.T. *Arthritis Rheum.* **1962**, *5*, 502-512.
7. Clark, P.; Casas, E.; Tugwell, P.; Medina, C.; Gheno, C.; Tenorio, G.; Orozco, J.A. *Ann. Intern. Med.* **1993**, *119*, 1067-71.
8. HERA Study Group, *Am. J. Med.* **1995**, *98*, 156-68.
9. Harada, A.; Kataoka, K. *Macromolecules* **1995**, *28*, 5294-5299.
10. Itaka, K.; Harada, A.; Nakamura, K.; Kawaguchi, H.; Kataoka, K. *Biomacromol.* **2002**, *3*, 841-5.
11. Itaka, K.; Yamauchi, K.; Harada, A.; Nakamura, K.; Kawaguchi, H.; Kataoka, K., *Unpublished*.
12. Tett, S.E.; Cutler, D.J.; Beck, C.; Day, R.O. *J. Rheumatol.* **2000**, *27*, 1656-60.

Chapter 12

Ultrasound Interactions with Polymeric Micelles and Viable Cells

Natalya Rapoport

Department of Bioengineering, University of Utah, Salt Lake City, UT 84112 (email: rapoportnatalia@netscape.net)

A new modality of drug targeting to tumors is based on drug encapsulation in polymeric micelles followed by a localized release at the tumor site, triggered by focused ultrasound. Ultrasound-induced drug release from micelles proceeds without power density threshold, indicating that this process does not require transient cavitation. In contrast, cell sonolysis proceeds only above the cavitation threshold. This difference provides a window of power densities, inside which effective drug release from micelles is not accompanied by significant mechanical damage of the cells. Hence, this window could be used in clinical applications of the technique.

Introduction

Polymeric micelles as drug delivery vehicles provide a number of advantages. Drug encapsulation in micelles decreases systemic concentration of a drug, diminishes intracellular drug uptake by normal cells, and provides for a passive drug targeting to tumors, thus reducing unwanted drug inter-actions with healthy tissues. *(1-17)* In addition, polymeric micelles sensitize multidrug resistant (MDR) cells to the action of drugs. *(9-14)*

Amphiphilic block copolymers self-assemble above a critical micellization concentration (CMC) into spherical micelles, whose size in the tens of nanometer range prevents renal clearance and extravasation through the normal blood vessels in healthy tissue. *(18)* However, micelles of this size penetrate through the leakier blood vessels of a tumor and gradually accumulate in the tumor tissue, resulting in passive tumor targeting of the micelle-encapsulated drug.

Encapsulation of drugs into polymeric micelles substantially reduces drug uptake by both normal and cancerous cells. *(1,2,5,13,14,20)* To enhance the drug uptake by tumor cells, we apply ultrasound that i) partially releases a drug from the micelles; ii) enhances the uptake of a micelle-encapsulated drug; and iii) enhances the micelle extravasation. These factors result in a localized and effective drug delivery to solid tumors. The main advantage of ultrasound is its non-invasive nature. The transducer is placed in contact with a water-based gel or water layer on the skin, and no insertion or surgery is required. However, high-power ultrasound may cause a severe mechanical damage to tissue cells, which would exert a deleterious effect on the surrounding tissue due to a massive release of lysosomal enzymes, causing tissue inflammation. In clinical applications of therapeutic ultrasound, this situation should be avoided. On the other hand, the presence of polymeric surfactants and drugs may affect ultrasound action upon the cells.

Here we report the results of our study of the mechanisms of ultrasound-induced drug release from micelles and cell sonolysis.

Materials and Methods

Transient cavitation. To characterize the intensity of transient cavitation under sonication, hydroxyl radicals generated upon the collapse of cavitation bubbles were trapped using the nitron spin trap 5,5-dimethyl-1-pyrroline-N-oxide (DMPO). This radical-trap forms relatively stable adducts with hydroxyl radicals. *(19)* DMPO was dissolved in phosphate buffered saline (PBS, pH 7.4) at a concentration of 0.1 M. The insonation was performed in darkness. Upon termination of the insonation, an aliquot of the solution was immediately frozen and kept in liquid nitrogen until recording of the radical production. The intensity of radical production was measured by electron paramagnetic resonance (EPR) spectroscopy, using an X-band Bruker ER-200 SRC spectrometer.

Cell lines. Promyelocytic leukemia HL-60 cells grown in suspensions were used in this study. The intensity of radical production as measured by EPR spectroscopy was correlated with the degree of cell sonolysis.

Micelle-forming polymer. The amphiphilic block copolymer used in this study, Pluronic P-105, has an average molecular weight of 6500. It comprises of 56 propylene oxide (PO) units as the central block and 37 ethylene oxide (EO) units each as the two side blocks. The critical micelle concentration measured for P-105 is close to 1 % at room temperature and close to 0.1 % at 37 °C. *(18)* Pluronic P-105 was kindly supplied by BASF Corporation.

Drug. Doxorubicin (DOX) was supplied in a 1:5 mixture with lactose by the University Hospital, Salt Lake City, Utah. Pure DOX was bought from Sigma, St. Louis, MO. Stock solutions of DOX were kept frozen.

Drug encapsulation in Pluronic micelles. DOX was introduced into PBS or Pluronic solution from a stock solution in PBS to produce a desired final concentration of 5.0 to 6.7 µg/ml, followed by an approx. 15 s sonication in a sonication bath operating at 90 kHz to facilitate drug encapsulation.

Optison microbubbles. Albumin-stabilized microbubbles were bought from Mallinckrodt Inc., St. Louis, MO.

Sonication. Sonication of HL-60 cells at 20 kHz was performed either in test tubes inserted into a cup horn apparatus, or in test tubes with an inserted ultrasound probe (Sonics and Materials, Newton, CT). Sonication at 67 kHz was performed in test tubes inserted into a bath sonicator (Sonicor Instruments, Copaique, NY).

Measuring drug release from micelles. The anthraquinone part of DOX molecules is inherently fluorescent when excited at a wavelength of 488 nm, making it an effective fluorescent probe. DOX fluorescence is quenched by collisions with water molecules (dynamic quenching). However, when DOX molecules are prevented from collisions with water, for instance by their encapsulation in the hydrophobic core of micelles, their fluorescence increases two- to three-fold. *(3)* This feature was used to measure drug release from micelles under the action of ultrasound. Real-time measurements of drug release were performed using a specially designed ultrasonic exposure chamber with fluorescence detection described in details elsewhere. *(6)*

Results and Discussion

Transient Cavitation

An example of the electron paramagnetic resonance (EPR) spectrum recorded upon sonication of a DMPO-containing PBS solution is shown in Figure 1a. The four-line spectrum is that of the DMPO adduct with hydroxyl radicals. *(19)* Factors affecting the intensity of transient cavitation are briefly discussed below and were recently reported in detail. *(20)*

Effect of doxorubicin (DOX). Introduction of DOX into solutions of PBS or the culture medium RPMI-1640 substantially enhanced radical production, implying enhanced transient cavitation (Table 1). The radical production was observed at lower power densities than without DOX, suggesting a decrease of the cavitation threshold. Since DOX is an amphiphilic molecule, this effect might be caused by DOX adsorption onto the air/water interface, facilitating bubble generation by weakening the boundary layer. This enhanced radical production in the presence of DOX is an important finding. Chemotherapy using DOX combined with focusing ultrasound on the tumor will produce active hydroxyl radicals in the tumor tissue, which will enhance the cytotoxic action of the drug via a radical damage of DNA. *(21,22)*

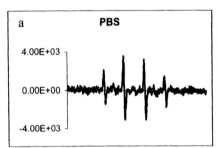
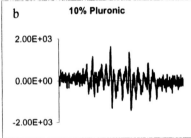

Figure 1. EPR spectra of DMPO-OH adducts formed upon sonication in PBS buffer (a) and Pluronic P-105 micellar solution (10% w/v) (b). Ultrasound frequency 20 kHz; instrument amplitude setting 2%; sample volume 1 ml. The ultrasound probe was inserted into the test tube. (Copyright 2002 Euromed Scientific Ltd.) (Reproduced with permission of the publishers of Drug Delivery Systems and Sciences **2002**, *2 (2), 37–46. Copyright 2002 Euromed Scientific Ltd..)*

Effect of Pluronic micelles. Sonication in the presence of Pluronic P-105 at concentrations above the CMC substantially decreased the radical production (Figure 1b; Table I), indicating an increase of the cavitation threshold.

Effect of DOX encapsulation into Pluronic micelles. Addition of DOX encapsulated into Pluronic micelles did not noticeably increase the radical production. We hypothesize that in the presence of Pluronic micelles, cavitation bubbles form and oscillate inside the micellar core, which creates a barrier to bubble expansion, this way increasing the cavitation threshold. Other factors may be involved in the reduced radical production, i.e. a "cage effect" (fast radical recombination in a "cage" created by a viscous medium before radicals are trapped by a trap), and hydroxyl radical scavenging by reaction with propylene oxide units of the micellar core. Based on the EPR measurements, the microviscosity within the core of Pluronic micelles was about an order of magnitude higher than the viscosity outside the micelles, which favors radical recombination. *(1)* While the relative importance of these factors remains to be explored, the substantially reduced cell sonolysis observed in the presence of Pluronic micelles (see below) suggests a significantly reduced transient cavitation.

Effect of Optison microbubbles. The concentration of dissolved gases is known to affect transient cavitation. We addressed this problem by introducing albumin-stabilized microbubbles into PBS and P-105 micellar solutions in the absence and presence of DOX (Table I). The burst of Optison microbubbles prevailed over their regeneration in all experiments performed at 20 kHz and 67 kHz at all power densities, as judged by a substantial decrease of the opacity of the sonicated samples. This observation indicates that microbubbles served as pre-formed nuclei of transient cavitations. The introduction of microbubbles into PBS and RPMI-1640 solutions resulted in a substantially increased radical production as shown for PBS in Table 1, while radical production in degassed samples was reduced (data not shown). The presence of Pluronic micelles substantially reduced but not completely eliminated the radical production induced by Optison microbubbles (Table 1).

Table 1. Hydroxyl radical production under sonication: Effect of DOX, Optison microbubbles, and Pluronic P-105 micelles. Ultrasound frequency 67 kHz; power density 2.4 W/cm^2; sonication duration 5 min; DOX concentration 50 μg/ml; concentration of Optison microbubbles (1 – 2) x10^8 bubbles/ml.

Sonicated system	Radical concentration [relative units]
PBS	0.8
PBS + DOX	1.6
PBS + DOX + OPTISON	4.0
10% P-105	Traces
10% P-105 + DOX	Traces
10% P-105 + DOX + Optison	0.5

Summarizing, transient cavitation was increased in the presence of DOX and microbubbles and decreased in the presence of Pluronic micelles.

Correlation between Transient Cavitation and Cell Lysis

The degree of cell lysis correlated well with the radical production, suggesting the important role of transient cavitation in cell sonolysis (Figure 2). The degree of cell lysis increased with increasing concentration of DOX in the incubation medium (Figure 3) and significantly dropped in the presence of Pluronic micelles (Figure 4). DOX encapsulated inside Pluronic micelles did not increase cell lysis. In contrast to Pluronic micelles, the introduction of Optison microbubbles into cell suspensions increased cell lysis (Figure 2). In all instances, the degree of cell sonolysis correlated well with the intensity of transient cavitation, implying that transient cavitation was responsible for cell lysis by mechanically damaging the cell membranes and releasing lysosomal enzymes.

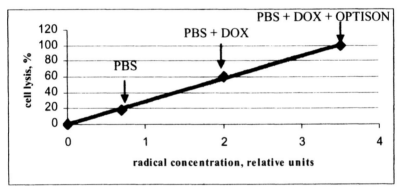

Figure 2. Correlation between radical generation under ultrasound and sonolysis of HL-60 cells. Ultrasound frequency 67 kHz; power density 4.3 W/cm[2]; duration 3 minutes. (Reproduced with permission of the publishers of Drug Delivery Systems and Sciences *2002, 2 (2), 37–46. Copyright 2002 Euromed Scientific Ltd..)*

Drug Release from Pluronic Micelles: Effect of Ultrasound

Drug release from micelles under continuous wave (CW) and pulsed ultrasound in the frequency range of 20 to 90 kHz was measured using an ultrasonic exposure chamber with real-time fluorescence detection. Examples of

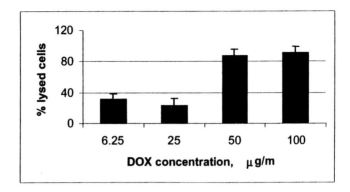

*Figure 3. Effect of DOX concentration in PBS on the sonolysis of HL-60 cells.
Ultrasound frequency 20 kHz; power density 0.06 W/cm²; duration 3 minutes.
Differences between DOX concentrations of 6.25 and 25 µg/ml are not
statistically significant, while those for DOX concentrations of 25 and 50 and 25
and 100 µg/ml are statistically significant (p << 0.05).* (Reproduced with
permission of the publishers of Drug Delivery Systems and Sciences **2002**, 2
(2), 37–46. Copyright 2002 Euromed Scientific Ltd..)

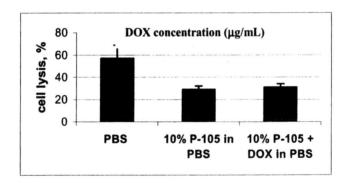

*Figure 4. Effect of Pluronic micelles on HL-60 cell sonolysis. Ultrasound
frequency 20 kHz; power density 0.09 W/cm²; duration 3 minutes; DOX
concentration 50 µg/ml (average values ± SD of at least four independent
experiments are shown).* (Reproduced with permission of the publishers of
Drug Delivery Systems and Sciences **2002**, 2 (2), 37–46. Copyright 2002
Euromed Scientific Ltd..)

drug release profiles from 10% Pluronic micelles are shown in Figure 5 for DOX at 20-kHz sonication. Both, CW and pulsed ultrasound with various duty cycles were explored. The drop in fluorescence intensity during the "ultra-sound on" phase indicated spontaneous drug release from the hydrophobic environment of micellar cores into the aqueous environment, caused either by ultrasound-induced drug diffusion out of micelles or micelle degradation under sonication. The fast increase in fluorescence intensity during the "ultrasound off" phase of pulsed ultrasound indicated fast re-encapsulation of released drug. This fast re-encapsulation suggests a very low concentration of free drug (non-extravasated and non-internalized), thus reducing unwanted interactions with normal tissues. The stationary level of drug release in CW experiments (i.e. constant fluorescence intensity in Figure 5a) results from an equilibrium bet-ween drug release and re-encapsulation. *(22)*

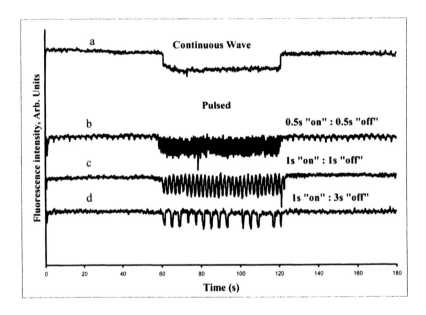

Figure 5. DOX (1.7 µg/ml) release profiles from Pluronic P-105 micelles (10%) under continuous wave and pulsed (20 kHz) ultrasound at a power density of 0.058 W/cm^2 at various duration of ultrasound pulses and inter-pulse intervals. The fluorescence intensity decreases when DOX is transferred from the hydrophobic environment of micelle cores into the aqueous bulk.
(Reproduced with permission of the publishers of Drug Delivery Systems and Sciences *2002*, 2 (2), 37–46. Copyright 2002 Euromed Scientific Ltd..)

The degree of drug release is affected by the following factors:
- Ultrasound frequency (higher release at lower frequencies);
- Power density (higher release at higher power);
- Ultrasound pulse duration (higher release at pulses longer than 0.5 s)
- Drug/micelle interaction (higher release of more hydrophilic drugs);
- micelle concentration (higher release at lower micelle concentrations);
- Drug concentration inside micelles (higher release at higher drug loading).

A higher drug release at low polymer concentrations is likely caused by a reduced re-encapsulation rate in the presence of fewer micelles, while a higher drug release at high loading results from replacing strong drug/polymer interactions within the micelle cores by weaker drug/drug interactions. *(6)*

Mechanism of Drug Release from Micelles

The degree of drug release under ultrasound was measured at DOX concentrations for which a linear dependence between fluorescence intensity and concentration was observed. *(6)* The left curve in Figure 6a illustrates the dependence of drug release from polymeric micelles on ultrasound power. The intersection of this curve at the coordinate origin ("0") when projected onto the power density axis indicates that there is no power density threshold for this release mechanism. Since transient cavitation proceeds above some power density threshold, these data suggest that a process other than transient cavitation was responsible for the drug release. In contrast, the curve showing the dependence between the degree of cell sonolysis and power density intersects the power density axis at about 0.05 W/cm^2, indicating a distinct power threshold and suggesting that transient cavitation is the underlying process (Figure 6a, right curve). This conclusion is supported by the good correlation between degree of cell sonolysis and concentration of trapped hydroxyl radicals formed upon collapse of cavitation bubbles (see Figure 2).

The different dependence of drug release and cell sonolysis on power density provides a window of power densities, inside which a noticeable drug release from micelles is not accompanied by substantial cell lysis. This window is marked by double-arrows in Figure 6. Position and width of this window depend on the ultrasound frequency, as illustrated in Figure 6b for a frequency of 67 kHz. Although both curves appear to be similar to the curves shown in Figure 6a, they are significantly shifted to higher power densities. This window between sufficient drug release from micelles and negligible cell lysis could be used in clinical applications, i.e. for the treatment of cancers.

Conclusions

Drug encapsulation in polymeric micelles combined with ultrasonic irra-diation is a promising new approach to drug targeting to tumor cells. Ultra-

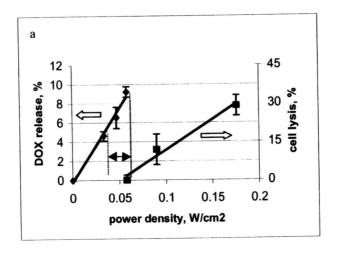

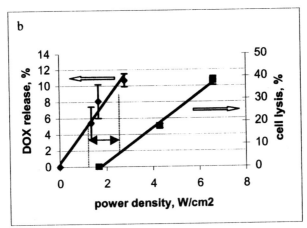

Figure 6. Dependence of drug release from 10% Pluronic P-105 micelles (left curves) and HL-60 cell sonolysis (right curves) on ultrasound power densities at frequencies of 20 kHz (a) and 67 kHz (b). DOX concentration is 10 μg/ml. The black double-arrows mark the windows between sufficient drug release and negligible cell lysis.
(Reproduced with permission of the publishers of Drug Delivery Systems and Sciences **2002**, 2 (2), 37–46. *Copyright 2002 Euromed Scientific Ltd..)*

sound not only triggers drug release from micelles but also enhances the uptake of micelle-encapsulated drugs. *(23-25)* These observations may be important factors in the observed dramatic sensitization of multidrug resistant cancerous cells to the action of conventional drugs encapsulated into Pluronic micelles. Animal tests have been initiated to verify and optimize the ultrasound technique *in vivo*.

Acknowledgment

This work was supported by the NIH grant R01 CA76562.

References

1. Rapoport, N. Stabilization and activation of Pluronic micelles for tumor-targeted drug delivery. *Colloids and Surface B: Biointerfaces* **1999**, *16*, 93-111.
2. Rapoport, N.; Munshi, N.; Pitina, L.; Pitt, W.G. Pluronic micelles as vehicles for tumor-specific delivery of two anticancer drugs to HL-60 cells using acoustic activation. *Polymer Preprints* **1997**, *38*, 620-621.
3. Rapoport, N.; Pitina, L. Intracellular distribution and intracellular dynamics of a spin-labeled analogue of doxorubicin by fluorescence and EPR spectroscopy. *J. Pharmaceutical Sci.* **1998**, *87*, 321-325.
4. Munshi, N.; Rapoport, N.; Pitt. W. G. Ultrasonic activated drug delivery from Pluronic P-105 micelles. *Cancer Letters* **1997**, *118*, 13-19.
5. Rapoport, N.Y.; Herron, J.N.; Pitt, W.G.; Pitina, L. Micellar delivery of doxorubicin and its paramagnetic analog, ruboxyl, to HL-60: effect of micelle structure and ultrasound on the intracellular drug uptake. *J. Control. Rel.* **1999**, *58*, 153-162.
6. Husseni, G.A.; Myrup, G.D.; Pitt, W.G.; Christensen, D.A.; Rapoport, N.Y. Factor affecting acoustically triggered release of drugs from polymeric micelles. *J. Control. Rel.* **2000**, *69*, 43-52.
7. Kwon, G.S.; Kataoka, K. Block copolymer micelles as long circulating drug vehicles. *Adv. Drug Deliv. Rev.* **1995**, *16*, 295-309.
8. Yu, B.G.; Okano, T.; Kataoka, K.; Kwon, G. Polymeric micelles for drug delivery: solubilization and hemolytic activity of amphotericin B. *J. Control Release* **1998**, *53*, 131-136.
9. Alakhov, V.Y.; Moskaleva, E.Y.; Batrakova, E.V.; Kabanov, A.V. Hypersensitization of multidrug resistant human ovarian carcinoma cells by Pluronic P85 block copolymer. *Bioconjugate Chem.* **1996**, *7*, 209-216.

172

10. Venne, A.; Li, S.; Mandeville, R.; Kabanov, A.V.; Alakhov. V.Y. Hypersensitizing effect of Pluronic L61 on cytotoxic activity, transport and subcellular distribution of doxorubicin in multiple drug-resistant cells. *Cancer Res.*, **1996**, *56*, 3626-3629.

11. Batrakova, E.V.; Li, S.; Miller, D.W.; Kabanov, A.V. Pluronic P85 increases permeability of a broad spectrum of drugs in polarized BBMEC and Caco-2 cell monolayers. *Pharm. Res.* **1999**, *16*, 1366-1372.

12. Batrakova, E.V.; Lee, S., Li, S.; Venne, A.; Alakhov, V.Y.; Kabanov, A.V. Fundamental relationships between the composition of pluronic block copolymers and their hypersensitization effect in MDR cancer cells. *Pharm. Res.* **1999**, *16*, 1373-1379.

13. Rapoport, N; Marin, A.; Luo, Y.; Prestwich, G.; Muniruzzaman, M. Intracellular Uptake and Trafficking of Pluronic Micelles in Drug-Sensitive and MDR Cells: Effect on the Intracellular Drug Localization. *J. Pharm. Sci.* **2002**, *91*, 157-170.

14. Rapoport, N. Controlled Drug Delivery to Drug-Sensitive and Multidrug Resistant Cells: Effects of Pluronic Micelles and Ultrasound. In *Advances in Controlled Drug Delivery*, Dinh, S., Ed.; ACS Symposium Series; American Chemical Society: Washington, DC, **2003**; *In print*.

15. Uhrich, K.E.; Cannizzaro, S.M.; Langer, R.S.; Shakesheff, K.M. Polymeric systems for controlled drug release. *Chem. Rev.* **1999**, *99*, 3181-3198.

16. Maeda, H.; Seymour, L.M.; Miyamoto, Y. Conjugates of anticancer agents and polymers: advantages of macromolecular therapeutics in vivo. *Bioconjugate Chem.* **1992**, *3*, 351-362.

17. Kataoka, K.; Matsumoto, T.; Yokoyama, M.; Okano, T.; Sakurai, Y.; Fukushima, S.; Okamoto, K.; Kwon, G.S. Doxorubicin-loaded poly(ethylene glycol)-poly(b-benzyl-L-aspartate) copolymer micelles: their pharmaceutical characteristics and biological significance. *J. Control. Rel.* **2000**, *64*, 143-153.

18. Alexandridis, P.; Holzwarth, J.F.; Hatton, T.A. Micellization of poly(ethylene oxide)-poly(propylene oxide)-poly(ethylene oxide) triblock copolymers in aqueous solutions: Thermodynamics of copolymer association. *Macromolecules* **1994**, *27*, 2414-2425.

19. Christman, C.L.; Carmichael, A.J.; Mossaba, M.M.; and Riesz, P. Evidence for free radical produced in aqueous solutions by diagnostic ultrasound. *Ultrasonics* **1987**, *25*, 31-34.

20. Rapoport, N.; Marin, A.; and Christensen, D.A. Ultrasound-Activated Micellar Drug Delivery. *Drug Delivery Systems and Sciences* **2002**, *2*, 37-46.

21. Roots R.; Okada S. Protection of DNA molecules in cultured mammalian cells from radiation-induced single-strand scissions by various alcohols and SH compounds. *Int. J. Radiol. Biol.* **1972**, *21*, 329-342.

22. Roots R.; Okada S. Estimation of life-times and diffusion distances of radicals involved in X-ray induced DNA strand breaks or killing of mammalian cells. *Radiat. Res.* **1995**, *64*, 306-320.

23. Husseini, G.A., Rapoport, N.Y., Christensen, D.A., Pruitt, J.D., Pitt, W.G. Kinetics of ultrasonic release of Doxorubicin from Pluronic P-105 micelles. *Colloids and Surfaces B: Biointerfaces* **2002**, *24*, 253-264.

24. Marin, A., Muniruzzaman, M., Rapoport, N. Acoustic activation of drug delivery from polymeric micelles: effect of pulsed ultrasound. *J. Control. Rel.* **2001**, *71*, 239-249.

25. Marin, A., Muniruzzaman, M., Rapoport, N. Mechanism of the ultrasonic activation of micellar drug delivery. *J. Control. Rel.* **2001**, *75*, 69-81.

Micro- and Nanoparticulate Carriers

Chapter 13

Lipids: An Alternative Material for Protein and Peptide Release

A. Maschke[1], A. Lucke[1,2], W. Vogelhuber[1], C. Fischbach[1], B. Appel[1], T. Blunk[1], and A. Göpferich[1,*]

[1]Department of Pharmaceutical Technology, University of Regensburg, 93040 Regensburg, Germany
[2]Aventis Pharma Deutschland GmbH, Frankfurt am Main, Germany
*Corresponding author: email: achim.goepferich@chemie.uni-regensburg.de

Many drug delivery technologies for parenteral protein and peptide delivery rely on biodegradable polymers. However, protein stability during release from these systems can be critical due to chemical and physical instabilities. Lipids such as triglycerides represent an interesting alternative material. It is the goal of this chapter to substantiate this hypothesis. After a brief overview on the polymer/protein interactions, a brief introduction into the use of lipids for protein and peptide release is given. Examples are given that demonstrate the ability of triglyceride matrices and microparticles to release peptides and proteins over a span of longer than two months. For insulin it is shown that stability and biological activity are preserved during release from triglyceride matrices.

Introduction

Due to the progress in biotechnology numerous therapeutically interesting proteins and peptides have been identified in recent years. A good example are growth factors that allow control of cell behavior and are a useful tool in tissue engineering applications. Unfortunately, proteins are usually not suitable candidates for oral administration, the route of application with a maximum of patient compliance. One reason is their rapid enzymatic degradation in the gastrointestinal tract. Despite extensive research efforts devoted to the development of oral protein and peptide delivery systems, this application route is currently limited to substances which possess special properties such as enhanced stability and sufficient bioavailability. *(1)* As a result, the majority of proteins and peptides are usually applied parenterally. Due to their short biological half-life, even after parenteral application, repeated injections or administration via infusions are necessary to obtain a therapeutical effect. As the compliance is usually low for both types of administration, numerous controlled release systems for parenteral protein and peptide release have been developed to reduce the application frequency. Another advantage of these systems is that they allow for site specific local protein delivery, which is in many cases necessary to avoid adverse effects when proteins are applied that elicit side effects after distribution throughout the body via the systemic circulation.

A classical technology that allows the delivery of these fragile compounds parenterally involves the use of degradable polymers. These materials have the advantage that they protect proteins from inactivation, circumvent post-application removal and concomitantly allow for controlled release. Most of today's parenteral drug delivery systems for protein and peptide drugs rely on this successful and well established principle. However, degradable polymers are sophisticated materials that bear some intrinsic problems. Among them is the difficulty of controlling drug release, which may be a complex mixture of swelling, erosion and diffusion phenomena that make it hard to obtain full control over the release process. *(2)* Furthermore, the degradation and erosion of the polymer constantly changes the physico-chemical environment inside a polymer matrix, which may expose protein and peptide drugs to detrimental effects. Controlled release systems already on the market are made of hydrophobic biodegradable polymers such as poly(α-hydroxyesters) with an excellent safety and biocompatibility record. However, these polymers are known to provide a micro-environment that may have detrimental effects on the stability of incorporated peptides or proteins especially during polymer erosion. *(3)* This observation illustrates that despite the success of degradable polymers, alternative delivery concepts would increase the availability of protein and peptide drugs for therapeutic applications.

Well established alternatives to lipophilic biodegradable polymers include hydrogels for sustained release. Some of these materials are excellent for the release of proteins and peptides over short periods of time, such as a few days. Many of these systems are, however, less suited for long term drug delivery unless chemically modified by methods such as cross-linking. In addition, the release mechanism can again be a complex mixture of swelling diffusion and degradation processes. In contrast to hydrogels, the potential of lipids for sustained release of insoluble substances or proteins has been explored extensively only for special cases. Among them are liposomes and solid lipid nanoparticles (SLN). *(4,5)* Although these systems are excellent drug carriers, their manufacture frequently requires factors known for their negative impact on protein and peptide stability, such as the use of organic solvent/water mixtures or shear forces. In contrast to these well investigated systems, pure lipid matrices in the form of monolithic matrices or microparticles have hardly been explored. The great advantage of such systems is that they obviate the need for many detrimental techniques and adjuvants. *(6)* Thus the use of organic solvents, for example, can be avoided altogether.

It is the goal of this review to illustrate the potential of triglyceride matrices to serve as a carrier for the controlled parenteral release of protein and peptide drugs. For a better comparison of the potential of triglycerides with that of biodegradable polymers to serve as drug delivery systems, the next section will focus on stability problems with proteins and peptides in biodegradable polymers. Thereafter, a short overview on lipid-based delivery systems will be given, as well as a report on the first results of the biocompatibility studies on selected triglycerides. Finally, the potential of triglyceride matrices for protein and peptide release will be presented. At the end of the paper we will illustrate that triglyceride matrices are suitable carriers for the release of proteins and peptides in cell culture.

Results and Discussion

Biodegradable Polymers for Controlled Drug Delivery

The most widely used class of biodegradable polymer for parenteral release of proteins and peptides are poly(α-hydroxy esters) such as poly(lactic acid) (PLA) and poly(lactic-*co*-glycolic acid) (PLGA). Their popularity stems not only from their ability to provide a depot that allows to deliver drugs for weeks, but also from their well characterized and widely accepted biocompatibility. *(7)* Furthermore, their properties have been reviewed in numerous publications, which provides a vast information source. *(8-10)* Among the remarkable properties it should be noted that the release profile of delivery devices made of PLA and PLGA can be controlled by the molecular weight and the copolymer composition. For example, PLA made of high contents of one stereoisomer (either D- or L lactic acid) tend to be more resistant to degradation compared to PLA made of racemic lactic acid. Higher concentrations of glycolic acid in PLGA lead to an increase of the degradation rate. *(11)* Therefore, a broad time window of degradation can be covered depending on the polymer composition. One can summarize that PLA and PLGA are widely used in drug delivery for their well characterized release behavior, biocompatibility and biodegradation. *(7)* The outstanding argument, however, is the fact that these polymers have been approved by the health authorities for numerous medical and drug delivery devices, which accelerates the development of new systems based on these materials tremendously.

Despite their numerous advantages, PLA and PLGA are sophisticated materials due to their complex degradation behavior. *(12)* While biodegradable polymers ideally loose mass continuously from their surface (surface erosion), poly(α-hydroxy esters) erode all over their cross section (bulk erosion). *(13)* Despite the hydrolytic degradation of the polymer backbone in an aqueous environment, PLA and PLGA matrices do not erode unless a critical degree of degradation is reached. This leads automatically to the accumulation of degra- dation products, i.e., lactic- and glycolic acid oligomers and monomers, inside the matrices. It is obvious that this can give rise to a number of adverse effects on sensitive drugs such as proteins and peptides, which will be discussed in the next section.

Stability of Proteins and Peptides inside PLA and PLGA

The stability of proteins and peptides inside biodegradable polymers depends on the manufacturing process as well as the conditions that prevail during polymer erosion and drug release. *(14)* The manufacturing protocol threatens the stability of proteins and peptides irrespective of the nature of the polymer. Common manufacturing techniques for implants include melt molding and extrusion. Microspheres are prepared using emulsion techniques such as solvent evaporation, spray drying, or supercritical fluid techniques. Certain preparation steps may have a negative impact on protein stability in any polymer, such as the use of organic solvents in emulsions, high temperature, ultrasound, high pressure, shear forces, or drying conditions. *(15)* Therefore, the critical manufacturing steps have to be reviewed with respect to protein stability. This may require specific measures for any drug/polymer combination. During protein release, the degradation and erosion mechanism may have a specific impact on protein and peptide stability that depends strongly on the polymer type and composition. Changes in protein structure frequently lead to aggregation and result in a loss of bioactivity. Protein adsorption can cause unfolding of tertiary structures and thus lead again to activity losses. *(6)* Apart from a complete inactivation, a change of protein structure by chemical instabilities may be of concern with respect to receptor specificity, receptor affinity, as well as immunogenecity. *(3)*

During PLA and PLGA erosion, a microclimate develops inside the swollen polymer matrix with pH values as low as 1.5 that stems from lactic or glycolic acid monomers and oligomers created during polymer degradation. *(16)* Concomitantly, non-physiological values of increased osmotic pressure have been reported. *(17)* It is obvious that these extreme conditions may have an impact on the stability of proteins and peptides in general. More recently it was reported that the pH inside polymer matrices in combination with degradation products can also lead to chemical changes in peptide structure. *(3)* These results were obtained when salmon calcitonin (sCT) and human atrial natriuretic peptide (ANP) were encapsulated in PLGA and PLA microspheres and subjected to erosion in phosphate buffer pH 7.4. The peptides were extracted from the microparticles at regular time intervals and subjected to a combined analysis of HPLC and mass spectrometry (HPLC-MS). Figure 1a shows a chromatogram that was obtained for ANP extracted from the particles prior to erosion. ANP gave rise to a single signal at a retention time of 9.11 minutes. When mass spectra were recorded from the eluted fraction at that retention time, they displayed three signals for ANP at m/z 789.1 $[(ANP+4H)^{4+}]$, 1051.8 $[(ANP+3H)^{3+}]$, and 1577.3 $[(ANP+2H)^{2+}]$, depending on the number of protons and the number of charges on the molecule (Figure 1b). After 21 days of incubation the chromatograms and mass spectra of extracted peptides changed significantly. The chromatograms contained an additional peak at 9.53 minutes (Figure 1c), the corresponding signals of which in the mass spectra shifted to higher values (Figure 1d). This observation indicated that the peptide's molecular mass had increased during incubation. The mass differences pointed towards the covalent attachment of lactate to the peptide structure. *(3)* The reaction sites in hANP and sCT were determined by enzymatic dissection of the peptide chain and subsequent HPLC-MS analysis. These studies revealed that hydroxy and primary amine groups are the main target of the reaction. *(3)* To determine the extent of acylation, the amount of acylated ANP (ANP-LA) and acylated sCT (sCT-LA) inside PLA and inside PLGA micropsheres was measured over a 28-day period (Figure 2). While the amount of acylated peptides increased continuously, the content of unaltered peptide decreased in an inverse manner. Finally 60% of the ANP and 7% of the sCT residing inside PLA microspheres were acylated, while only slightly lower values were obtained for PLGA. These findings correlate well with experiments indicating that the velocity of the chemical reaction depends on pH as well as on the lactic acid content. *(3)*

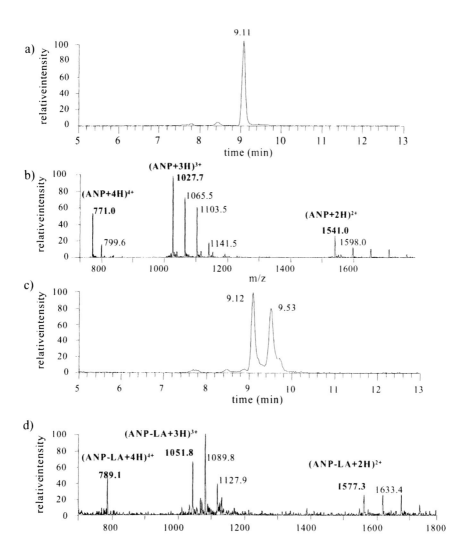

Figure 1. (a) HPLC-MS total ion chromatogram and (b) electrospray mass spectrum (retention time 9.1 min.) of native ANP extracted from PLA microspheres after manufacturing; (c) HPLC-MS total ion chromatogram and (d) electrospray mass spectrum (retention time of 9.5 min.) of acylated ANP from PLA microspheres after 21 days of degradation. (Reproduced with permission from Reference (3). Copyright 2002).

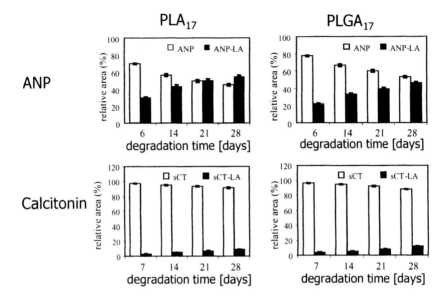

Figure 2. ANP and sCT stability in PLA (Mw 17,000) and PLGA (Mw 17,000) microspheres. (Reproduced with permission from Reference (3). Copyright 2002).

Those results make it obvious that precautions have to be taken to provide an environment inside PLA and PLGA microspheres that prevents chemical reactions between incorporated proteins and peptides and polymer degradation products. There are some possibilities to protect the peptide against acylation such as the introduction of hydrophilic porogens, i.e., PEG, to achieve fast release of degradation products from the matrices or increasing the pH inside the microspheres by adding basic substances. *(3,18,19)* Both approaches, however, must be further investigated since the reaction may be driven not only by degradation products but also by an acylation of peptides and proteins at the polymer/water interface.

Despite their intrinsic problems, biodegradable polymers have a long history of use, excellent biocompatibility and world-wide approval by numerous drug authorities. However, in cases where they fail for the reasons outlined above, it would be highly desirable to have alternative materials available that allow for the safe release of protein and peptide drugs. Among the numerous carriers that offer tremendous possibilities for protein and peptide release, hydrogels represent a potent class of materials for the manufacture of controlled release systems. A plethora of natural or synthetic materials such as cellulose derivatives, hyaluronic acid derivatives, alginate, collagen, gelatin, starch, dextran, and fibrin have been proposed as matrix materials to mention only a few. *(20)* Many proteins have been incorporated and monitored for their *in vitro* release from such systems. *(21)* Despite their definite advantages, especially with respect to maintaining the stability of protein and peptide drugs, the release from hydrogels can be substantially faster than from degradable polymers such as PLA and PLGA and is usually a matter of hours or a few days. Polyionic complexation or cross-linking of the polymer can immobilize the protein and thus reduce protein release rates but may also have an impact on protein stability. *(22)* The application of hydrogels *in vivo* can change their release behavior compared to *in vitro* significantly due to the active role of enzymes in degradation and erosion depending on the chemical structure of the hydrogel. Therefore, alternative technologies are desirable that obviate the need for cross-linking to release protein and peptide drugs over extended periods of time. One way to achieve this goal is by reducing the effective surface area of a hydrogel available for drug release. This can be achieved by embedding the protein or peptide into a matrix material in which it is insoluble and can only be released via a network of pores. Lipids such as triglycerides are such a class of material. In the next section we will, therefore, briefly review drug delivery systems based on lipids to illustrate their potential for controlled protein and peptide release.

Drug Delivery Systems based on Lipids

There are numerous examples for lipid derived drug delivery systems such as emulsions or liposomes. Other concepts that have been proposed are multi-vesicular liposome preparations, cubic phase gels, hollow porous microparticles, and hollow lipid microcylinders. *(23-26)* Lipid microcylinders are 0.5 µm diameter hollow open-ended tubes that consist of one or two lipid bilayers. The release of encapsulated substances such as tetracycline, 2-methoxynaphtalene, and TGF-beta has been reported to proceed primarily via diffusion out of the open ends. *(27-29)* Microcylinders loaded with albumin released approximately 50% of the protein within eight days. Cubic phase gels are another interesting drug delivery system. A considerable number of proteins and peptides such as somatostatin, vasopressin, lysozym, desmopressin, and insulin have already been incorporated into these systems. Release from cubic phase gels can be maintained over 3-4 days *in vitro* and 6-9 hours *in vivo*, respectively.

Despite their advantages, the systems outlined above have no matrix-type character. Therefore, their principle of release is different from that of a solid matrix that relies on aqueous release pathways. This usually leads to an *in vitro* release that is complete within days. The first approach that relied on the release of proteins via the pores of an impermeable matrix other than that of a degradable polymer was made by preparing pellets for retarding drug release after oral administration. *(30)* For parenteral drug administration lipid microparticles have been proposed. *(31)* Composed of substances such as tri-glycerides, monoglycerides, and emulsifiers, they can be prepared using solvent evaporation, melt dispersion, or spray drying techniques. *(32)* Lipophilic as well as hydrophilic substances have been incorporated in these systems such as cytostatics, vaccines, and non-steroidal antiinflammatoric substances. *(33-36)* For intravenous application, solid lipid nanoparticles (SLN) have been developed. *(5)* SLN can be produced using spraying techniques or high pressure homogenization of lipid emulsions. *(37,38)* They are composed of solid lipids and, depending on the manufacturing procedure, emulsifiers that are needed for the emulsification process. Lipophilic as well as hydrophilic drugs have been incorporated. *(39)* Due to their small size in combination with the crystallization behavior of the lipid matrix, the incorporation of drugs and the improvement of drug release control is still under investigation. *(40)*

All delivery systems mentioned above have some disadvantages regarding drug incorporation and stability. In some cases organic solvents have to be used, which may pose a problem when they have a toxic potential. In the case of SLN the loading capacity for proteins can be considered a problem. Surfactants needed for emulsification can be a threat to protein and peptide stability. Furthermore, the duration of drug release is limited. To overcome the afore-mentioned problems and to achieve a long lasting sustained release, we became interested in lipid matrices made of pure triglycerides. Our goal was to gain control over drug release via a small effective release area. In the first step towards the development of such release systems, we were interested in the compatibility of the material with biological systems.

Compatibility of Triglycerides with Mammalian Cells

To determine any toxic or apoptotic effects of triglycerides, we investigated their compatibility in a cell culture system. It is generally well accepted that material characteristics such as chemical composition, hydrophobicity, and topography of materials strongly influence cell properties during cultivation. *(41)* Accordingly, the extent of cell adhesion, their subsequent proliferation capacity, and terminal differentiation have been reported to be affected by the material surface on which they are cultured. We, therefore, investigated if there were any major differences in the cell/material interactions between poly(α-hydroxyesters) and triglycerides. To assess their compatibility with cells, glyceryl tripalmitate and PLGA films were prepared by spin casting and seeded with 3T3-L1 pre-adipocytes. The cells were proliferated, differentiated to adipocytes and, after nine days, the phenotype of cells was investigated by red oil O-staining of intracellular lipid droplets. Concomitantly, the activity of glycerol-3-phosphate dehydrogenase (GPDH) was assessed as a key enzyme involved in triacylglycerol biosynthesis. Conventional tissue culture polystyrene (TCPS) served as a control.

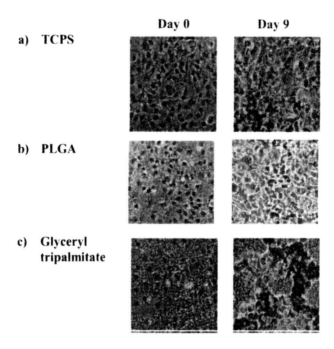

Figure 3. 3T3-L1 cells on a) TCPS, b) PLGA, and c) glyceryl tripalmitate. Day 0 immediately after cell seeding, day 9 after differentiation to adipocytes and red oil O-staining of intracellular lipid droplets. (See page 6 of color insert.)

Figure 3 shows that cells adhered well to all three materials throughout the experiment. The time course of lipid accumulation on glyceryl tripalmitate films was neither distinguishable from PLGA films nor from TCPS. Furthermore, the lipid droplet size as well as the staining intensity could be shown to be comparable on surfaces of all investigated materials. The increase of specific GDPH activity of 3T3-L1 cells on glyceryl tripalmitate, PLGA, and TCPS surfaces with time was essentially the same. No significant differences in cellular enzyme activity could be detected between the applied materials (Figure 4). These results indicate that triglycerides like glyceryl tripalmitate seem to be suited for 3T3-L1 cultivation in the same manner as PLGA and conventional cell culture materials. The surface properties of the material did not negatively influence adhesion, proliferation, and subsequent differentiation of the cells, which led us to the conclusion that triglycerides are biocompatible in this test system. These results are in good agreement with early data obtained from

186

biocompatibility tests with triglycerides after subcutaneous application in mice indicating that the material is well tolerated. *(42)*

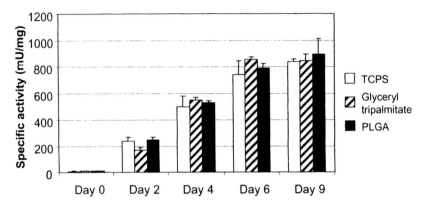

Figure 4. Specific GPDH activity of 3T3-L1 cells differentiated on glyceryl tripalmitate, TCPS, and PLGA surfaces.

Controlled Drug Release from Triglyceride Matrix Cylinders

After we had shown their compatibility with a biological system, we explored the potential of triglyceride matrices for drug release. Therefore, we manufactured small cylindrical monolithic matrices (2mm diameter, 2 mm height) by compression. *(43)* Matrices made of glyceryl trilaurinate, glyceryl trimiyristate, glyceryl tripalmitate, or glyceryl tristearate were loaded with pyranine, the release of which was monitored over a period of 120 days. *(43)* As triglycerides can crystallize in three different modifications (α-, β'- or the most stable β-modification), which may be associated with different drug release properties, differential scanning calorimetry (DSC) thermograms of the matrices were recorded prior to the investigation of release. The data suggested that the lipid modification was not changed during the manufacturing process. *(43)*

Figure 5 shows the release behavior over a time period of 120 days. During the first 24 hours a moderate burst release of approximately 15-20% dye could be observed, followed by a concave release profile indicative of diffusion-controlled release. An increase of the fatty acid chain length led to slower release of the incorporated compound in the homologous series. With all investigated triglycerides, pyranine can be released for several weeks. Glyceryl tristearate matrices can release pyranine for even more than 120 days. These results demonstrate the potential of triglyceride matrices to release substances in a controlled way over extended periods of time. As pyranine is essentially insoluble in the matrix one can assume that it is released via a network of pores from the matrices.

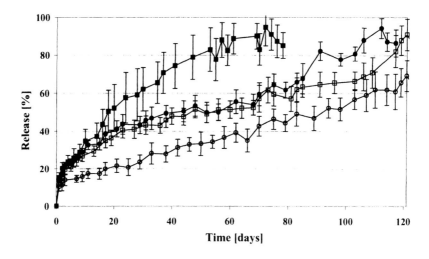

Figure 5. In vitro release of pyranine from different triglyceride matrices: (■) glyceryl trilaurinate, (●) glyceryl trimyristate, (□) glyceryl tripalmitate, and (○) glyceryl tristearate. (Reproduced with permission from Reference (43). Copyright 2002 Elsevier).

For some applications, the release kinetics may be too slow. It would, therefore, be desirable to identify strategies that allow to accelerate the release from these matrices. One technique involves the introduction of hydrophilic porogens such as gelatin that form or increase the diameter of pores inside the lipid matrix during erosion, increasing the diffusional flux of drug out of the matrix. The validity of this concept was proven by loading lipid matrices with a freeze dried gelatin gel. *(42)* When matrices were charged with gelatin contents increasing from 1 to 20%, the release of pyranine accelerated significantly (Figure 6).

Although the release of pyranine as hydrophilic model substance gave useful insight into the release behavior of monolithic triglyceride matrices, it is a low molecular weight compound, the release of which may differ significantly from that of a protein or a peptide. We, therefore, tested the potential of glyceryl tripalmitate to control the release of insulin as a model protein. *(44)* 1% (w/w) insulin was incorporated as a solid by mixing triglyceride powder in a mortar prior to compression. The investigation of lipid matrices by light microscopy revealed that they had a well defined geometry and a smooth surface (Figure 7).

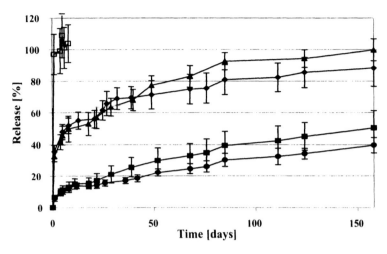

Figure 6. Drug release of pyranine from glyceryl trimyristate matrices as a function of gelatin content; (●) 0%, (■) 1%, (▲)5%, (◆) 10%, and (□) 20% (w/w) gelatin. (Reprinted from Reference (42). Courtesy of Marcel Dekker, Inc.).

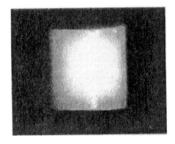

Figure 7. Light microscope picture of a glyceryl tripalmitate matrix (size 2x2 mm; weight 7mg).

DSC thermograms recorded of the matrices contained again only one endothermic transition that stemmed from the stable ß-modification, demonstrating that no modification changes occurred during the manufacturing process (Figure 8). During the *in vitro* release, protein residing inside the matrices was extracted from samples and analyzed by HPLC. After an insignificantly small burst release within the first 96 hours, an almost linear release profile was obtained. After 56 days 42.6% of insulin had been released (Figure 9).

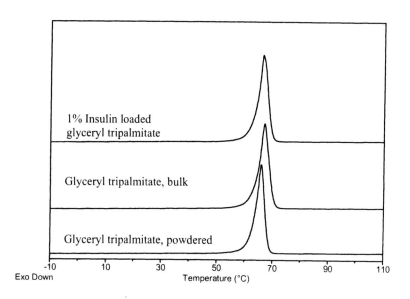

Figure 8. DSC-Thermograms of bulk lipid, pure lipid matrix, and peptide loaded lipid matrices. Only one single endothermic peak of the β-modification could be detected in each case.

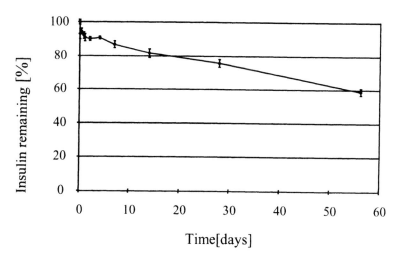

Figure 9. Insulin release from a glyceryl tripalmitate matrix (Dynasan 116; 1% Insulin) over a period of 56 days.

Scanning electron micrographs (SEM) of the lipid matrices revealed that its structure was preserved during two months of incubation in the release medium (Figure 10). While at lower magnification the surface had a smooth appearance, pores became visible at higher magnification. When the insulin residing inside the matrices was investigated for chemical changes using HPLC-MS or for the formation of dimers using size exclusion chromatography, no changes were observed (data not shown). These encouraging results suggest that triglycerides have a tremendous potential as a material for the control of protein and peptide release. Concomitantly, these lipids seem to preserve the chemical integrity of insulin during release, which is of utmost significance for controlled release applications in which proteins and peptides are involved.

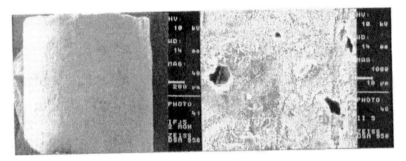

Figure 10. Scanning electron micrographs of insulin-loaded glyceryl tripalmitate matrices after incubation in PBS buffer for 56 days (left), and surface of a matrix incubated for 28 days (right).

Drug Release from Lipid Microparticles

Disadvantages of macroscopic lipid matrices are their limited suitability for parenteral application via injection and their potential to provoke adverse reactions by the body. To overcome these potential problems and to offer the possibility for a simple and economical fabrication process, triglyceride microparticles for the controlled release of peptides and proteins have been developed. Lipid microparticles can be prepared by different methods, such as solvent evaporation, melt dispersion, spray drying, or spray congealing. *(45-48)* Manufacturing by melt dispersion techniques obviates the need for organic solvents and is, therefore, particularly attractive.

To examine protein and peptide release from triglyceride microparticles, systems loaded with insulin, thymocartin or somatostatin were prepared using solvent evaporation or melt dispersion techniques. *(49,50,51)* The drug was incorporated as a solid or solution by vigorous vortex-mixing or ultrasonication. The microparticles were characterized with regard to particle size, lipid modify-cation, morphology, and drug loading. *In vitro* release was monitored over 14 days (PBS-buffer pH 7,4, 22°C, shaking water bath). While particles prepared by solvent evaporation crystallized exclusively in the stable β-modification, particles prepared by other methods also contained lipid in the α-modification. Data obtained for insulin-loaded glyceryl tripalmitate microparticles reveal the potential of this technology as well as some of the challenges that have to be met in order to take full advantage of it. *(52)* Due to the instability of insulin in solution under these conditions, the release data are shown as the residual protein content inside the microparticles over time. Microparticles loaded with insulin by melt dispersion showed a rapid burst release within the first day of incubation (Figure 11). Micrographs of these particles reveal the presence of insulin crystals on the surface, which were probably created by expulsion of the protein during lipid crystallization. Removal of surface bound drug by washing with water or 0.1 M hydrochloric acid suppressed the burst release significantly (Figure 11) and insulin was released continuously over 2 weeks.

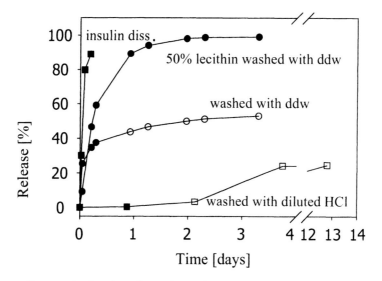

Figure 11. Insulin release from glyceryl tripalmitate microparticles.

To asses the impact of molecular weight on an incorporated protein or peptide, the release of somatostatin from triglyceride microparticles was investigated as well. Somatostatin microparticles were prepared by solvent evaporation and melt dispersion with 2%, 4,5% and 9.3% (w/w) loading. The microparticles showed no burst release and approximately 80% of the peptide was released within 13 days. *(50)* The release of somatostatin was faster than that of insulin, indicating that incorporation of smaller molecules may lead to enhanced release.

However, this interpretation has to be taken with some caution as besides the molecular weight physical properties of the incorporated protein/peptide such as hydrophobicity, and secondary and tertiary structures affect the release kinetics as well. The above results well illustrate the potential of triglyceride microspheres to control the release of proteins and peptides. However, despite their advantage for parenteral application, the reduced dimensions of microparticles compared to a monolithic matrix can lead to a partial loss of control over protein release caused by burst phenomena.

Drug Release from Lipid Matrices in Cell Culture

Although the chemical integrity of proteins after encapsulation in lipid matrices and lipid microparticles was confirmed by HPLC-MS analysis (44), changes in bioactivity may occur, which are not detectable by this method as they can be related to changes of secondary or higher structures. Thus, it is of fundamental importance to prove that a protein incorporated into a matrix retains its bioactivity during manufacturing process and release. Concomitantly, we were interested to study if triglycerides could be used for the release of proteins in cell and tissue cultures. Therefore, insulin-loaded sterile lipid matrices were prepared and tested in an insulin-sensitive three-dimensional bovine chondrocyte cell culture model. The system has been recently proposed as an adequate method for investigating sustained release of insulin. (53) The manufacturing of sterile matrices was accomplished by sterilization of glyceryl tripalmitate at 160°C for 2 hours. The molten lipid was then tempered to allow for a crystallization in the stable β'-modification. Insulin was sterilized by filtration of its aqueous solution through a 0.22μm pore-size membrane filter and lyophilization under aseptic conditions. The triglyceride was powdered, mixed with the lyophilized protein in a mortar, and compressed to matrices under aseptic conditions. Bovine articular chondrocytes were seeded onto biodegradable polyglycolic acid scaffolds and cell-polymer constructs were cultured for two weeks in tissue culture plates on an orbital shaker. Lipid matrices containing 2.08% (w/w) insulin were incubated together with the cell culture constructs for two weeks. Cell-loaded scaffolds cultured either under supplementation with insulin every 2-3 days or insulin free served as controls. The effect of released insulin on the quality of tissue-engineered cartilage was assessed by histology and biochemical analysis of extracellular matrix components such as glucosaminoglycanes (GAG) and collagen. Histological cross-sections showed a more mature cartilagenous tissue as well as a higher content and more even distribution of GAG in all cell-polymer constructs supplemented with insulin loaded triglyceride matrices as compared to constructs receiving no insulin (Figure 12). Furthermore, released insulin had effects on cartilage structure, appearance, and composition comparable to cartilage supplemented exogenously with insulin

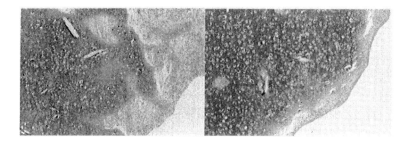

Figure 12. Effect of insulin lipid matrices on tissue-engineered cartilage. Higher content and a more even distribution of glucosaminoglycanes (GAG) was detected in cell-polymer constructs, cultivated in the presence of insulin lipid matrices (right), as compared with control constructs receiving no insulin (left). GAG was stained red with safranin O, causing the dark grey areas in this black and white print.

(data not shown). These findings support the conclusion that insulin released from these lipid matrices retained its bioactivity during fabrication and release.

Conclusions

The release of proteins and peptides from biodegradable polymers can be accompanied by substantial stability problems. During the erosion of PLA and PLGA, for example, the acidic microclimate combined with an accumulation of degradation products can lead to protein and peptide acylation. Although these polymers are well tolerated and approved for many applications by health authorities, it is desirable to have alternative materials for parentral protein and peptide release. The ability of triglycerides to release a variety of different peptides and proteins has been demonstrated for somatostatin, insulin, and thymocartin. Triglyceride matrices are able to release encapsulated proteins for 2-3 months. The release rate can be controlled by the fatty acid chain length and can be increased by incorporation of hydrophilic porogens such as gelatin. The application of insulin loaded triglyceride matrices in a 3-D cartilage cell culture model has proven that the integrity and bioactivity of insulin was preserved during manufacturing and release. The compatibility with cells *in vitro* and *in vivo* indicate that triglycerides are well tolerated and, therefore, a promising material for the manufacture of protein and peptide drug delivery systems.

Acknowledgements

Part of this work was sponsored by the 'German Ministry of Commerce (BMWi)' through the 'Forschungsvereinung der Arzneimittelhersteller'(FAH) Grant No. 12711 N. Thanks are due to Aventis for providing us with insulin.

References

1. Humberstone, A. J.; Charman, W. N. *Adv. Drug Delivery Rev.* **1997**, *25*, 103-128.
2. Göpferich, A. *Europ. J. Pharm. Biopharm.* **1996**, *42*, 1-11.
3. Lucke, A.; Kiermaier, J.; Göpferich, A. *Pharm. Res.* **2002**, *19*, 175-181.
4. Crommelin, D. J. A.; Daemen, T.; Scherphof, G. L.; Vingerhoeds, M. H.; Heeremans, J. L. M.; Kluft, C.; Storm, G. *J. Controlled Release* **1997**, *46*, 165-175.
5. Müller, R. H.; Mäder, K.; Gohla, S. *Europ. J. Pharm. Biopharm.* **2000**, *50*, 161-177.
6. Lefebvre, J.; Relkin, P. In *Surface Activity of Proteins*; Magdassi, S., Ed.; Marcel Dekker: New York (NY), 1996; 181-236.
7. Anderson, J. M.; Shive, M. S. *Adv. Drug Delivery Rev* **1997**, *28*, 5-24.
8. Vert, M.; Mauduit, J.; Li, S. *Biomaterials* **1994**, *15*, 1209-1213.
9. Vert, M.; Li, S.; Garreau, H. *Macromol.Symp.* **1995**, 633-642.
10. Mauduit, J.; Vert, M. *S.T.P.Pharma Sci.* **1993**, *3*, 197-212.
11. Göpferich, A. *Biomaterials* **1996** , *17*, 103-114.
12. Göpferich, A. *Macromolecules* **1997**, *30*, 2598-2604.
13. von Burkersroda, F.; Schedl, L.; Göpferich, A. *Biomaterials* **2002**, *23*, 4221-4231.
14. Perez, C.; Castellanos, I. J.; Costantino, H. R.; Al-Azzam, W.; Griebenow, K. *J. Pharm. Pharmakol.* **2002**, *54*, 301-313.
15. van de Weert, M.; Hennink, W. E.; Jiskoot, W. *Pharm. Res.* **2000**, *17*, 1159-1167.
16. Fu, K.; Pack, D. W.; Klibanov, A. M.; Langer, R. *Pharm. Res.* **2000**, *17*, 100-106.
17. Brunner, A.; Mader, K.; Göpferich, A. *Pharm. Res.* **1999**, *16*, 847-853.
18. Jiang, W.; Schwendeman, S. P. *Pharm. Res.* **2001**, *18*, 878-885.
19. Zhu, G.; Schwendeman, S. P. *Pharm. Res.* **2000**, *17*, 351-357.
20. Lee, K. Y.; Mooney, D. J. *Chem. Rev.* **2001**, *101*, 1869-1879.
21. Gombotz, W. R.; Wee, S. *Adv. Drug Delivery Rev.* **1998**, *31*, 267-285.
22. Tabata, Y.; Ikada, Y. *Adv. Drug Delivery Rev.* **1998**, *31*, 287-301.
23. Ye, Q.; Asherman, J.; Stevenson, M.; Brownson, E.; Katre, N. V. *J.Controlled Release.* **2000**, *64*, 155-166.

24. Shah, J. C.; Sadhale, Y.; Chilukuri, D. M. *Adv.Drug Delivery Rev.* **2001**, *47*, 229-250.
25. Bot, A. I.; Tarara, T. E.; Smith, D. J.; Bot, S. R.; Woods, C. M.; Weers, J. G. *Pharm.Res.* **2000**, *17*, 275-283.
26. Meilander, N. J.; Yu, X.; Ziats, N. P.; Bellamkonda, R. V *J.Controlled Release* **2001**, *71*, 141-152.
27. Price, R.; Patchan, M. *J.Microencapsulation* **1991**, *8*, 301-306.
28. Schnur, J. M.; Price, R.; Rudolph, A. S. *J. Controlled Release* **1994**, *28*, 3-13.
29. Spargo, B. J.; Cliff, R. O.; Rollwagen, F. M.; Rudolph, A. S. *J.Microencapsulation* **1995**, *12*, 247-254.
30. Bergauer, R.; Lutz, O.; Speiser, P. *Pharm.Ind.* **1977**, *39*, 1274-1278.
31. Cortesi, R.; Esposito, E.; Luca, G.; Nastruzzi, C. *Biomaterials* **2002**, *23*, 2283-2294.
32. Domb, A. J.; Bergelson, L.; Amselem, S. In *Microencapsulation*; Benita, S., Ed.; Drugs Pharm. Sci.; Marcel Dekker: New York (NY), 1996; Vol. 73, 377-410.
33. Takenaga, M. *Adv.Drug Delivery Rev.* **1996**, *20*, 209-219.
34. Amselem, S.; Alving, C. R.; Domb, A. J. In *Microparticulate Systems for the Delivery of Proteins and Vaccines*; Cohen, S.; Bernstein, H., Eds.; Drugs Pharm. Sci.; Marcel Dekker: New York (NY), 1996; Vol. 77, 149-168.
35. Ohmukai, O. *Adv.Drug Delivery Rev.* **1996**, *20*, 203-207.
36. Kurozumi, S.; Araki, H.; Tanabe, H.; Kiyoki, M. *Adv.Drug Delivery Rev.* **1996**, *20*, 181-187.
37. Freitas, C.; Mullera, R. H. *Europ. J. Pharm. Biopharm.* **1998**, *46*, 145-151.
38. Zimmermann, E.; Scholer, N.; Katzfey, U.; Muller, R. H.; Hahn, H.; Liesenfeld, O. *Proc.Int.Symp.Controlled Release Bioact.Mater.* **1999**, 593-594.
39. Mehnert, W.; Mader, K. *Adv.Drug Delivery Rev.* **2001**, *47*, 165-196.
40. Jenning, V.; Schafer-Korting, M.; Gohla, S. *J. Controlled Release* **2000**, *66*, 115-126.
41. Fischbach, C.; Seufert, J.; Neubauer, M.; Lazariotou, M.; Göpferich, A.; Blunk, T. *Keystone symposia: Molecular Control of Adipogenesis and Obesity* **2002**, 72.
42. Vogelhuber, W.; Magni, E.; Mouro, M.; Spruss, T.; Gazzaniga, A.; Göpferich, A. *Pharm.Develop.Technol* **2003**, *8*, 77-85.
43. Vogelhuber, W.; Magni, E.; Gazzaniga, A.; Göpferich, A. *Eur.J.Pharm.Biopharm.* **2002**, in press.
44. Maschke, A.; Guse, C.; Herrmann, J.; Göpferich, A. 4th *World Congreß on Pharmaceutics and Biopharmaceutics* **2002**, 891-892
45. Bodmeier, R.; Wang, J.; Bhagwatwar, H. *J.Microencapsulation* **1992**, *9*, 89-98.

196

46. Bodmeier, R.; Wang, J.; Bhagwatwar, H. *J.Microencapsulation* **1992**, *9*, 99-107.
47. Eldem, T.; Speiser, P.; Hincal, A. *Pharm.Res.* **1991**, *8*, 47-54.
48. Yajima, T.; Umeki, N.; Itai, S. *Chem. Pharm. Bull.* **1999**, *47*, 220-225.
49. Reithmeier, H.; Göpferich, A.; Herrmann, J. *Proc.Int.Symp.Controlled Release Bioact.Mater.* **1999**, *26*, 681-682.
50. Reithmeier, H.; Herrmann, J.; Göpferich, A. *Int.J.Pharm.* **2001**, *218*, 133-143.
51. Reithmeier, H.; Herrmann, J.; Göpferich, A *J. Controlled Release* **2001**, *73*, 339-350.
52. Reithmeier, H Ph.D. thesis, University of Regensburg, Regensburg, GE, **1999**.
53. Kellner, K.; Schulz, M. B.; Göpferich, A.; Blunk, T. *J. Drug Targ.* **2001**, *9*, 439-448.

Chapter 14

Precision Polymer Microparticles for Controlled-Release Drug Delivery

Cory Berkland[1], Kyekyoon (Kevin) Kim[2], and Daniel W. Pack[1,*]

[1]**Department of Chemical and Biomolecular Engineering, University of Illinois, Urbana, IL 61801**
[2]**Department of Electrical and Computer Engineering, University of Illinois, Urbana, IL 61801**
*Corresponding author: email: dpack@uiuc.edu

Fabrication of biodegradable polymer microparticles with precise size control provides a means for enhanced control of drug delivery rates. The ability to control delivery kinetics is important for many applications. For example, the frequent administrations needed for highly potent drugs with narrow therapeutic windows could be reduced with a system capable of delivering the drug at a constant rate for a prolonged time. We have developed a precision particle fabrication (PPF) methodology that generates monodisperse microdroplets comprising a variety of materials. We have fabricated poly(lactide-*co*-glycolide) (PLG) particles of precisely 10, 50, and 100 µm in diameter, encapsulating the model compound piroxicam. We show that drug release rates and the shape of the drug release profile depend strongly on the particle diameter. Further, combinations of microparticles of appropriate sizes and in appropriate ratios release the drug at a constant rate (zero-order release) for 14 days. We have also fabricated PLG microcapsules with unprecedented control of the polymer shell thickness. These unique technologies may provide improved methods to tailor drug release kinetics from simple, biodegradable polymer microparticles.

Introduction

Controlled-release technologies provide continuous delivery of pharmaceuticals for prolonged durations (hours, days, or weeks, depending on the application) following a single administration of a drug-loaded device. Such devices include miniature pumps, multi-layered tablets/capsules, and polymeric structures such as microparticles, rods, disks, and pellets. Controlled release technology has been developed to address formulation problems stemming from drug instability, short *in vivo* half-life, the need for local administration due to systemic toxicity and/or the need for high local concentrations, drugs for which compliance is a nuisance or difficult to achieve, highly potent drugs which exhibit severe peak-concentration-related side effects, etc. These needs are growing more urgent as an increasing fraction of pharmaceuticals comprise peptides, proteins, and nucleic acids, which most often require frequent injections or infusions due to their instability in the gastrointestinal system, short half-lives, and high potency.

Biodegradable microspheres have been one of the most studied controlled release systems due to their relatively simple fabrication, versatility, and facile administration to a variety of locations. Early studies focused on the mechanisms and kinetics of polymer degradation and drug release. A combination of experiments and theory has led to an excellent understanding of the various effects of polymer composition and molecular weight, device shape and size, and the presence of excipients, in order to allow design of delivery systems with desirable properties for a given application. *(1-4)* Another focus of research has been the instability of therapeutic proteins during device fabrication, storage, and delivery, and these issues are being addressed for many important systems. *(5-9)*

A key limitation that remains is the lack of true control of drug release rates and the shapes of the release rate profiles. Release from matrix-type microspheres is governed largely by the diameter of the particles, the drug loading (i.e., concentration within the microsphere), the size of the encapsulated molecule (governing its rate of diffusion through the device), and degradation kinetics of the microsphere-forming polymer. A variety of polymers with varying molecular weight and comonomer ratios exhibiting different degradation kinetics is available commercially. For example, poly(lactide-*co*-glycolide) (PLG) ranging in molecular weight from several thousand to over one hundred thousand, and comprising lactide/glycolide ratios from 100/0 to 50/50, can be purchased from several manufacturers. These polymer choices allow some control of the release rates, especially the duration. However, drug is released most commonly *via* diffusion through the device – either through the polymer matrix or through aqueous pores within the device. As a result, drug release profiles are generally concave downward, with the highest release rates at t = 0 and decreasing rates thereafter. Some drugs, including proteins and plasmid DNA, often exhibit a "burst" at early times followed by a lag phase wherein very little drug is released, and a subsequent concave downward release profile. In contrast, zero-order (linear) release is most desirable for many applications, while pulsatile release – in which drug is released in given amounts after predefined periods of little or no release – is needed for some indications including for many vaccines. Both zero-order and pulsatile release have been difficult to achieve with simple polymer microsphere devices.

Enhanced control of microparticle morphology may provide more precise control of release rates. Certainly, precise control of particle size can afford better control of drug release as size is a critical factor; smaller particles release drug at a faster rate than larger particles, all other parameters being equal, due to the increase in surface area/volume ratio with decreasing particle size. Furthermore, multi-wall particles, consisting of a core of one material (aqueous or polymeric) surrounded by one or more shells of a second material, provide another means for enhanced control of drug release. In these particles, not only the overall size, but also the thickness of the shells, will critically impact the drug release rates. Current particle manufacturing techniques typically produce particles exhibiting reproducible but broad size distributions with little control over shell thickness. Thus, control of drug release rates is limited.

We are developing a precision particle fabrication (PPF) methodology that provides unprecedented control of particle size, size distribution, and shell thickness. (10,11) PPF is a spraying technology in which a solution of polymer, with entrained drug (codissolved, as a particle suspension, or as an aqueous-in-oil emulsion) is extruded through a small nozzle to form a stable laminar jet. This stream is disrupted into uniformly sized microdroplets by acoustic excitation of the apparatus. Thus, the particle size is controlled by the size of the nozzle opening, the solution flow rate, and the vibration frequency. Droplets can be "hardened" to form particles by a variety of methods such as spray drying, spray freezing, or phase inversion in a non-solvent phase. Here we describe the PPF methodology and its use to fabricate uniform PLG particles encapsulating model drug compounds. In addition, we will describe how precise control of particle size can translate into control of drug release rates.

Materials and Methods

Overview Of The Precision Particle Fabrication Technology

The PPF technique consists of modifications and novel combinations of methods originally developed for fabrication of micro- and nanoparticles comprising various materials. *(10,12-16)* The main apparatus (Figure 1) is based on extruding a solution containing the sphere material through a small nozzle or other orifice to form a stable, laminar jet. To break the fluid into droplets, the nozzle is vibrated at a chosen frequency, launching a wave of acoustic energy along the liquid jet and generating periodic instabilities that break the stream into a train of monodisperse droplets.

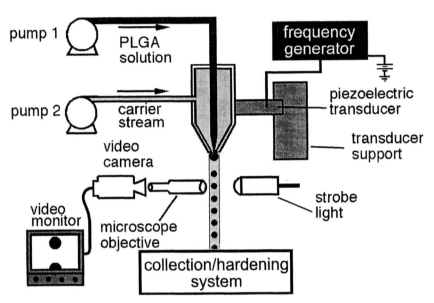

Figure 1. Schematic diagram of the precision particle fabrication apparatus.

The basic PPF methodology has been used for several years to form particles of various sizes and morphologies from a variety of materials and for diverse applications. For example, uniform particles have been fabricated from silica, iron oxide, tantalum oxide, barium-titanium oxide, elemental silver and frozen hydrogen in sizes ranging from 10 nm to 2 mm in diameter. In our recent work, we have extended the PPF techniques to fabrication of particles comprising biomedical materials, most notably biodegradable polymers. *(10,11)*

We can reduce droplet size, and in fact form droplets smaller than the nozzle opening, by employing an annular flow of a non-solvent phase around the polymer jet, termed a "carrier stream". The carrier stream is pumped at a linear velocity greater than that of the polymer stream. Thus, frictional contact between the two streams generates a downward force that effectively "pulls" the polymer solution away from the tip of the nozzle. The polymer stream is accelerated by this force and, therefore, thinned to a degree depending on the difference in linear velocities of the two streams. Finally, we may employ electrohydrodynamic forces to further reduce the jet size, allowing us to generate polymer nanoparticles as well.

Formation of uniform microdroplets and control of their size can be predicted by theory. A stream of liquid under the influence of surface tension alone is dynamically unstable and will naturally break into random-sized droplets. Rayleigh first derived the jet instability equations for a cylindrical, inviscid jet subject to disturbances from the equilibrium configuration. *(17)* Although additional work has since been carried out on this problem, his work still stands as the foundation of jet instability studies. Lord Rayleigh found that the most unstable wavelength (λ_{max}) of a disturbance imposed on the jet surface, giving rise to maximum growth rate and consequently in breakup of the jet into uniform droplets, is 9.016 times the radius of the unperturbed jet, r_j. However, a range of wavelengths around this maximum can be used to generate uniform droplets, and typically the practical range is given in Equation (1). *(18)*

$$7\,r_j < \lambda < 36\,r_j \qquad (1)$$

The reason for the upper limit on λ is that above this value the instability growth is so small that random noise near the wavelength of the applied acoustic wave causes random breakup of the jet. The upper and lower limits may vary somewhat from system to system since they depend on the noise level and the amplitude of the acoustic wave.

In the PPF apparatus, the acoustic excitation frequency is related to the wavelength according to $f = v_j / \lambda$, where v_j is the velocity of the liquid jet. Assuming the volume of the resulting sphere should be equal to the volume of a cylindrical element of the jet, the height of which is defined by the ultrasonic wavelength, we find that the drop radius, r_d, is given by

$$r_d = (3r_j^2 v_j /4f)^{1/3} \qquad (2)$$

and at the optimum wavelength, $r_d = 1.891 \cdot r_j$. Thus, by imposing a uniform, high-amplitude oscillation on the nozzle, which will dominate the random, natural instability, we can control the breakup of the stream into droplets. Equation 2 predicts the relationship between the controllable primary experimental parameters and allows us to choose conditions to generate a pre-defined microsphere size.

To test the theory, we extruded PLG solutions in solvents such as methylene chloride or ethyl acetate through 40- to 100-μm diameter orifices and disrupted the streams at various fixed frequencies. The emerging micro-droplets were imaged by video microscopy immediately downstream of the region of jet breakup (Figure 2a,b). As predicted by theory, the droplet size increased with increasing PLG solution flow rate and decreased with increasing vibration frequency. Furthermore, the droplet radius was proportional to $(1/f)^{1/3}$ as predicted (Figure 2c).

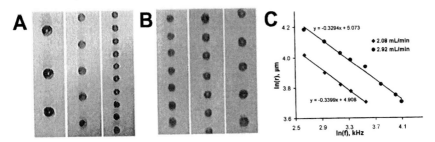

Figure 2. Video micrographs showing PLG microdroplets (i.v. 0.19 dL/g; 50/50 lactide/glycolide) dissolved in methylene chloride (5% w/v) falling from the PPF nozzle at constant flow rate with increasing acoustic frequency (A) and at constant acoustic frequency and increasing flow rate (B). Log-log plots of droplet diameter versus acoustic frequency at two different flow rates reveal slopes of the lines equaling –1/3 as predicted by equation 2 (C).

Fabrication Of Uniform Microspheres

PLG microparticles have been generated using the PPF apparatus most commonly using both acoustic excitation and a non-solvent carrier stream to control the particle size. The nascent PLG/solvent droplets were captured in a non-solvent bath (1% poly(vinyl alcohol), PVA, in water) and hardened by allowing for extraction and evaporation of the solvent. During the hardening process (typically lasting 3 hours), care was taken to ensure that the size of the microdroplets was not disturbed. The resulting particles are spherical, and their surfaces are smooth (Figure 3a,b). Further, the interior of the polymer matrix appears dense and non-porous (Figure 3c).

We have reported the generation of uniform PLG microparticles from 5-500 μm in diameter (Figure 4). For the formation of microparticles down to 25 μm, size can be controlled by varying the orifice diameter, the PLG solution flow rate, and the acoustic frequency. As the microparticle size decreases, however, the difficulty in fabrication of small nozzles, increase in the pressure drop at the nozzle orifice, and increased risk of nozzle clogging become problematic. Thus, employing a combination of acoustic excitation and a carrier stream is preferred for fabrication of particles smaller than ~30 μm.

The size uniformity of PPF microparticles approaches that of commercially available size standards. While the particle uniformity can be perceived in the micrographs, size distributions comprising greater than 5,000 particles provide a means for quantitative analysis of the uniformity. In general, at least 95% of

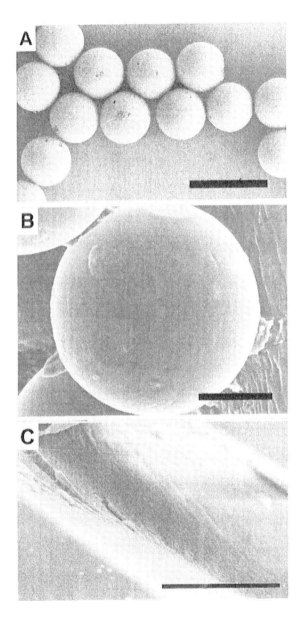

Figure 3. Scanning electron micrographs of PLG microparticles (i.v. 0.19 dL/g; 50/50 lactide/glycolide) formed via PPF. Uniform 65-μm microspheres; scale bar = 100 μm (A). Close up of particle surface; scale bar = 50 μm (B). Interior of fractured PLG microsphere; scale bar = 10 μm (C).

.the microspheres exhibit diameters that are within 1.0-1.5 µm of the average diameter. The size distributions appear narrower for the 10-µm diameter particles than for the larger particles. However, PPF-fabricated particles typically exhibit a polydispersity – defined as the ratio of the volume-average diameter and the number-average diameter – between 1.002 and 1.015, regardless of their size.

Encapsulation And Release Of Piroxicam

We have demonstrated the use of the PPF methodology to control drug release rates using a model compound, piroxicam. Piroxicam is a non-steroidal anti-inflammatory drug (NSAID) used to treat osteo- and rheumatoid arthritis. It has a molecular weight of 331 g/mole and is poorly soluble in water (53.3 µg/mL at pH 7). The commercially available piroxicam formulation is orally administered, in the form of 10- and 20-mg capsules, once or twice per day. The drug has a long plasma half-life (~50 h), and as a result steady-state blood levels are not achieved until 7-12 days after the start of treatment. Thus, although therapeutic effects may become evident earlier in treatment, the physician cannot assess the effectiveness of therapy until at least two weeks after treatment has begun. Meanwhile, as with other NSAIDs, side effects include gastrointestinal toxicity such as inflammation, ulceration, bleeding, and perforation, which can be serious especially in patients with a history of ulcers or gastrointestinal bleeding. As a result, there is interest in development of a controlled release formulation that could be administered locally in the affected joints rapidly resulting in high local concentrations of the drug.

As a first step, we investigated the effect of uniform microsphere size on the release rate of piroxicam. (11) Piroxicam was encapsulated in PLG microspheres in the PPF process by codissolving the drug with the polymer in methylene chloride. *In vitro* release experiments showed that the overall rate of release decreased with increasing microsphere size (Figure 5a). This is expected due to the decrease in surface area/volume ratio with increasing microsphere diameter. A more interesting result was the change in shape of the release profile. The smallest, 10 µm particles exhibited a concave downward shape typical of diffusion-controlled release. Release profiles from larger particles, in contrast, showed a sigmoidal shape. Similar results were obtained at several different loadings of piroxicam (mass drug/mass PLG), as well as for a water-soluble model compound, rhodamine B. (11)

Varying the piroxicam loading in the microspheres also had an effect on the piroxicam release rates. The release rate decreased with increasing loading (Figure 5b). For diffusion-controlled release, no dependence of the release rate (in terms of percent of total drug released per unit time) on loading is expected. The decreased release rate observed may be the result of retarded water uptake

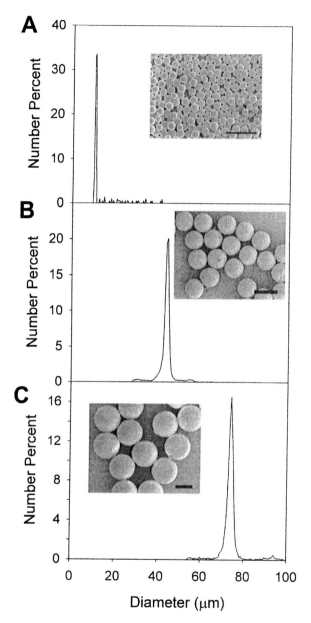

Figure 4. Size distributions of uniform PLG microspheres (i.v. 0.19 dL/g; 50/50 lactide/glycolide) fabricated using the PPF apparatus. Inset: scanning electron micrographs of the same particles; scale bars = 50 μm.

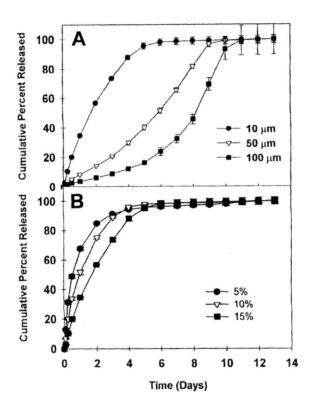

Figure 5. In vitro piroxicam release profiles showing the effect of PLG micro-sphere size (i.v. 0.19 dL/g; 50/50 lactide/glycolide; piroxicam loading = 15%) (A), and piroxicam loading (10-µm PLG particles) (B) on the release rates.

and drug solubilization due to the hydrophobic piroxicam or buffering of the intrapolymer pH environment, and thus slowing of the polymer degradation rate by piroxicam (pK_a 5.1 and 2.3). Another possibility is that the piroxicam is non-uniformly distributed in the polymer, and as loading is increased the distribution changes; i.e., a smaller fraction of the total drug may be located at/near the particle surface. However, no evidence for non-uniform piroxicam distribution has been observed and, in fact, by fluorescence microscopy the drug appears to be well dispersed throughout the particles.

In order to extend the duration of piroxicam release from uniform PLG microspheres, we examined the effects of polymer molecular weight (reported as intrinsic viscosity; i.v.), on the release rate profiles. Piroxicam was encapsulated in 50-μm diameter particles using the PPF apparatus, at theoretical loading of 15% w/w, in the same manner as in the experiments described above. For PLG from i.v. = 0.39 to 1.08 dL/g, the release profiles exhibited the same sigmoidal shape (Figure 6). Importantly, initial rates decreased and total duration of release increased with increasing molecular weight. While release was complete in less than 14 days for the microspheres made with i.v. 0.19 dL/g PLG (Figure 5a), the microspheres made with higher molecular weight polymers release piroxicam over the course of 30-40 days.

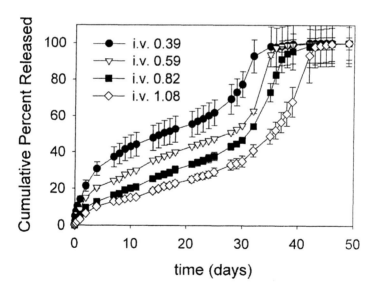

Figure 6. The effect of PLG intrinsic viscosity (i.e., molecular weight) on the release rates of piroxicam from uniform 50-μm microspheres fabricated with the PPF technology.

Mathematical Model of Piroxicam Release From PLG Microspheres

Release of piroxicam from PLG microspheres can be described using a model comprising Fickian diffusion of the drug from the spherical particles with a time-dependent diffusivity. The rate of drug release by Fickian diffusion from a spherical particle can be predicted according to

$$\frac{M_t}{M_\infty} = 1 - \frac{6}{\pi^2} \sum_{j=1}^{\infty} \frac{\exp\left[- j^2 \pi^2 D_{eff} / r^2\right]}{j^2} \tag{3}$$

where M_t/M_∞ is the fraction of drug released from the particle after time t, D_{eff} is the effective diffusivity characterizing transport of drug through the polymer matrix, and r is the radius of the particle. *(19)* It is not known whether piroxicam is released by transport directly through the PLG matrix or through water-filled pores in the polymer. Regardless, the concave upward release profiles observed for piroxicam cannot be described by equation 3 and, thus, cannot result from diffusion alone.

The increasing release rates could result from several mechanisms. For example, increasing water uptake may solubilize the drug increasing the driving force for diffusion, and/or swell the polymer matrix increasing the effective diffusivity of drug through the polymer. However, the kinetics of water penetration are likely to be too fast to explain the phenomenon observed here. Another possible explanation is that polymer degradation, which would be expected to result in both increasing diffusivity of drug through the polymer matrix and an increase in the size of aqueous pores in the polymer (also potentially leading to an increase in the effective diffusivity), is playing an important role. Several researchers have shown that polymer degradation typically proceeds exponentially according to $M_n(t) = M_n(0)\cdot\exp(-kt)$, where $M_n(t)$ is the polymer molecular weight after time t and $M_n(0)$ is the initial molecular weight. As a result, it has been suggested that the effective drug diffusivity may be given by $D_{eff} = D_{eff}(0)\cdot\exp(kt)$. Incorporating this time-dependent diffusivity, the fractional drug release can be found according to

$$\frac{M_t}{M_\infty} = 1 - \frac{6}{\pi^2} \sum_{j=1}^{\infty} \frac{\exp\left[- j^2 \pi^2 D_{eff}(0)\left(e^{kt} - 1\right)/ kr^2\right]}{j^2} \tag{4}$$

where $D_{eff}(0)$ is the initial effective diffusivity of drug through the polymer before any degradation has occurred and k is the rate constant for polymer degradation. Equation 4 predicts the change in shape of the piroxicam release profiles with increasing microsphere size reasonably well with $D_{eff}(0) = \sim 6\text{-}10$ x

10^{-14} cm^2/sec and k from 0.02-0.05 h^{-1} (Figure 7). This analysis suggests that polymer degradation may be a major factor leading to the sigmoidal release profiles. Direct measurements of water uptake rates, effective diffusivities, and polymer degradation rates will be necessary to prove this hypothesis.

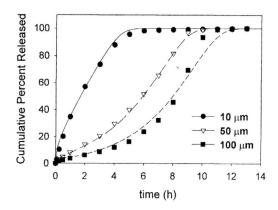

Figure 7. Drug release profiles predicted according to Equation 4 (lines) show an excellent fit to experimentally determined piroxicam release rates (symbols). For all three curves, $D_{eff}(0) = 3 \times 10^{-14}$ cm^2/sec; $k = 0.03$ h^{-1}.

Zero-Order Release Profiles From Mixtures Of Uniform Microspheres

A variety of applications require, or at the least benefit from, zero-order drug delivery kinetics. For example, given simple first-order clearance of drug from the circulation, nearly constant blood concentrations can be achieved with a constant rate of drug delivery. Such a system is particularly important for delivery of highly potent drugs and those with narrow therapeutic windows. Several types of devices can provide zero-order release. Pumps are commercially available that can be programmed to deliver drugs at predefined rates through a surgically implanted tube. Also, non-porous, hemispherical microparticles with a small orifice in the flat face have been shown to provide an optimum geometry for zero-order drug release. *(20)* However, most of these types of devices have distinct disadvantages in comparison to microspheres, including in particular the difficulty in their manufacture and/or administration.

The precise control of delivery rates afforded by uniform microspheres provides a new mechanism for generating predefined release profiles including zero-order release. Drug release from mixtures of uniform microspheres is simply a drug-mass weighted average of the release rates from the individual microspheres. Thus, given the concave downward and sigmoidal piroxicam release profiles from small and large PLG microspheres, respectively, mixtures of such microspheres would be expected to result in an intermediate release profile. Using the weighted averages, we predicted release profiles for various mixtures of 10-, 50-, and 100-μm PLG microspheres loaded with 5-20% w/w piroxicam/PLG from the individual microsphere release profiles determined experimentally.

Several combinations were predicted to provide zero-order piroxicam release. Two examples employing mixtures of 10- and 50-μm particles are shown in Figure 8. By varying the ratios of the two sizes, zero-order piroxicam release can be achieved at different rates for approximately 2 weeks. Similar results were obtained to generate zero-order release of rhodamine B from mixtures of uniform microspheres. *(11)*

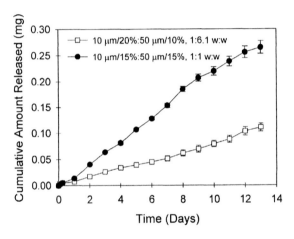

Figure 8. Zero-order release of piroxicam from mixtures of uniform PLG (i.v. 0.19 dL/g; 50/50 lactide/glycolide) microspheres in the ratios indicated in the figure legend.

Polymer Microcapsules With Controlled Shell Thickness

The PPF methodology can be adapted to fabricate polymer microcapsules by using a system of multiple, co-axial nozzles in addition to the carrier stream and acoustic excitation. The material that will form the core – gas, aqueous solution, oil, or polymer solution – is extruded through the innermost nozzle while the shell-forming material – generally a polymer solution – is passed through the surrounding nozzle. Drug can be selectively loaded into the core or shell phases by including them in the appropriate fluids, either as solutions, emulsions, or particulate suspensions. As with uniform, solid microspheres, we can control the overall microcapsule size very precisely by controlling the flow rates and acoustic frequency. Also, we have unique control of the shell thickness through controlling the relative flow rates of the core and shell phases.

To demonstrate control of microcapsule shell thickness, streams of PLG microcapsules with an oil core were photographed as they fell from the PPF apparatus. By holding the core-phase flow rate constant and increasing the shell–phase flow rate, the shell thickness was steadily increased (Figure 9a). Similarly, the core size could be controlled by increasing the core-phase flow rate while maintaining a constant shell-phase flow rate (not shown). These microcapsule droplets can be hardened by various methods as with the solid microspheres. Extraction of the solvent in 1% PVA in water results in solid, hollow microcapsules as desired. The polymer shell is dense and non-porous (Figure 9b). The shells can be made surprisingly thin; the microcapsule in Figure 9c has a shell only 1.6 µm thick.

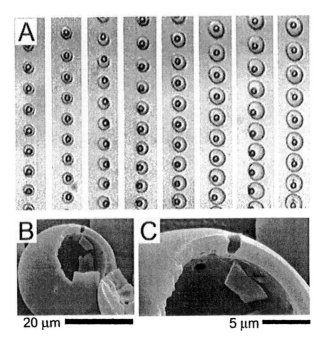

Figure 9. Video micrographs of microcapsule droplets with vegetable oil core and PLG/methylene chloride shell falling from the PPF apparatus (A). The core-phase flow is constant while the PLG solution is increased from left to right in the series of images. Scanning electron micrographs showing a hardened (B) and fractured (C) PLG microcapsule. The PLG shell is ~1.6 µm thick.

Conclusions

The ability to fabricate polymer microparticles with precise control of their size and morphology may have important effects in controlled release drug delivery. We have demonstrated that the PPF technology can provide enhanced control of drug release kinetics from simple microspheres. Indeed, we have generated a microsphere system capable of zero-order release of a small-molecule model compound. Further, the microcapsule fabrication technology may permit similar control of release kinetics for various types of drugs including peptides, proteins, and nucleic acids via unprecedented control of the microcapsule shell thickness. Thus, through advanced control of microparticle fabrication, the PPF methodology may provide a tool to push forward the boundaries of controlled release drug delivery.

References

1. Bawa, R.; Siegel, R.A.; Marasca, B.; Karel, M.; Langer, R. *J. Controlled Rel.* **1985**, *1*, 259-267.
2. Siegel, R.A.; Langer, R. *Pharm. Res.* **1984**, *1*, 2-10.
3. Park, T.G.; Lu, W.; Crotts, G. *J. Controlled Rel.* **1995**, *33*, 211-222.
4. Rafati, H.; Coombes, A.G.A.; Adler, J.; Holland, J.; Davis, S.S. *J. Controlled Rel.* **1997**, *43*, 89-102.
5. Krewson, C.E.; Dause, R.; Mark, M.; Saltzman, W.M. *J. Biomater. Sci.* **1996**, *8*, 103-117.
6. Costantino, H.R.; Langer, R.; Klibanov, A.M. *Bio/Technol.* **1995**, *13*, 493-496.
7. Costantino, H.R.; Langer, R.; Klibanov, A.M. *J. Pharm. Sci.* **1994**, *83*, 1662-1669.
8. Cleland, J.; Langer, R. *ACS Symp. Ser.* **1994**, *567*, 1-19.
9. Zhu, G.Z.; Mallery, S.R.; Schwendeman, S.P. *Nat. Biotechnol.* **2000**, *18*, 52-57.
10. Berkland, C.; Kim, K.; Pack, D.W. *J. Controlled Rel.* **2001**, *73*, 59-74.
11. Berkland, C.; King, M.; Cox, A.; Kim, K.; Pack, D.W. *J. Controlled Release* **2002**, *82*, 137-147.
12. Kim, N.K.; Kim, K.; Payne, D.A.; Upadhye, R.S. *J. Vac. Sci., Technol. A* **1989**, *7*, 1181-1184.
13. Kim, K.; Jang, K.Y.; Upadhye, R.S. *J. Am. Ceram. Soc.* **1991**, *74*, 1987-1992.

14. Jang, K.Y.; Kim, K. *J. Vac. Sci., Technol. A* **1992,** *10***,** 1152-1157.

15. Jang, K.Y.; Kim, K.; Upadhye, R.S. *J. Vac. Sci., Technol. A* **1990,** *8***,** 1732-1735.

16. Kim, K.; Ryu, C.K. *Nanostructured Materials* **1994,** *4***,** 597-602.

17. Rayleigh, L. *Proc. London Math. Soc.* **1879,** *10***,** 4.

18. Schneider, J.M.; Lindblad, N.R.; Hendricks, J.C.D.; Crowley, J.M. *J. Appl. Phys.* **1967,** *38***,** 2599.

19. Carslaw, H.S.; Jaeger, J.C. *Conduction of Heat in Solids*, 2nd Ed.; Oxford University Press: New York, 1986.

20. Hsieh, D.S.T.; Rhine, W.D.; Langer, R. *J. Pharm. Sci.* **1983,** *72***,** 17-22.

Chapter 15

A Novel Mechanism for Spontaneous Encapsulation of Active Agents: Phase Inversion Nanoencapsulation

Jules S. Jacob[1] and Edith Mathiowitz[2,*]

[1]Spherics, Inc., 701 George Washington Highway, Lincoln, RI 02865
[2]Department of Molecular Pharmacology, Physiology and Biotechnology, Brown University, Providence, RI 02912 (email: Edith_Mathiowitz@Brown.edu)

A common means of purifying polymers is by precipitation of concentrated polymer solutions with excess non-solvent, typically resulting in a solid matrix or gel. Interestingly enough, "phase inversion" of dilute polymer solutions in a narrow concentration range, with an optimal ratio of solvent to non-solvent, brought about the spontaneous formation of discrete nanospheres or microspheres that have great potential for use as drug delivery and imaging vehicles. The process, dubbed "phase inversion nanoencapsulation" or "PIN" differs from existing methods of encapsulation in that it is nearly instantaneous. The size of the final spheres is determined by polymer viscosity and not by the mixing rate of the initial emulsion, as with traditional microencapsulation techniques.

Introduction

Microencapsulation techniques are widespread and varied. *(1-5)* Methods typically involve solidification of a pre-existing emulsion of polymer or polymer solution, by changing temperature, evaporating solvent, or adding chemical cross-linking agents. Physical and chemical properties of the material to be encapsulated dictate the suitable methods of encapsulation. Phase inversion is a term used to describe the physical phenomena by which a polymer dissolved in a continuous phase solvent system coalesces into a solid macromolecular network in which the polymer is the continuous phase. *(6)* This event can be induced through several means, such as removal of solvent (e.g. evaporation), addition of another species, addition of a non-solvent, or addition to a non-solvent (wet process). In the latter, the polymer solution can be poured or extruded into a non-solvent bath. The process is thought to occur in the following manner. A polymer in solution undergoes a transition from a single phase homogeneous solution to an unstable two phase mixture composed of polymer-rich and polymer-poor fractions. Spherical droplets or micelles of non-solvent in the polymer-rich phase serve as nucleation sites and become coated with polymer. At a critical concentration, the polymer droplets precipitate from solution and solidify. Given favorable surface energy, viscosity, and polymer concentrations, the micelles coalesce and precipitate to form a continuous polymer network.

Phase inversion phenomena have been applied to produce macro- and microporous polymer membranes, and hollow fibers used in gas separation, ultrafiltration, ion exchange, and reverse osmosis. *(7)* Structural integrity and morphological properties of these membranes are functions of polymer molecular weight, polymer concentration, solution viscosity, temperature, and solubility parameters (of polymer, solvent and non-solvent). For wet process phase inversion, polymer viscosities must be greater than approximately 10,000 centipoises to maintain membrane integrity. *(6)* Lower viscosity solutions may produce fragmented polymer particles as opposed to a continuous system. Furthermore, it is known that faster precipitation results in membranes with finer porosity. (8)

Materials and Methods

Materials. Poly (lactic acid) or PLA 24 kDa and poly(lactide-*co*-glycolide) or PLGA in molar ratios of 50:50 and 75:25 were purchased from Birmingham Polymers, Inc., Birmingham, AL; polyanhydrides, such as poly(fumaric-*co*-sebacic) acid or P(FA:SA) in molar ratios of 20:80 and 50:50, poly-(carboxyphenoxypropane-*co*-sebacic) acid or P(CPP:SA) in molar ratio of 20:80 were synthesized in house *(9-11)*; polycaprolactone or PCL and polystyrene 50 kDA or PS with molecular weights ranging from 1-112,000 kDa were purchased from Scientific Polymers, Inc., and Polysciences, Inc. Zink insulin was purchased from Blue Ridge Pharmaceuticals, Greensbors, MI. Methylene chloride was purchased from Burdick +Jackson, Maskeqon, MI. Ethanol was purchased from Pharmes, Inc., Brookfeild, PA.

Nanosphere Fabrication. PIN nanospheres were fabricated in a one-step process by preparing a polymeric solution of polystyrene (PS) in methylene chloride and dispersing the polymer solution into a non-solvent, using a 1:40 solvent (methylene chloride) to non-solvent (petroleum ether) ratio. The nanospheres were collected by either filtration or centrifugation and air-dried. The initial concentration of polymer was varied to produce four formulations, 1%, 5%, 10%, 20% PS (w/v). PIN nanospheres fabricated from polystyrene (MW = 50 kDa) using a 1:40 solvent (methylene chloride) to non-solvent (ethanol) ratio were also fabricated. The initial concentration of polymer was varied to produce two formulations, 1% and 10% PS (w/v).

Scanning electron microscopy (SEM). Microspheres were applied to a carbon-adhesive tab, mounted on an aluminum stub and sputter-coated with Au-Pd using a Polaron Sputter Coater. Samples were examined at 8 kV accelerating voltage with a Hitachi S2600 SEM.

Transmission electron microscopy (TEM). Microspheres were infiltrated with LR white embedding resin (EM Sciences, Inc.) and cured at 37°C for 3 days. 80 nm sections were cut with a diamond knife and collected on Formvar-coated 200 mesh grids. Sections were stained with osmium tetroxide vapor for 30 minutes in sealed containers and examined at 80 kV using a Phillips EM 300 TEM.

Results and Discussion

We found it interesting that "phase inversion" of dilute polymer solutions in a narrow concentration range, with an optimal ratio of solvent to non-solvent, caused the spontaneous formation of discrete nanospheres. The process, dubbed "phase inversion nanoencapsulation" or "PIN" differs from existing methods of encapsulation in that it is a one-step process, nearly instantaneous and determined by polymer viscosity and not by the mixing rate of the initial emulsion, as with traditional microencapsulation techniques, e.g., solvent evaporation, solvent removal, or hot melt. In a typical process, a dilute polymer solution is poured into a non-solvent and, under conditions described in Table I, nanospheres or microspheres are formed. A variety of polymers have been used to fabricate "PIN" nanospheres including polyesters, such as poly(lactic acid), poly(lactide-*co*-glycolide) in molar ratios of 50:50 and 75:25, polycaprolactone, poly-anhydrides, such as poly(fumaric-*co*-sebacic) acid in molar ratios of 20:80 and 50:50, poly(carboxyphenoxypropane-*co*-sebacic) acid in molar ratio of 20:80, and polystyrenes. Polymers with molecular weights ranging from 1-112,000 kDa have been successfully used to fabricate nanospheres (Table I).

Table I. *Summary of phase in version experiments (for details see text).*

Polymer	MW [kDa]	Conc. [%] (w/v)	Visc. [centi- poise]	Solvent	Non- Solvent	Product
polystyrene	50	1		CH_2Cl_2	PE	500 nm - 2 µm
polystyrene	50	3		CH_2Cl_2	PE	1 - 2 µm
polystyrene	50	5		CH_2Cl_2	PE	1 - 4 µm
polystyrene	50	10		CH_2Cl_2	PE	1 - 5 µm
polystyrene	50	15		CH_2Cl_2	PE	1 - 10 µm + aggregates
polystyrene	50	20		CH_2Cl_2	PE	large aggregates
polystyrene	50	1		CH_2Cl_2	EtOHI	<100 nm
polystyrene	50	5		CH_2Cl_2	EtOH	<100 nm
polystyrene	50	10		CH_2Cl_2	EtOH	100 nm - 3 µm
polycaprolactone	72	1	3.188	CH_2Cl_2	PE	1 - 3 µm
polycaprolactone	72	5	7.634	CH_2Cl_2	PE	large aggregates
polycaprolactone	112	1	4.344	CH_2Cl_2	PE	aggregates
polycaprolactone	112	5		CH_2Cl_2	EtOH	large aggregates
polyvinylphenol	1.5-7	1		Acetone	PE	250 nm - 1 µm
polyvinylphenol	1.5-7	5		Acetone	PE	1 - 2 µm
polyvinylphenol	1.5-7	10		Acetone	PE	1 - 5 µm
polyvinylphenol	9-11	1		Acetone	PE	100 nm - 2 µm
polyvinylphenol	9-11	5		Acetone	PE	250 nm - 2.5 µm
polyvinylphenol	9-11	10		Acetone	PE	500 nm - 10 µm
polylactic acid	2	1	0.088	CH_2Cl_2	PE	100 nm
polylactic acid	2	5	1.143	CH_2Cl_2	PE	500 nm - 2 µm
polylactic acid	2	10	2.299	CH_2Cl_2	PE	1 – 10 µm
polylactic acid	24	1	1.765	CH_2Cl_2	PE	100 nm
polylactic acid	24	5	2.654	CH_2Cl_2	PE	500 nm - 1 µm
polylactic acid	24	10	3.722	CH_2Cl_2	PE	10 µm + aggregates
polylactic acid	100	1	2.566	CH_2Cl_2	PE	100 nm
polylactic acid	100	5	4.433	CH_2Cl_2	PE	0.5 - 2 µm + aggregates
polylactic acid	100	10	8.256	CH_2Cl_2	PE	film + aggregates
ethylenevinyl acetate	55	1		CH_2Cl_2	PE	Globular strands
ethylenevinyl acetate	55	5		CH_2Cl_2	PE	Coalesced strands
ethylenevinyl acetate	55	10		CH_2Cl_2	PE	Continuous sheet
poly(acrylonitrile-co-vinyl chloride)	>100	1	2.566	Acetone	PE	1 - 20 µm
poly(acrylonitrile-co-vinyl chloride)	>100	5	15.9	Acetone	PE	100 µm + aggregates

CH_2CL_2 methylene chloride; PE petroleum ether; EtOH ethanol.

Nanospheres and microspheres in the range of 10 nm to 10 µm can be produced by controlling the initial polymer concentration and indirectly the solution viscosity (Figure 1). Using initial polymer concentrations in the range of 1-2% (w/v) and solution viscosities of 1-2 cps, with a "good" solvent such as methylene chloride and a strong non-solvent such as petroleum ether or hexane, in an optimal 1:100 ratio, generates particles with sizes ranging from 100-500 nm. Under similar conditions (see Table 1), initial polymer concentrations of 2-5% (w/v) and solution viscosities of 2-3 cps, typically produce particles with sizes of 500-3000 nm. Using very low molecular weight polymers (less than 5 kDa), the viscosity of the initial solution may be low enough to enable the use of 10% (w/v) initial polymer concentrations which generally result in microspheres with sizes ranging from 1-10 µm (see Table 1). Above concentrations of 15% (w/v) and solution viscosities greater than approximately 3.5 cps, microspheres irreversibly coalesce into intricate, interconnecting fibrillar networks with micron-thickness dimensions.

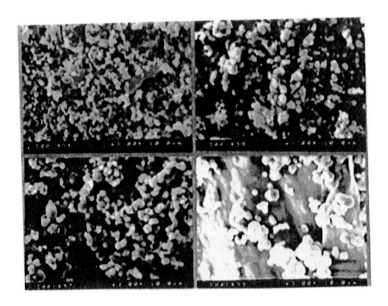

Figure 1. Scanning electron micrographs (SEM) of PIN nanospheres fabricated from polystyrene (MW=50 kDa) using a 1:40 solvent (methylene chloride):non-solvent (petroleum ether) ratio. The initial concentration of polymer was varied to produce four formulations: (a) 1% PS (w/v) - discrete particles with smooth, roughly spherical morphology ranging in size from 0.5-1 µm; (b) 5% PS (w/v) - particles with larger size range of 1-4 µm; (c) 10% PS (w/v) - particles with diameters ranging from 1-6 µm and coarser aggregates; and (d) 20% PS (w/v) - particles with the same size range as the 10% group, but also a dense sheet-like aggregate of coalesced polymer (background).

An important finding was the miscibility of the solvent in the non-solvent (or solvent extraction), which is essential for the formation of precipitation nuclei. These nuclei ultimately serve as seed for further particle growth. Alternatively, if a polymer solution is totally immiscible in the non-solvent then solvent extraction is not possible and no nanoparticles are formed.

Surprisingly, it was found that nanospheres generated with "hydrophilic" solvent/non-solvent pairs (e.g., polymer dissolved in methylene chloride with ethanol as non-solvent; see Figure 2) yielded approximately 100% smaller particles than the same concentration of polymer used with "hydrophobic" solvent/non-solvent pairs (e.g., polymer dissolved in methylene chloride with hexane as non-solvent). The explanation may be that ethanol was a better non-solvent for the polymer than hexane thus creating nucleation and precipitation in particles with size ranges similar to the primary particles proposed by the phase inversion theory. Similarly, the range of solvent to non-solvent ratios has been experimentally determined to be greater than 1:40 (minimally) and 1:100 for optimal efficiency. Mixing ratios less than 1:40 result in particle coalescence, presumably resulting from incomplete solvent extraction or a slower rate of solvent diffusion into the bulk non-solvent phase.

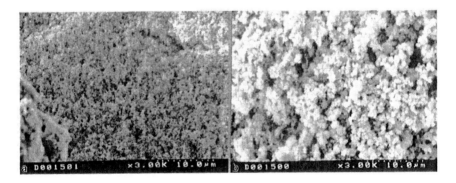

Figure 2. SEM of PIN nanospheres fabricated from polystyrene (MW=50 kDa) using a 1:40 solvent (methylene chloride) to non-solvent (ethanol) ratio. The initial concentration of polymer was varied to produce two formulations: (a) 1% PS (w/v) - discrete particles with smooth, roughly spherical morphology ranging in size from 0.01-0.1 μm, and (b) 10% PS (w/v) - particles with a larger size range of 0.5-1μm.

The theory of microphase separation phenomena as related to the formation of porous polymeric membranes is well developed. *(6, 12)* A prevalent theory supports the formation of "primary" particles of about 50 nm in diameter as the initial precipitation event resulting from solvent removal. (12) As the process continues, primary particles collide and coalesce forming "secondary" particles with dimensions of approximately 200 nm, which eventually join to form pores in the polymer matrix. Transmission electron microscopy (TEM) of PIN spheres, showing polymer inclusions in the size range of both primary and secondary particles, provides support for this theory (Figure 3).

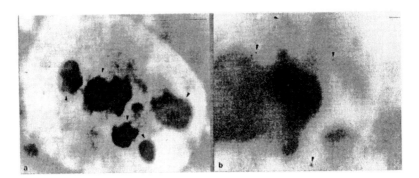

Figure 3. Transmission electron microscopy (TEM) of PIN nanospheres fabricated from PLA (MW 24 kDa); (a) a single nanosphere showing PLA morphology with white contrast and roughly circular inclusions (arrows) within the sphere having darker contrast (size marker = 1μm); (b) higher magnification of (a) showing the interface between voids and polymer matrix. The larger inclusions range in size from 0.3-1.0 μm and may well represent the coalescence of smaller inclusions (arrows) depicted in (b), which range in size from 15-30 nm. Size marker equals 0.1 μm.

An alternative hypothesis tenders "nucleation and growth" by precipitation of polymer around a core micellar structure, in contrast to coalescence of primary particles. *(13)* The observations that a very uniform size distribution of small particles forms at lower polymer concentrations (0.5-1%, see Figure 1a) as well as by using "hydrophilic" solvent to non-solvent pairs (see Figure 2a) without coalescence supports the nucleation and growth theory, while not excluding coalescence at higher polymer concentrations, (greater than 10% w/v) where larger particles are formed because of increased viscosity. The solvent would be extracted more slowly from larger particles, so that random collisions of the partially-solvated spheres would result in coalescence and, ultimately, formation of fibrous networks.

The phase inversion process can be used to encapsulate a wide variety of agents by including them in either micronized solid form or emulsified liquid form to the polymer solution. In the first scenario, the solid encapsulant acts as a core nucleus and polymer in solution precipitates and forms a continuous coating around the particle. The second case entails dispersion of concentrated encapsulant in aqueous solution into polymer solution in a hydrophobic solvent, typically using sonication to produce a fine (less than 1 μm), and stable emulsion. In this case, the emulsion droplet serves as the nucleus around which the polymer precipitates. The resulting nanospheres can be lyophilized to dehydrate the emulsion and precipitate the encapsulant as a solid particle within the polymer matrix.

Among the bioactive agents that have been encapsulated are dyes, such as rhodamine, antibiotics such as tetracycline, small water-insoluble drugs such as dicumarol *(14)*, proteins, such as insulin and bovine serum albumin, and plasmid DNA such as human CMV. An example of insulin release from PIN nanospheres composed of a 4:1 blend of PLA 24 kDa and poly(fumaric acid) is shown in Figure 4. Micronized zinc insulin (0.2-0.8 μm) was incorporated into a 5% (w/v) polymer solution in methylene chloride at a loading of 4.4 ± 0.7% (w/w), and PIN spheres were fabricated using petroleum ether as the non-solvent. The resulting PIN microspheres ranged in size from 0.5-1.5 μm as judged by scanning electron microscopy. Insulin release in phosphate-buffered saline (PBS) at pH 7.2 and 37°C was studied over a 22 hours time period. 20-50 mg of microspheres were aliquotted in triplicate and suspended in 1 ml of PBS in microfuge tubes.

At each time point, samples were pelleted by centrifugation at 6 G for 5 minutes, the release fluid was removed for analysis and replaced with 1 ml of fresh PBS. Microspheres were re-suspended in PBS by 15-30 sec of vortex agitation. After 1 hour, approximately 24% of the total insulin was released, and at the end of 5 hours nearly 45% of the drug had left the particles. Further drug release occurred at a slower rate over the time period from 5 to 22 hours. At the end of the experiment 53% of the initial loading, as determined by extraction, remained encapsulated in the PIN spheres. The efficiency of encap-sulation was judged to be 85-90%. This drug will eventually be released after complete degradation of the polymer matrix occurs.

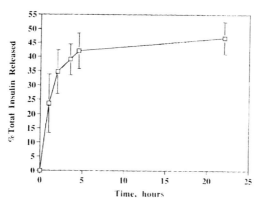

Figure 4. *Insulin release from PIN nanospheres composed of a 4:1 blend of PLA 24 kDa and poly (fumaric acid). Micronized zinc insulin was incorporated into a 5% (w/v) polymer solution in methylene chloride at a loading of 4.4 ± 0.7% (w/w), and PIN spheres were fabricated using petroleum ether as the non-solvent.*

Conclusions

The PIN process offers important advantages over existing encapsulation methodologies, especially with respect to the control of nanosphere sizes. Clearly, the delivery of encapsulated drugs in nanometer-size vehicles is of great value for intravenous and imaging applications, but also for administration by oral and inhalation routes. Studies are currently ongoing that use PIN nanospheres to bypass the GI barrier and deliver drugs, proteins, and plasmid DNA for therapeutic benefits.

Acknowledgements

This research was supported by NIH grant GM 4767601.

References

1. Beck, L.R., et al., *A New Long-Acting Injectable Micro-Capsule System for the Administration of Progesterone.* Fertility and Sterility, 1979. **31**: p. 545-551.
2. Mathiowitz, E., et al., *Polyanhydride Microspheres as Drug Carriers. II. Microencapsulation by Solvent Removal.* Journal of Applied Polymer Sciences, 1988. **35**: p. 755-774.
3. Mathiowitz, E. and R. Langer, *Polyanhydride Microspheres as Drug Carriers. I. Hot Melt Microencapsulation.* Journal of Controlled Release, 1987. **5**: p. 13-22.
4. Mathiowitz, E., et al., *Polyanhydride Microspheres as Drug Carriers. IV. Morphological Characterization of Microspheres by Spray Drying.* Journal of Applied Polymer Science, 1992. **45**: p. 125-134.
5. Lim, F. and D. Moss, *Microencapsulation of Living Cells and Tissues.* Journal of Pharmaceutical Sciences, 1981. **70**: p. 351-354.
6. Kesting, R.E., *Phase Inversion Membranes*, in *Materials Science of Synthetic Membranes*, D.R. Loyd, Editor. 1985, American Chemical Society: St. Louis. p. 132-164.
7. Michaels, S., *High Flow Membrane.* 1971.
8. Michaels, S., *High Flow Membrane.* 1971: USA.
9. Mathiowitz, E., et al., *Bioadhesive Drug Delivery Systems*, in *Encyclopedia of Controlled Drug Delivery,*, E. Mathiowitz, Editor. 1999, Jhon Willy.
10. Domb, A., et al., *Polyanhydrides. IV. Unsaturated Polymers Composed of Fumaric Acid.* Journal of Polymer Science, 1991. **29**(4): p. 571-579.

11. Mathiowitz, E., et al., *Biologically Erodible Microspheres as Potetial Oral Drug Delivery Systems.* Nature, 1997. **386**: p. 410-414.

12. Kamide, K. and S.-I. Manabe, *Role of Microphase Separation Phenomena in the Formation of Porous Polymeric Membranes*, in *Materials Science of Synthetic Membranes*, D.R. Lloyd, Editor. 1985, American Chemical Society: Washington, DC. p. 492.

13. Sperling, L.H., *Introduction to physical Polymer Science.* Second Edition ed. 1992, New York: John Wiley & Sons, Inc. 594.

14. Chickering, D.E.I., J.S. Jacob, and E. Mathiowitz, *Poly (Fumaric-co-Sebacic) Microspheres as Oral Drug Delivery Systems.* Biotechnology and Bioengineering, 1996. **52**.

Chapter 16

Polymer Nanocontainers for Drug Delivery

Marc Sauer and Wolfgang Meier*

Department of Chemistry, University of Basel, CH–4056 Basel, Switzerland
*Corresponding author: email: wolfgang.meier@unibas.ch

Vesicle-templated nanocontainers prepared from ABA triblock copolymers possess great potential for applications in areas such as drug delivery or pharmacology. For example, PMOXA-PDMS-PMOXA copolymers self-aggregate in water to form vesicles in a size range from 50 nm up to 100 μm. Intravesicular crosslinking of polymerizable end groups transforms the vesicles into solid-like nanocontainers. The permeability of these nanocontainers can be controlled either by attachment of stimuli-responsive groups or by reconstitution of membrane proteins within the container shells. These functionalizations can be used to prepare responsive load-and-release systems and biomimetic hybrid materials such as responsive nanoreactors or DNA-loaded nanoparticles with outstanding properties. Potential applications such as enzyme encapsulation and gene transfection will be discussed and illustrated using model systems.

Introduction

In recent years materials with well-defined structures in the submicron range have attracted increasing interest. Tailoring the composition, structure, and function of these materials at the nanometer level in a controlled manner may lead to new properties for well-known materials and, hence, to new applications. This concept has largely been inspired by biomineralization, where a few inorganic minerals molded into an appropriate shape lead to a large variety of different material properties. *(1)* As in Nature, one has to develop preparative procedures that allow precise control over structure and morphology formation. Self-assembled superstructures of surfactants and/or polymers have proven to be a valuable tool, providing compartmentalization on the nanometer scale, which can be used as a structural template for newly formed materials. Hollow spheres with dimensions in the submicrometer range are of particular interest due to their potential for encapsulation of large quantities of guest molecules or large-sized guests within their inner cores. These systems can be useful for applications in areas as diverse as biological chemistry, synthesis, and catalysis. For example, the use of polymeric nano-containers as confined reaction vessels, protective shells for enzymes and cells, transfection vectors in gene therapy, and drug carriers has been proposed. *(2)*

Naturally occurring nanometer-sized structures such as micelles and vesicles are already being used in biological systems, performing tasks still too complex to be completely understood. *(3)* Although they are perfectly designed to fulfill their operations in a biological environment, their direct use in many technical applications is often limited. Formed mostly by non-covalent inter-actions, these objects are of limited stability and easily undergo structural changes. *(4)* Within the last years, great efforts have been devoted to the design of mechanically stable polymeric nanocontainers. *(5-18)* The high mechanical stability of such nanocontainers, however, often becomes a major drawback due to the limited permeability of these rigid structures. *(19,20)* Loading guest molecules into these capsules after their formation or releasing substances from the capsules' interior in a controlled way at a desired target location becomes very challenging. To address this challenge, promising approaches have been presented very recently allowing control over the wall permeability of poly-meric capsules. This control was achieved by (i) a pH-dependent switch of the structure of polyelectrolyte multilayer shells, (ii) varying the solvent quality for crosslinked block copolymer shells, and (iii) reversible pH-induced swelling of crosslinked polyelectrolyte nanocontainers. *(21-23)* Following, we summarize our efforts to provide alternative routes achieving control of the permeability of polymeric nanocapsules.

Materials and Methods

Formation Of Triblock Copolymer Vesicles

Amphiphilic block copolymers are one of the most promising materials for preparing well-defined nanocontainers with outstanding properties due to the high diversity of block copolymer chemistry, allowing the synthesis of polymers with properties optimized for the desired application. *(24)* Amphiphilic block copolymers self-assemble in solution into nanometer-sized superstructures in the same way as low molecular weight amphiphiles such as surfactants and lipids. Based on their hydrophilic-hydrophobic character, they form micelles, vesicles, and, at higher concentrations, liquid crystalline phases (Figure 1).

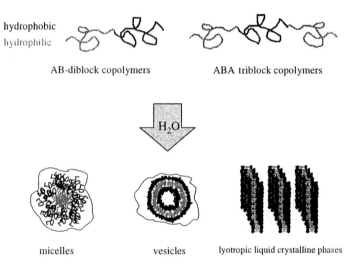

Figure 1. Schematic illustration of block copolymer self-assembly in aqueous solution.

Recently, we introduced a new type of reactive amphiphilic ABA triblock copolymer consisting of a flexible hydrophobic poly(dimethylsiloxane) (PDMS) middle block and two hydrophilic poly(2-methyloxazoline) (PMOXA) end blocks, which carry additionally polymerizable methacrylate groups at their ends. *(25)* The phase behavior in aqueous solution of such ABA triblock copolymers is shown schematically in Figure 2. Depending on the experimental conditions and the constitution of the polymer, one observes nanotubes, freestanding films, and vesicular structures. Above a polymer concentration of 50 wt%, the system forms homogeneous lamellar or bicontinuous cubic crystalline phases.

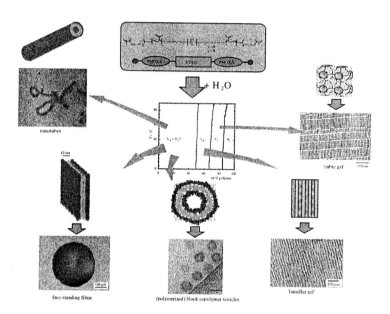

Figure 2. Phase behavior of a PMOXA-PDMS-PMOXA triblock copolymer.

The size of the block copolymer vesicles can be controlled in a range from 50 nm up to 100 μm, depending on the preparation method. These vesicles are significantly more stable than those formed by conventional low molecular weight lipids. They can be further stabilized by intravesicular crosslinking of the block copolymers, i.e. via UV-initiated polymerization of reactive methacrylate end groups. *(25)* These crosslinked particles possess solid-state properties with respect to their size and shape persistence, and they do not disintegrate upon dilution. Crosslinked vesicles even remain intact after isolation from aqueous solution and redispersion in organic solvents. However, they can be physically disrupted by strong shear forces, which is characteristic for solid state materials. Water-soluble substances can be encapsulated within these structures during their formation (Figure 3). But similar to other capsules that consist of crosslinked polymer shells, these particles have a rather low shell wall permeability. Following we will present two different approaches on how to achieve control over the particles´ permeability.

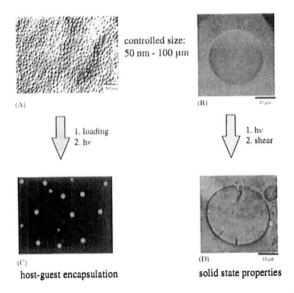

Figure 3. Microscopy images of ABA triblock copolymer vesicles. Transmission electron micrographs (TEM) of small unilamellar vesicles (A) and a giant vesicle (B); confocal fluorescence microscopy image of small unilamellar vesicles loaded with fluorescent dye (C); and TEM of a physically disrupted polymerized giant vesicle (D).

Controlling The Vesicle Wall Permeability

In the first approach, stimuli-responsive groups directly connected to the particles' surface were utilized to receive an immediate response towards a given stimulus, triggering the desired change of the wall permeability. PH-sensitive groups were attached only to the inner side of the container walls by encapsulation of sodium acrylate monomers within the vesicles interior during their formation (Figure 4). UV-induced polymerization applied after removal of extravesicular monomers crosslinked not only the block copolymers within the respective superstructure but linked also the newly formed polyacrylate chains to the inner side of the membranes. With increasing pH, the electrostatic repulsion between identically charged carboxylate anions along the polyacrylate chains was expected to induce an increase of the particle dimensions and/or the membrane permeability. Unfortunately, due to the low permeability of the polymer membrane only a few hydroxy ions were able to permeate per time unit, delaying the particles response.

In a first set of experiments, the pH-sensitivity of the particle dimensions was investigated. The vesicle radius remained unaffected between pH 4 and 10. A few hours after adjusting the pH to 11, however, a tremendous increase in radius of vesicles functionalized with 10 wt% acrylate with respect to the block copolymer concentration was observed. For example, in aqueous solution at pH 6.8 particles with an average diameter of about 30 nm were present. Twelve hours after changing the pH to about 11, most particles were disrupted and the few remaining ones had grown in radius by about a factor of ten, resulting in an increase of the encapsulated volume by a factor of about 1000.

In order to study the membrane permeability under physiological conditions, the fluorescent dye FITC-dextrin was encapsulated within vesicles functionalized with 0.1 wt% acrylate with respect to the block copolymer concentration. The dye was encapsulated at a concentration where it was self-quenching but would show a detectable fluorescence intensity after its release from the vesicles interior into the surrounding bulk water. As shown in Figure 5, no dye molecules were released from the vesicles within 30 hours at pH < 7. Two hours after raising the pH to 7, however, the fluorescence intensity increased at a constant rate for about 20 hours. At pH 8, all dye molecules were released within 12 hours. These results clearly demonstrate the ability to control the release and release rate by pH adjustment.

The attachment of stimuli-responsive functional groups represents only one possibility to control the permeability of these particles. A completely different approach would be the insertion of bacterial membrane proteins into the artificial triblock copolymer membranes, mimicking biological systems, where specific or unspecific channel proteins are responsible for the transport of various substances across lipid membranes. *(26)* These biomimetic hybrid

230

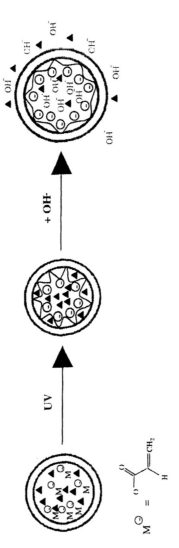

Figure 4. Schematic illustration of pH-sensitive nanocontainers.

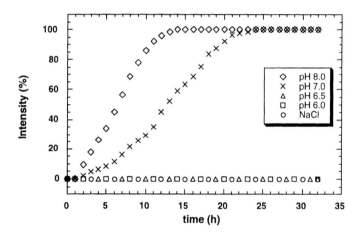

Figure 5. Fluorescence intensity versus time curves showing the pH-dependent release of the fluorescent dye FITC-dextrin from functionalized block copolymer vesicles (0.1 wt% polyacrylate with respect to the block copolymer).

materials could then be used to prepare responsive nanoreactors. This goal was achieved by encapsulation of the enzyme β-lactamase, which is able to hydrolyze β-lactam antibiotics like penicillin inside the vesicles interior (Figure 6a).

The bacterial membrane protein OmpF was incorporated into the vesicular membrane to achieve control over the particle wall permeability. In biological systems, this protein enables the intrusion of β-lactam antibiotics into bacteria. In this artificial system, the channel protein allows the transport of penicillin into the vesicles´ interior, where it is subsequently hydrolyzed to penicillinoic acid. Penicillinoic acid can leave the vesicular nanoreactor through the same channels, and can be quantified by iodometry in the bulk water phase. In contrast to penicillin, penicillinoic acid reduces iodine to iodide, and this conversion can readily be monitored by decolorization of the starch-iodine complex (Figure 6b). The absorbance of the starch-iodine complex remained constant on the time scale of the experiment for nanocapsules prepared in the absence of membrane proteins. As expected, the penicillin was not able to diffuse across the triblock copolymer shells and could, therefore, not be hydrolyzed by the enzyme. The absorbance of the complex decreased after insertion of membrane proteins into the vesicular membranes due to the reduction of iodine, clearly indicating that the encapsulated enzyme and incorporated channel proteins remained functional within the artificial polymer matrix. However, the activity of the encapsulated enzyme seemed to be rather low when compared to free enzyme. This difference could be the result of a low penicillin concentration inside the containers if the diffusion of penicillin and penicillinoic acid through the container walls was the rate-determining step. Indeed, increasing the diffusion rate by increasing the bulk penicillin concentration or increasing the number of OmpF channels in the nanoreactor walls resulted in a higher production of penicillinoic acid. Therefore it is save to assume that enzymes encapsulated in nanoreactors show essentially the same activity as free enzymes.

Responsive Nanoreactors For Encapsulation And Delivery

These channel proteins have two interesting features. Besides the fact that they exclude molecules with a molecular weight higher than 400 g/mole from diffusion across the membrane, rendering these membranes semipermeable, the proteins also close above a critical transmembrane potential. This voltage gating can be used as a switch to activate or deactivate the nanoreactors. Addition of a polyelectrolyte such as sodium polystyrene sulfonate gives rise to a Donnan-potential across the membrane. The polyelectrolyte is too large to enter the interior of the vesicles, causing an unequal concentration of ions

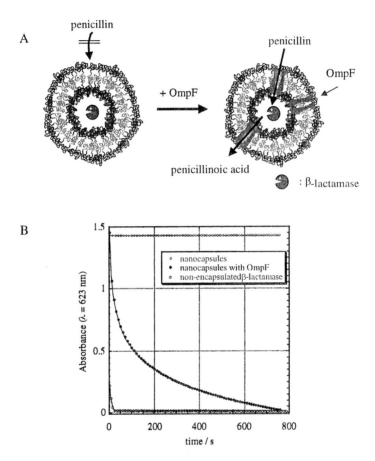

Figure 6. Schematic illustration of a block copolymer nanoreactor (A). Absorbance of starch-iodine complex in the presence of block copolymer nanocapsules, nanoreactors, and free enzyme (B).

inside and outside the containers and creating the desired Donnan-potential. The channel proteins close above a potential of about 100 mV and the nanoreactors are 'switched off' (Figure 7). The closure is fully reversible, and decreasing the potential below 100 mV reactivates the nanoreactors. This reactivation can be achieved by diluting the system with additional buffer or by increasing the ionic strength of the milieu through addition of sodium chloride.

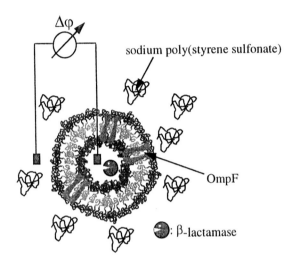

Figure 7. Schematic illustration of a switchable nanoreactor.

The ability to trigger the activation/deactivation of the nanoreactors is particularly interesting for practical applications, since it allows a local and temporal control on the uptake and release of substrates. Moreover, enzymes located inside these containers are fully protected against degradation by proteases or self-denaturation.

Another important aspect of these triblock copolymer nanocontainers is the observation that hydrophilic PMOXA end blocks of certain lengths prevent un-specific protein adsorption. This observation could be particularly interesting for use of such nanocapsules as an intravenous drug delivery system that is not recognized by the immune system. The protective feature of PMOXA requires a minimum length of the hydrophilic blocks because the layer formed by short PMOXA blocks is too thin to prevent interactions between external ligands and incorporated receptors and proteins. To verify this observation, the bacterial membrane protein LamB was used as a model system (Figure 8). This protein forms trimeric channels in the outer cell wall of bacteria, allowing a specific transport of maltodextrins. In addition, it serves as a receptor for lambda phages and has been proposed as the major intrusion path for viral DNA during infection.

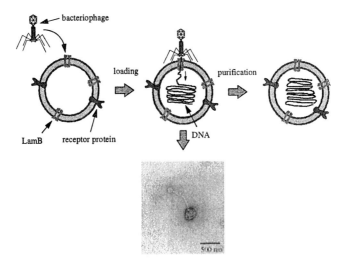

Figure 8. Schematic illustration and transmission electron micrograph of virus-assisted loading of block copolymer nanocontainers.

The LamB protein was reconstituted into the membranes of triblock copolymer vesicles. Nonincorporated proteins were removed by gel-filtration to avoid interaction between free protein and phages. In order to probe whether the phages are still able to bind to the incorporated LamB, we incubated the particles with lambda phages. The transmission electron micrograph shown in Figure 8 clearly demonstrates binding of the phages to the protein in the nanocontainer walls via their tails. Moreover, the enormous size difference between the phage and the LamB protein/vesicle complex suggests a rather strong interaction between both structures. Interestingly, the functionality of the receptor protein is fully preserved in the artificial block copolymer membranes. The protein is still able to induce the intrusion of viral DNA into the nanocontainers. *(27)*

The potential of this system as a new gene vector is obvious. Particularly the small size of around 200 nm and the electrically neutral shell of the containers could be useful for delivery applications. In addition, other receptor molecules can be inserted into the container walls, allowing a specific transport of genes into desired target cells and making the nanocontainers a versatile delivery system.

The well-known biotin-streptavidin interaction was utilized as a primitive model to demonstrate the potential of this delivery system. Nanocontainers were prepared, in which about 1 mole% of the underlying block copolymers had been modified with biotin groups at their ends. These containers were then loaded with fluorescently labeled DNA. Simultaneously, a micropatterned surface was prepared by microcontact printing, consisting of a regular array of parallel streptavidin coated stripes with a diameter of about 7 μm. This surface was incubated with the nanocontainer dispersion, washed with buffer, and observed through a confocal fluorescence microscope (Figure 9). The micrograph clearly demonstrates immobilization of the intact DNA-nanocontainers only at surface areas that had been modified with streptavidin. Streptavidin-free surface areas where no receptor-ligand interactions were possible remained essentially free of nanocontainers.

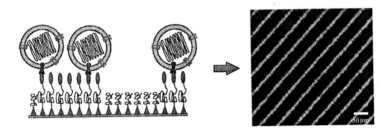

Figure 9. Schematic illustration and confocal fluorescence micrograph image of nanocontainers filled with fluorescently labeled DNA that are immobilized at a micropatterned surface.

Conclusions

The investigations described above show that vesicles prepared from ABA triblock copolymer molecules possess great potential for applications in areas such as drug delivery or pharmacology. Their permeability can be triggered by attachment of stimuli-responsive groups or by reconstitution of membrane proteins within the vesicular shells. This functionalization can be used to prepare responsive load-and-release systems or biomimetic hybrid materials, i.e. responsive nanoreactors or DNA-loaded nanoparticles.

References

1. Mann, S. *Biomimetic Materials Chemistry*; VCH: New York, 1996.
2. Meier, W. *Chem. Soc. Rev.* **2000**, *5*, 295.
3. Niemeyer, C. *Angew. Chem. Int. Ed.* **2001**, *40*, 4128.
4. Lasic, D.D. *Liposomes from Physics to Applications*; Elsevier: Amsterdam, 1993.
5. Ringsdorf, H.; Schlarb, B.; Venzmer, J. *Angew. Chemie* **1988**, *100*, 117.
6. Selb, J.; Gullot, Y.; Goodamann, F. *Developments in Block Copolymers*; Elsevier: Amsterdam, 1985.

7. Mann, S. *J. Chem. Soc. Dalton Trans.* **1997**, 3953.
8. Meier, W. *Curr. Opin. Colloid Interface Sci.* **1999**, *4*, 6.
9. Newkome, G.R.; Moorefield, C.N.; Vögtle, F. *Dendritic Molecules: Concepts, Synthesis, Perspectives*; VCH: Weinheim, 1986.
10. Qinggao, M.; Remsen, E.E.; Clark Jr., C.G.; Kowalewski, T.; Wooley, K.L. *Proceedings of the National Academic of Sciences USA* **2002**, *99*, 5058.
11. Sanji, T.; Nahatsuka, Y.; Onishi, S.; Sakewai, H. *Macromolecules* **2000**, *33*, 8524.
12. Caruso, F.; Caruso, R.A.; Möhwald, H. *Science* **1998**, *282*, 1111.
13. Barthelet, C.; Armes, S.P.; Lascelle, S.F.; Luk, S.Y.; Stanley, H.M.E. *Langmuir* **1988**, *14*, 2032.
14. Marinakos, M.; Novak, J.P.; Brouseau III, L.C.; House, A.B.; Edeki, E.M.; Feldhaus, J.C.; Feldheim, D.L. *J. Am. Chem. Soc.* **1999**, *121*, 8518.
15. Kong, X.Z.; Kan, C.Y.; Li, H.H.; Yu, D.Q.; Juan, Q. *Polym. Adv. Technol.* **1997**, *8*, 627.
16. Emmerich, O.; Hugenberg, N.; Schmidt, M.; Sheikov, S.S.; Baumann, F.; Deubzer, B.; Weiss, J.; Ebenhoch, J. *Adv. Mater.* **1999**, *11*, 1299.
17. Okubo, M.; Konishi, Y.; Minami, H. *Colloid Polym. Sci.* **1988**, *276*, 638.
18. Landfester, K. *Adv. Mater.* **2001**, *13*, 765.
19. Discher, B.M.; Hammer, D.A.; Bates, F.S.; Discher, D.E. *Curr. Opin. Colloid Interface Sci.* **2000**, *5*, 125.
20. Discher, B.M.; Won, Y.Y.; Ege, D.S.; Lee, J.C.M.; Bates, F.S.; Discher, D.E.; Hammer, D.A. *Science* **1999**, *284*, 1143.
21. Stewart, S.; Liu, G.J. *Chem. Mater.* **1999**, *11*, 1048.
22. Sukhorukov, G.B.; Antipov, A.A.; Voigt, A.; Donath, E.; Möhwald, H. *Macromol. Rapid Commun.* **2001**, *22*, 44.
23. Sauer, M.; Meier, W. *Chem. Commun.* **2001**, 55.
24. Hadjichristidis, N. *Block Copolymers: Synthetic Strategies, Physical Properties, Applications*; Wiley: New York, 2002.
25. Nardin, C.; Hirt, T.; Leukel, J.; Meier, W. *Langmuir* **2000**, *16*, 1035.
26. Meier, W.; Nardin, C.; Winterhalter, M. *Angew. Chem. Int. Ed.* **2000**, *39*, 4599.
27. Graff, A.; Sauer, M.; Van Gelder, P.; Meier, W. *Proceedings of the National Academic of Sciences USA* **2002**, *99*, 5064.

Chapter 17

Nanocapsules from Liposomal Templates

Gerold Endert, Silke Lutz, Frank Essler, Doris Schoffnegger, and Steffen Panzner*

Novosom AG, Weinbergweg 22, D–06120 Halle, Germany
*Corresponding author: email: steffen.panzner@novosom.com

We here for the first time describe the encapsulation of single liposomes within ultrathin networks made from poly-electrolytes. Prevention of aggregate formation and encapsulation of single liposomes were achieved using a titration approach, where limited amounts of polyelectrolyte were added to the liposome suspension. The lipid bilayer was found to be stable during the coating procedure. True formation of cage-like structures was verified by detergent treatment, encapsulation of macromolecules, and electron microscopy. Solubilization of the inner liposomes allows gentle removal of the templating core, leaving unaffected hollow shell structures behind. Polymer encapsulated lipo-somes can be manufactured from synthetic and natural polymers, and even proteins, and constitute a novel bio-material with promising characteristics. The entire structure can be constructed from biological materials or other substances that are generally regarded as being safe, a parti-cular advantage for biomedical applications. These capsules are expected to be useful in the development of novel oral drug delivery systems that are well suited for the transport of biological macromolecules, i.e. DNA, proteins, and peptides.

Introduction

Liposomes are well-described structures consisting of a phospholipid bilayer membrane that spherically encloses an aqueous inner core. As the membrane is impermeable for almost any hydrophilic molecule, liposomes are being used as biocompatible packaging devices. In fact, drugs of almost any kind as well as a great many of biologics ranging from simple metabolites to the most complex macromolecules can be loaded into liposomes. The liposomal membrane protects the cargo against detrimental effects coming from the environment. *(1)*.

The versatility of liposomes, however, is greatly diminished by their biological and mechanical instability. We, therefore, set out to encapsulate individual liposomes into a stable polymer network. During the last years, a novel technique for the formation of hollow spheres in the nanometer and micrometer scale was developed. In brief, colloidal templates were coated with alternating layers of oppositely charged polyeletrolytes. *(2,3)* This layer-by-layer (LbL) technique was established for a number of templates and polyelectrolytes, the most frequently used ones being polystyrene or melamine, coated with alternating layers of polyamines and polysulfonic acids. *(4,5)* Functional molecules such as dyes, enzymes, or nucleic acids were incorporated in the interior or in the wall of these structures. *(6-9)* After formation of several layers, the templates were destroyed by heat or hydrolysis, leaving the intact shell structures behind. *(10)*

Despite of being an attractive template, the use of liposomes as a core material has not been reported so far. *(11)* In fact, binding of a first polyelectrolyte to the liposomal membrane was shown to promote cargo efflux or even complete disappearance of the vesicular structure. *(12)* Furthermore, binding of a second polyelectrolyte on top of the first resulted in removal of the first polymer from the membrane rather than in the formation of a polyelectrolyte mesh. *(13)*

We here present a method to circumvent these problems. Liposomal nanocapsules were successfully prepared from a number of polymer systems. These novel structures were characterized with respect to their stability against detergent and serum components, and possible applications are discussed.

Materials and Methods

Adsorption procedure. 1 mL of a dipalmitoylphosphatidylcholine (DPPC)/ dipalmitoylphosphatidylglycerol (DPPG) liposome suspension (90/10 mol%) in buffer (10 mM HEPES, pH 7.5) was rapidly mixed with defined amounts of polymer solution (1 mg/mL stock in buffer). After a few minutes, particle size and zeta potential of the mixture were recorded using a Malvern Zetasizer 3000HSA with dynamic light scattering (DLS). The endpoint of the titration was reached when particle size and zeta potential remained constant upon addition of further polymer.

Shell permeability. FITC-labeled dextrins of different molecular weights (4, 19.5, 42, 77, and 2000 kD) were encapsulated into liposomes by hydration of the lipid films with 25 mg/mL of the respective dextrin solution in buffer (10 mM HEPES, 150 mM NaCl at pH 7.5). Non-encapsulated material was removed by flotation, and four or six alternating polylysine and alginic acid layers were adsorbed onto the liposomes. The permeability of the shell structures was assayed after solubilization of the inner liposome templates with 0.2% Triton X-100. In particular, shell remnants were sedimented at 500,000 g for 120 minutes, and fluorescence intensities were recorded for the pellets and supernatants.

Serum protection. Liposomes (60% DPPG, 40% DPPC) were prepared in the presence of 100 mM carboxyfluorescein (CF). Non-incorporated CF was removed by gel filtration, and the liposomes were coated with albumin and heparin at pH 4.0. After adsorption of the fourth layer, 0.12% glutaraldehyde was added, and the shells were crosslinked overnight. Excess glutaraldehyde was removed by extensive dialysis against buffer (10 mM HEPES, 150 mM NaCl at pH 7.5), and the suspension was concentrated to 10 mM lipid by ultrafiltration. 10 µl liposomes or liposomal nanocapsules were mixed with 1 ml human serum and incubated at 37 °C. Samples were taken at defined time points and immediately diluted with buffer.

Results and Discussion

Capsule Formation on Liposomal Templates

Charged liposomes made of 90% DPPC and 10% DPPG were used for the preparation of polyelectrolyte nanocapsules. Titration of the negatively charged liposomes with increasing amounts of polylysine first resulted in a loss of net surface charge, accompanied by the formation of aggregates. At higher polylysine concentrations, however, complete charge reversal of the colloid occurred. Under these conditions, binding of the polymer molecules to the liposome surface was sufficiently stable to prevent aggregate formation (Figure 1). As little as 30 µg of the polymer was found to be sufficient for complete charge reversal of 1 mg of liposomes.

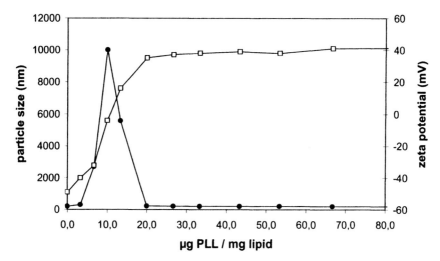

Figure 1. Titration curve of negatively charged DPPC/DPPG liposomes. Dependence of particle size (filled circles) and zeta potential (hollow squares) on poly-L-lysine (PLL) concentration.

Complete and saturable binding of polylysine was confirmed by titration of liposomes using FITC-labeled polylysine and subsequent separation of the unbound polymer. As long as the zeta potential had not reached its plateau, all polylysine was found in the upper flotating phase, giving evidence of its complete binding to the liposomes. Overtitration, however, resulted in the presence of free polymer in the subphase (data not shown). These results encouraged us to adopt the titration approach to form multilayers of oppositely charged polyelectrolytes. The amount necessary for the formation of a particular layer was determined by titration in individual small-scale experiments. Based on these results, larger batches of up to 100 mL were prepared with the desired polymer-to-lipid ratio. Up to 8 layers of oppositely charged polyelectrolytes could be adsorbed onto liposomal templates (Figure 2).

The zeta potential and, therefore, surface charge of the particles alternated from positive to negative dependent on the deposited polymer. The particle size increased with each additional layer, suggesting a multilayer deposition rather than a removal of prebound material. The formation of liposomal nanocapsules is possible using a wide range of shell materials and lipid compositions. To name a few, shells were successfully prepared from synthetic polymers such as poly(acrylic acid), poly(allylamine), poly(dimethyldiallyl) ammonium chloride, and polylysine, from natural materials such as alginic acid, heparin, modified dextrins and chitosan, and even from proteins such as albumin and hemoglobin.

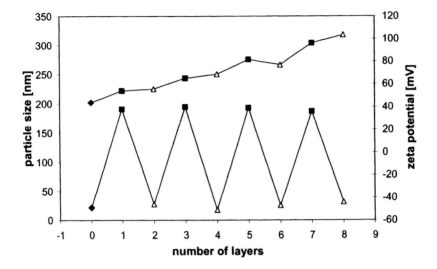

Figure 2. Layer-by-layer adsorption of polylysine (filled squares) and sodium alginate (open triangles) onto charged liposomes. Particle size and zeta potential as measured with DLS versus number of adsorbed layers.

Evidence for Capsule Formation

To truly show the formation of polymer shells around the liposomes, the stability of these novel structures against detergent was determined. Different liposomal nanocapsules with zero to six layers were generated using albumin and heparin or polylysine and alginate, respectively. After completion of shell formation, the templating liposomes were solubilized by treatment with Triton X-100. Delipidation and formation of stable nanocapsules from liposomal templates were demonstrated by three independent sets of experiments. First, it was shown that changes in particle size before and after treatment with detergent decreased as the number of polymer layers increased (Figure 3). A minimum of 3 to 4 layers was found to be sufficient for the generation of stable nanocapsule shells. The same observation was made using changes in the intensity of scattered light as measured by DLS as the probe (data not shown).

Second, the buoyant density of the delipidated nanocapsules was found to be much higher than that for the core containing structures, indicating a loss of the low density bearing lipids (data not shown).

Third, we determined the ability of these nanocapsules to retain macro-molecular probes. Closed shells should allow the encapsulation of macro-molecules even after removal of the lipids. Liposomes themselves are often used for the encapsulation of large macromolecules and, therefore, provide excellent tools for the determination of the shell permeability. FITC-labeled dextrins of different sizes were loaded into liposomes, and nanocapsules were formed from

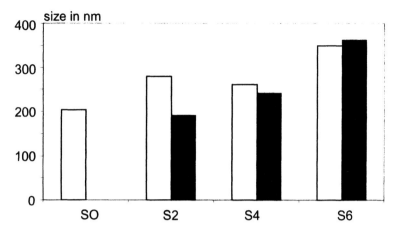

Figure 3.   Stability against detergent.   The size of uncoated liposomes or liposomes coated with up to six layers of albumin/heparin (S0 to S6) was determined in the absence (open bars) or presence (filled bars) of detergent.

these templates. The lipid membranes were then solubilized with detergent, and the distribution of dextrins was measured after sedimentation of the shells (Figure 4).   Shell walls made from polylysine and alginate were found to be surprisingly permeable towards dextrins smaller than about 40 kDa. However, they clearly retained dextrin probes with a molecular mass larger than 70 kDa, thus giving evidence of the formation of closed nanocapsules.

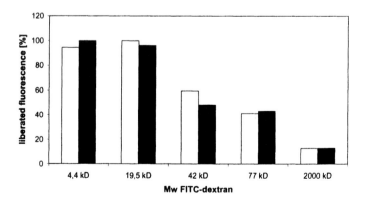

Figure 4. Permeability of nanocapsules against FITC-dextrins of different sizes after solubilization of their lipid core with Triton-X 100. Nanocapsules with 4 (open columns) or 6 (filled columns) alternating layers of polylysine and alginate were sedimented after detergent treatment, and the amount of FITC-dextrin in the supernatant was measured.

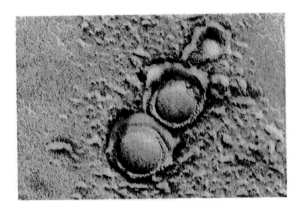

Figure 5. Freeze-fracture electron micrograph of liposomal nanocapsules of about 200 nm in diameter. A thin outer polymer layer that is rougher than expected from a lipid bilayer surrounds the smooth inner lipid membrane.

Eventually, we were able to visualise the presence of liposomal nano-capsules by freeze-fracture electron microscopy (Figure 5). Untreated liposomes would show a smooth and spherical surface. The liposomal nano-capsules, however, clearly posses a coat surrounding the liposomal core, showing a rough appearance at the cleavage site. These observations demonstrate that liposomes indeed are suitable templates for the fabrication of nanocapsules consisting of a novel, non-lipidic shell.

Protective Envelopes

Like any other foreign material that is brought into the body, liposomes are attacked by several defence systems. For example, serum components are specialised in permeabilizing membranes and have to be physically separated from the surface of liposomes to retain the liposomes' stability under physiological conditions. A narrow polymer meshwork of sufficient thickness as provided by the nanocapsules should give such protection. Unfortunately, capsules made from alternating polylysine/alginate layers have shown a comparatively high permeability even for large dextrin molecules. In fact, these capsules provided no protection of the liposomal membrane against human serum (data not shown). On the other hand, protein-containing shell structures were calculated to be much more tightly packed, based on the amount of adsorbed material. For example, albumin adsorbs with at least 200 µg per mg of lipid in a single layer. Assuming a monomolecular layer, the lateral spacing of these molecules is about 9 nm. Albumin itself has an ellipsoidal shape and is about 4x14 nm in size, therefore, the resulting pores or channels are no larger than a single protein molecule of average size. *(14)*

The albumin/heparin system was tested for its ability to protect the under-lying membrane. Liposomes were loaded with self-quenching amounts of carboxyfluorescein as a model cargo and covered with four layers of albumin/ heparin. The adsorption cycle was carried out at pH 4, using the albumin as the polycation. To later allow serum contact at pH 7, the shell was crosslinked with 0,12% glutaraldehyde. Excess glutaraldehyde and free carboxyfluorescein were carefully removed before incubation with serum. As shown in Figure 6, the uncoated liposomal membrane is readily perforated by the serum and carboxyfluorescein is released into the medium. In stark contrast, the coated liposomes are much more stable in human serum and slowly release their cargo.

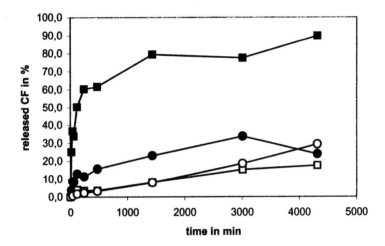

Figure 6. Release of carboxyfluorescein from liposomes (squares) and liposomal nanocapsules (circles). The liposomal nanocapsules were made from four crosslinked layers of albumin and heparin. Open symbols describe the release of cargo in buffer, filled symbols stand for the release in serum.

Cage-like and stable structures around liposomes are new. A number of technical challenges had to be overcome. First, true layer formation had to be achieved rather than polyelectrolyte competition. For example, binding of quarternized poly (4-vinylpyridinium) onto negatively charged liposomes was found to be stochiometric and saturable. However, after addition of poly(acrylic acid) as an anionic polymer to the polycation-liposome complexes, removal of the polycation was preferred over layer formation. A possible explanation for this behavior is the small size of the liposomes, having a mean diameter of about 50 nm. A single liposome, therefore, was much smaller than the contour length of the used polymer of about 300 nm. Liposomes were likely bound like pearls on a polyelectrolyte string, still allowing free access of the polyanion. Furthermore, the charge spacing of poly(acrylic acid) is narrow and equal to poly(vinylpyrinidinium), thus giving the interaction between both polymers a competitive edge over the liposome-polyelectrolyte interaction. *(13)*

Second, the permeability of the liposomal membranes had to remain unaltered upon binding of the shell material to it. Liposome permeabilization upon addition of polyelectrolytes of opposite charge had been reported, dependent on the amount of charged species in the bilayer, with a critical concentration of 30% found for cardiolipin. *(12)* A correlation between the charge content of a bilayer and the amount of adsorbed material was also observed in our experiments. However, we did not measure significant leakage of small solutes even at 60% molar fraction of the negatively charged DPPG in our lipid bilayers. Probably, permeabilization is a particular problem of the cardiolipin liposomes.

Third, the small size of the liposomes, which is comparable to the size of the polymers used for decoration, was a challenge for the routine production of these particles. The conventional scheme of excess polymer addition and subsequent removal of unbound polymer after each adsorption step results in long process times and low yields when applied to a liposomal system. More-over, excess alginate or polylysine could not be removed by filtration due to the strong tendency of these polymers to adsorb onto the filter membranes. As a consequence, complete binding of the added polyelectrolytes to the liposome surface was desirable. By using the titration approach, it was possible to identify conditions that allow complete binding of polymers to the colloidal templates and prevent aggregation of the liposomal templates.

Once established, the procedure is astonishingly simple. A number of coatings can be applied to colloidal particles by just adding a known amount of polymer to the suspension. The titration approach eliminated the need of washing steps during the preparation, thus gaining in process speed and simplicity. Careful titration allowed the formation of at least 8 layers without interruption of the process. As the binding is fast and purification of the intermediate particles is unnecessary, a continuous process for the coating of liposomes or other colloids was established in our lab.

Conclusions

True formation of cage-like structures by adsorption of alternating layers of oppositely charged polyelectrolytes around liposomal templates has been shown independently by detergent treatment, encapsulation of macromolecules, and visually by electron microscopy. Solubilization of the inner liposomes allows gentle removal of the templating core, leaving unaffected hollow shell structures behind. Shells constructed from four or more layers were found to be stable. Cargo molecules may be preloaded into the liposomes and are liberated upon detergent treatment. Using this approach, the permeability of the shell walls for enclosed materials was determined. These shell walls can be highly porous, thus facilitating the free exchange of solutes and solubilized components. The ease of core removal provides excellent means for the construction of hollow spheres containing sensitive components such as proteins.

Single encapsulation of liposomes in layered polymer networks generates a novel material with promising characteristics. The structures show a high degree of complexity, having an aqueous core surrounded by an almost impermeable lipid bilayer that in turn is packed into a meshlike and stable polymer network. The fact that the entire structure can be constructed from biological materials or other substances that are generally regarded as safe is of particular advantage for biomedical applications. Sufficiently dense shell walls have been found to protect the liposomal membrane against physiological destruction in serum. These structures, therefore, should allow use as a long-term depot for the sustained release of proteins, peptides, or other sensitive macromolecules. Shells of different thickness or composition will withstand physiological destruction for different periods of time, and will slowly expose the inner lipid membrane after erosion has progressed. Cargo molecules are protected and safe as long as this membrane poses the ultimate diffusion barrier. Such a depot will work similar to a secreting cell, bearing cargo filled vesicles inside the cytoplasm until a release signal is received.

The potential lack of toxicity together with ease of preparation and liberation of enclosed components will probably catalyze a number of further developments. Capsules are expected to be useful in the development of novel oral drug delivery systems that are particularly well suited for the transport of biological macromolecules such as DNA, proteins, and peptides. Other potential applications may lie in the fields of enzyme encapsulation or biosensor development.

References

1. Lasic, D.D. *Liposomes: From Physics to Applications*; Elsevier: Amsterdam, 1993.
2. Donath, E.; Sukhorukov, G.B.; Caruso, F.; Davies, S.A.; Möhwald, H. *Neuartige Polymerhohlkörper durch Selbstorganisation von Polyelektrolyten auf kolloidalen Templaten. Angew. Chem.* **1998**, *110*, 2323-2327.
3. Caruso, F.; Möhwald, H. *Preparation and Characterization of Ordered Nanoparticle and Composite Multilayers on Colloids. Langmuir* **1999**, *15*, 8276-8281.
4. Decher, G. *Fuzzy Nanoassemblies : Towards Layered Polymeric Multicomposites. Science* **1997**, *277*, 1232-1237.
5. Möhwald, H. *From Langmuir Monolayers to Nanocapsules. Colloids and Surfaces A* **2000**, *171*, 25-31.
6. Caruso, F.; Möhwald, H. *Protein Multilayer Formation on Colloids Through a Stepwise Self-Assembly Technique. J. Am. Chem. Soc.* **1999**, *121*, 6039-6046.

7. Sukhorukov, G.; Dähne, L.; Hartmann, J.; Donath, E.; Möhwald, H. *Controlled Precipitation of Dyes into Hollow Polyelectrolyte Capsules Based on Colloids and Biocolloids. Advanced Mater.* **2000**, *12*, 112-115.
8. Caruso, F.; Trau, D.; Möhwald, H.; Renneberg, R. *Enzyme Encapsulation in Layer-by-Layer Engineered Polymer Multilayer Capsules. Langmuir* **2000**, *16*, 1485-1488.
9. Lvov, Y.; Antipov, A.; Mamedov, A.; Möhwald, H.; Sukhorukov, G.B. *Urease Encapsulation in Nanoorganized Microshells. Nano Letters* **2001**, *1*, 125-128.
10. Caruso, F.; Caruso, R.A.; Möhwald, H. *Nanoengineering of Inorganic and Hybrid Hollow Spheres by Colloidal Templating. Science* **1999**, *282*, 1111-1114.
11. Zasadsinsky, J.A.; Kisak, E.; Evans, C. *Complex Vesicle Based Structures. Curr. Opin. Colloid Interface Sci.* **2001**, *6*, 85-90.
12. Yaroslavov, A.A.; Kiseliova, E.A.; Udalykh, O.Y.; Kabanov,V.A. *Integrity of Mixed Liposomes Contacting a Polycation Depends on the Negatively Charged Lipid Content. Langmuir* **1998**, *14*; 5160-5163.
13. Yaroslavov, A.A.; Efimova, A.A., Kulkov, V.E.; Kabonov, V.A. *Adsorption of Polycation on the Surface of Negatively Charged Liposomes: The Effect of Phase State of the Lipid Bilayer on the Composition of Polycation-Liposome Complex. Polymer Science* **1994**, *36*, 215-220.
14. Peters, T. Jr. *Serum Albumin. Adv. Prot. Chem.* **1985**, *37*, 161-245.

Chapter 18

From Polyelectrolyte Capsules to Drug Carriers

Gleb B. Sukhorukov

Max-Planck-Institute of Colloids and Interfaces, Golm, Potsdam, D–14424, Germany (email: gleb@mpikg-golm.mpg.de)

This paper describes a novel method for micro- and nano-encapsulation, consisting of a layer-by-layer adsorption of oppositely charged macromolecules onto colloidal particles that function as a template. Protein aggregates, emulsion droplets, biological cells, and drug nanocrystals can be utilized as templates, covering a size range from 50 nm to tens of microns. Synthetic and natural polyelectrolytes, multivalent dyes, and magnetic nanoparticles have been used as layer constituents to fabricate the shell. Some colloidal templates can be decomposed without affecting the polymer shell, leading to the formation of hollow capsules. The permeability through the capsule walls depends on the shell thickness and composition, and can be regulated by the pH and ionic strength of the solution, or by solvent exchange. Enzymes can be encapsulated by molecular weight-selective shells, trapping the enzymes but allowing small molecules to permeate through the capsule walls. The presence of poly-electrolytes on only one side of the capsule walls allows the formation of a pH gradient across the walls, which has been utilized to precipitate small molecules such as drugs within the restricted volume of the capsule interior.

Introduction

Designing functional colloidal particles is of highest interest to various research areas, such as medicine, biotechnology, catalysis, and ecology. In general, research on particle formation and encapsulation requires the ability to form a colloidal core of defined content and size, and a shell that provides stability, permeability to release core material, and catalytic or affinity properties. In order to develop functionalized colloids, tailoring the different components of one particle becomes important to combine several properties in one core-shell structure. The desired properties may be adjusted to facilitate the interaction of the core with the solvent or to add certain desired chemical properties. Moreover, the shell may exhibit magnetic, optical, conductive, or targeting properties for directing core forming bioactive materials. Delivery systems providing sustained release of bioactive materials form a major challenge in the development of advanced drug formulations. Most systems comprise polymer particles in the size range of 50nm to 100µm. Currently the drug molecules are either embedded in polymer matrices or encapsulated in core-shell structures. In the latter case, the shell permeability or degradation rate determine the release rate of the bioactive core material.

This paper is devoted to a recently introduced novel pathway fabricating nano-engineered core-shell structures based on a wide selection of materials. This method emanated from research on the formation of ultrathin polymer films using alternating adsorption of charged species on a macroscopic support. This approach was proposed by Iler in 1966 and later developed by Mallouk *et al.* *(1,2)* In 1991, Decher *et al.* proposed a method for forming polyelectrolyte films by using the alternating adsorption of polycations and polyanions *(3)*. A crucial factor for this polyionic layer-by-layer (LbL) assembly is the alternating change of the surface charge upon polyelectrolyte adsorption. Beginning in 1998, the concept of LbL-assembly of charged species was transferred to coat micron and sub-micron sized colloidal particles, as illustrated in Figure 1. *(4)* The idea was to utilize the nano-engineered properties of multilayers as shell structures formed around colloidal particles.

Results and Discussion

Multilayer Assembly on Colloidal Particles.
The main problem in transferring the layer-by-layer technology from flat surfaces to colloidal particles consists in the need to separate remaining free polyelectrolytes from the particles prior to performing the next deposition cycle. Several approaches have been studied to address this problem, including centrifugation, filtration, and so-called sequential addition of polyelectrolytes at matched concentration. *(4-6)* It should be mentioned that for scale-up purposes

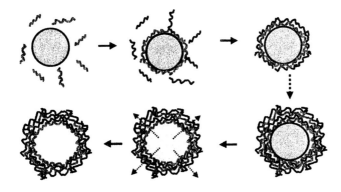

Figure 1. Consecutive adsorption of positively (gray) and negatively (black) charged polyelectrolytes onto negatively charged colloidal particles (a-d). After dissolution of the colloidal core (e), a suspension of polyelectrolyte capsules is obtained (f).

filtration often is the method of choice. *(6)* The progress of film formation, i.e. charge reversal and continuous layer growth, was monitored at each step by electrophoresis, dynamic light scattering, single particle light scattering (SPLS), and fluorescent intensity measurements. *(4,5)* For instance, changes in the particle charge (zeta-potential ξ) upon LbL-deposition of the polyanion/ polycation pair sodium poly(styrene sulfonate) (PSS) and poly(allylamine hydrochloride) (PAH) is illustrated in Figure 2. The ξ–potential alternates between positive and negative values, indicating the successful deposition of polyelectrolytes of opposite charges. The sequential layer growth has been verified using SPLS. (4,6)

In Figure 3, the intensity distribution of particles coated with 8 layers is compared to uncoated particles as the control. The adsorbed mass of the deposited layers can be derived from the peak shift in the intensity distribution. These data can be converted into a layer thickness of the adsorbed polyelectrolyte multilayers, assuming the refractive index is known. *(4)* The increase of the polyelectrolyte film thickness is proportional to the layer number (Figure 3). The mean polyelectrolyte layer thickness was found to be 1.5 nm in the case of PSS/PAH assembled from 0.5 M NaCl. It should be noted that the average layer thickness strongly depends upon both the polyelectrolytes being used and the salt concentration during the polyelectrolyte assembly. More rigid polymers and increasing salt concentrations lead to thicker adsorption layers.

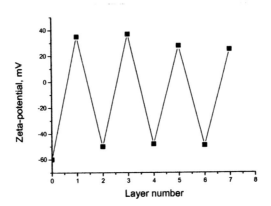

Figure 2. ξ-potential as a function of layer number for PSS/PAH coated poly-sterene latex particles. The particle diameter is 640 nm.

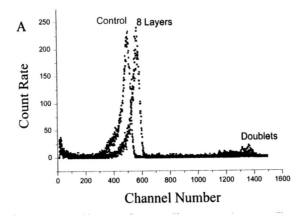

Figure 3. Normalized light scattering intensity distributions of PAH/PSS coated polysterene sulfate latex particles (diameter 640 nm). Particles with 8 layers are compared to uncoated ones (A). Shell thickness as a function of layer number (B).

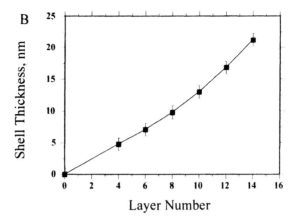

Figure 3. *Continued.*

LbL-Adsorption of Polyelectrolytes on Protein Aggregates and DNA Particles.

The multilayer assembly can be formed not only on solid particles like silica, polystyrene (PS) latex particles, or organic crystals, but also on "soft" particles formed just prior to the multilayer build-up, i.e. protein aggregates and compacted DNA. The use of micron-sized protein aggregates as templates for polyelectrolyte multilayer assembly was studied for lactate dehydrogenase, chemotrypsine, and catalyse microcrystals. *(7-9)* Polyelectrolyte multilayer coating of these aggregates captures the proteins inside the capsules and, in addition, provides a selective barrier for the diffusion of different species (substrates, inhibitors) from the exterior.

The general mechanism of protein encapsulation is illustrated in Figure 4, using the enzyme chymotrypsin, whose activity can be easily monitored, as the model protein. *(8)* In this case, the preformed protein aggregates serve as template for the multilayer formation instead of the solid colloidal particles shown earlier. Chymotrypsin precipitated immediately after mixing the enzyme with a saline solution, as monitored by the increasing turbidity of the suspension (Figure 4a,b). This aggregation process was reversible, depending on the NaCl concentration. Therefore, the enzyme precipitation could be easily optimized by varying the amount of sodium chloride. Due to the positive charge of chymotrypsin at pH 2.3, the negatively charged polyanion PSS was taken as the first layer of the multilayer assembly (Figure 4c), followed by PAH as the

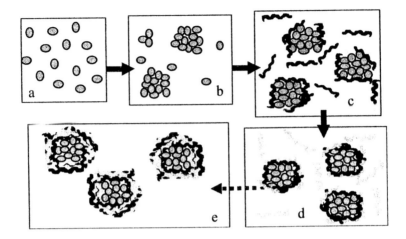

Figure 4. Scheme of layer-by-layer adsorption of polyelectrolytes onto protein aggregates formed in salt solution.

second, polycationic layer (Figure 4d), producing the multilayer aggregates displayed in Figure 4e.

A scanning electron micrograph of chymotrypsin aggregates coated with a (PSS/PAH/PSS) triple layer is shown in Figure 5. The morphology of the micron-sized aggregates appears to be amorphous. Each aggregate consists of smaller spherical protein particles, the so-called primary aggregates, with diameters in the order of 100-300 nm. Characteristic features of the aggregates are a very high surface area and the presence of pores. Such structures are assumed to form as a result of a secondary aggregation of the polyelectrolyte-coated primary aggregates. This secondary structure is preserved by the sequential deposition of additional polyelectrolyte layers. Generally, factors such as the duration of aggregate growth, the nature of the polyelectrolytes, and the number of layers will influence composition and morphology of these aggregates. Studies of the enzymatic activity revealed that encapsulated chymotrypsin retained about 70% of its original activity. The encapsulated enzyme is protected against high molecular weight inhibitors, which cannot permeate the capsule wall and influence the enzyme functionality. At pH > 8, chymotrypsin is released from the capsules due to the pH-dependent permeability change of the (PSS/PAH/PSS) triple layer. *(8)*

In addition to proteins, condensed DNA particles with a size range of about 50-100 nm have been encapsulated by a polyelectrolyte triple layer, producing

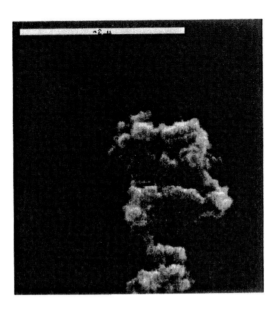

Figure 5. Scanning electron micrograph of protein aggregates covered by a PSS/PAH/PSS polyelectrolyte triple layer. Scale bar is 2μm.

stable suspensions. The uptake of these particles by biological cells was enhanced compared to naked DNA if the outer layer contained appropriate receptors as evidenced by sequential gene expression. *(10-12)*

Hollow polyelectrolyte capsules with a determined size, shape, and wall thickness will form if the cores of a shell-core aggregate can be decomposed without affecting the shell stability (Figure 1). To date, various organic and inorganic cores, i.e. melamine formaldehyde (MF) particles, organic crystals, carbonate particles, and biological cells were used as templates for the fabrication of these hollow capsules. Decomposition can be achieved by different processes, such as low pH for MF and carbonate particles, organic water-miscible solvents for organic crystals, and strong oxidizing agents (i.e. NaOCl) for biological cells. *(5,13-15)*

Capsule Wall Permeation of Small Molecules

Evaluation of the potential use of polyelectrolyte coatings in controlled drug release systems requires an understanding of the permeation of small polar molecules (molecular weights < 500 D) through the polyelectrolyte shells. It would be advantageous to be able to decrease the layer permeability for small molecules once they are encapsulated, i.e. by increasing the wall thickness through deposition of additional polyelectrolyte layers. This approach has been verified using the small polar fluorescent marker fluorescein as the model compound. *(16)* Microparticles of fluorescein with an average size of about 5 µm were coated with different numbers of PSS/PAH polyelectrolyte double layers at pH 2, where fluorescein is insoluble in water and both polyelectrolytes are strongly charged. Hence the resulting multilayer films contain the same amount of amino and sulfur groups (Figure 6a-d). After formation of the multilayer shells, the core was dissolved by increasing the pH from 2 to 8, where fluorescein particles rapidly dissolved (Figure 6e-g).

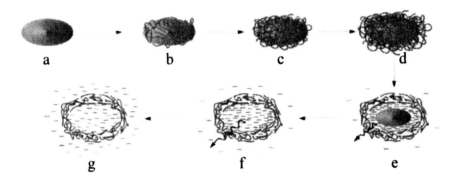

Figure 6. Scheme of the polyelectrolyte multilayer deposition process and subsequent core dissolution. The initial steps (a-d) involve stepwise shell formation on a fluorescein core. After the desired number of polyelectrolyte layers is deposited, the coated particles are exposed to pH 8 (e) and core dissolution with fluorescein penetration into the bulk is initiated, resulting in fully dissolved cores and empty capsules (f). (See page 7 of color insert.)

The release of fluorescein was monitored by increasing fluorescence in the bulk. Fluorescence spectroscopy is a convenient tool for the determination of the core dissolution rate because the fluorescence of dye molecules contained within the core is completely suppressed by self-quenching. Figure 7 displays typical time-dependent fluorescence curves of fluorescein particles covered with multilayers of different thickness (9, 13, 15, and 18 layers), obtained after switching the pH from 2 to 8. For comparison, the fluorescence curve for uncoated fluorescein particles (0 layer) is shown as well. After a comparatively short induction period, the fluorescence intensity increases at a constant rate and finally reaches a plateau. The initially slow fluorescence increase can be explained by the start of the core dissolution. At this stage of the process the structure of the polyelectrolyte multilayer may change because of the nascent osmotic pressure coming from dissolved fluorescein molecules. Shortly after the beginning of the core dissolution, the concentration of fluorescein inside the capsules becomes constant and almost saturated, since a steady state situation between progressing core dissolution and permeation is established. One may assume a constant concentration gradient between the shell interior and the bulk because the bulk solution can be considered as being infinitely diluted. Therefore, the rate of fluorescein penetration through the polyelectrolyte layers to the bulk becomes constant, resulting in the constant increase of the intensity curves. This state corresponds to the stage of dissolution depicted in Figure 6f. However, the slope of the linear region decreases with the number of polyelectrolyte layers, indicating reduced fluorescein permeation with increasing layer thickness. After complete core dissolution, the fluorescein concentration inside the shell equilibrates with the bulk. The driving force for diffusion decreases and the release levels off.

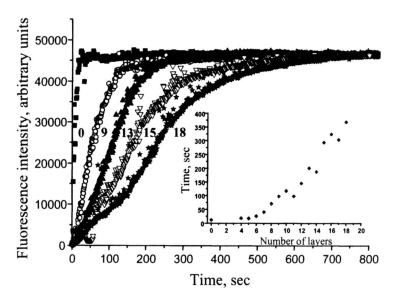

Figure 7. Release of fluorescein measured by fluorescence increase obtained by dissolving fluorescein particles covered with shells of different thickness (9, 13, 15, and 18 layers), compared with naked (0) fluorescein particles. The insert shows time of complete dissolution as a function of layer number.

The release of fluorescein can be discussed more quantitatively. *(16)* The permeation of fluorescein through the shell wall is described by its permeability. Equation (1) combines a flux (J) with parameters of the system and the rate of change of fluorescein concentration, c^e, in the bulk. When this rate is constant, one may easily calculate the permeability (P) from the slope of the fluorescence increase

$$\frac{dc^e}{dt}V_0 = J = P \cdot \left(c^i - c^e\right) \cdot S \qquad (1)$$

where V_0 is the volume of solution, J is the fluorescein flux through the capsule walls, S is the total surface area, and $\left(c^i - c^e\right)$ is the difference between the fluorescein concentration inside (c^i) and outside (c^e) the capsules.

The interior of the capsules contains a saturated fluorescein solution, c^s, at a concentration of 25 mg/ml. Hence, the concentration difference at the beginning of the process on the right side of Eq. 1 can be safely replaced by $c^i=c^s$. The capsules were assumed spherical with an average diameter of 5 μm. The permeability, P, can thus be calculated from

$$P = \frac{dc/dt \cdot V_0}{c^s \cdot S} \qquad (2)$$

The permeability for 8 to 18 layers was calculated to be approx. 10^{-8}m/s. Assuming a single polyelectrolyte layer thickness of 2 nm, the permeability can be converted into a diffusion coefficient (D) by means of multiplying the permeability with the shell wall thickness. The calculated diffusion coefficients are in the order of 10^{-15}m^2/s.

If the permeability of the polyelectrolyte multilayers is caused by diffusion through an entangled polymer network, it should scale with the inverse of the layer thickness. The time of complete release as a function of layer numbers is shown as insert in Figure 7. As can be seen, the diffusion properties of polyelectrolyte multilayers for small molecules become significant when the number of layers exceeds 8 or about 15-20 nm thickness. This result is supported by another study demonstrating that the conformation of the first eight layers differs from that of further assembled layers. (17) These thicker layers are more dense, resulting in a fivefold reduction of the estimated diffusion coefficient. These studies demonstrate the ability to control the penetration of small molecules by the layer thickness, although this observation has only been made for the system PSS/PAH and might be different for other polyelectrolyte capsules.

Polyelectrolyte complexes are known to be very sensitive to the presence of salt. (18) Therefore, the permeability coefficient of polyelectrolyte multilayers strongly depends on the ionic strength of the solution. Figure 8 shows the time-dependent change in fluorescence intensity of solutions containing increasing amounts of sodium chloride. The small salt ions partially form ion pairs with oppositely charged groups of the polyelectrolytes, making the polyelectrolyte multilayers more diffusive. (17) As shown in the insert of Figure 8, the permeability coefficient derived from the release curves shows a dramatic increase of one order of magnitude upon increasing the NaCl concentration from 1 to 500 mM.

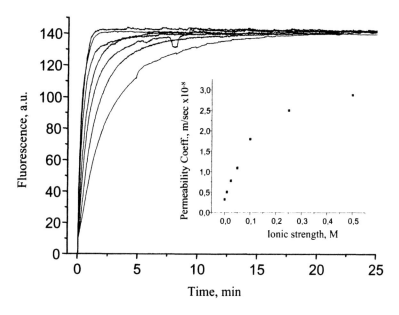

Figure 8. Fluorescein release profiles obtained at different NaCl concentrations (1, 10, 25, 50, 100, 250, 500 mM, bottom to top). The insert illustrates permeability coefficient dependence on ionic strengths.

In conclusion, polyelectrolyte multilayer shells of sufficient thickness (10-20 nm) assembled around cores consisting of low molecular weight compounds provide barrier properties for their release under conditions where the core is dissolved. Increasing the shell thickness above 20 nm, however, might cause difficulties for the release due to the density of these multilayer capsule walls. Nevertheless, multilayer coating of micro- and nanoparticles is a promising approach for fabrication of systems with prolonged and controlled release properties. The release can be adjusted by the number of assembled polyelectrolyte layers. A large variety of synthetic polyelectrolytes with different properties, polysaccharides, and other biopolymers used for multilayer assembly provide many possibilities to tune the release properties of the shells, ensure their biocompatibility, and allow finding the "best fitting" shells for the respective cores. The assembling of shells using the LbL technique opens new pathways for biotechnological applications, where controlled and sustained release of a substance is required. Many problems connected with drug formulation, release, and delivery, i.e. controlling the concentration in the organism and periodicity of its reception, might be resolved by the formation of shells on precipitates and nanocrystals. Adding targeting properties to poly-electrolyte layers seems to be feasible. This way the affinity of polyelectrolyte multilayer-coated drugs to specific tissues can be enhanced.

Encapsulation of Macromolecules

As discussed above, small molecules can permeate through polyelectrolyte multilayer shells if the film thickness is within the 10-20 nm range, while large molecular weight compounds are excluded. Hence, these polyelectrolyte capsules have semipermeable properties. However, several approaches have been developed that allow loading macromolecules into hollow polyelectrolyte capsules after the core has been decomposed. The first approach comprises controlled opening and closing of pores within the capsule walls. Pores can be created by segregation within polyelectrolyte multilayers, caused either by pH or solvent change. Polyelectrolyte multilayers undergo a transition at a pH close to the pK value of the respective polyelectrolytes. The accumulation of charge within the network of entangled polymers results in segregation and pore formation, large enough for macromolecules to permeate the capsule walls. This process is completely reversible upon changing the pH, allowing to trap macromolecules inside the capsules. Several macromolecules, such as albumin, chymotrypsin, and dextrin have been encapsulated by this protocol. *(19,20)* This reversible segregation within polyelectrolyte multilayers can also be introduced by adding another solvent to the aqueous solution, i.e. ethanol. Recently, urease encapsulation by solvent variation and its enzymatic activity has been studied. *(21)*

Another approach consists in the precipitation of macromolecules (or polymers) onto the surface of colloidal particles, encapsulation of the core/macromolecule complex with a LbL polyelectrolyte shell, and removal of the core, leaving the macromolecules dissolved within the capsule interior. An appropriate selection of particle concentration, polymers, and speed of deposition can achieve a smooth coverage of the core by macromolecules. The process is similar to the protein precipitation discussed earlier, with the exception that the precipitation now occurs in the presence of colloidal particles. The three stages of this process are shown in Figure 9: i) Precipitation of macromolecules (or polymers) on a colloidal surface (Figure 9a-c); ii) Encapsulation of precipitated macromolecules and colloidal particles within a stable polyelectrolyte shell (Figure 9d); and iii) Decomposition of the core and removal of the decomposition products by permeation through the capsule shell (Figure 9e), while the macromolecules dissolve and remain inside the capsule interior (Figure 9f-h). This approach has been tested for the encapsulation of non-ionic polysaccharides, i.e. dextrin, and the polyelectrolyte system PSS/PAH. *(22)* Dextrin was precipitated by dropwise addition of ethanol, while the shell formation was triggered by the presence of multivalent ions such as Me^{3+} and CO_3^{2-}, which form insoluble complexes with PSS and PAH, respectively. Some swelling of the capsules after polymer dissolution was observed due to osmotic pressure. The amount of polymer-load per capsule depends on the amount of added polymers divided by the number of colloidal particles harvesting the precipitating polymers. The possible loss of polymers due to breakage of some capsules did not exceed 10-15%. The simplicity of this procedure allows filling these capsules with very small, less than nanogram, quantities of polymers.

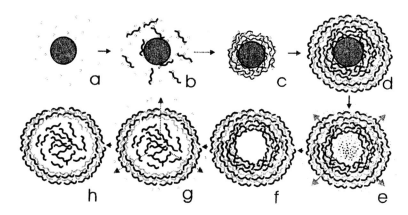

Figure 9. Schematic illustration of the preparation of capsules loaded with polyelectrolytes.

Additional advantages of this loading approach are: (i) The size distribution of the capsules is determined by the size distribution of the cores used as templates; (ii) The loaded polymers can be dosed easily and distributed homogeneously in each capsule; and (iii) There are possibilities to load the capsules with several different substances. The last point has not yet been proven, but it seems feasible to precipitate different macromolecules either sequentially or at the same time (if they precipitate under the same condition) on the surface of colloidal particles. The important issue here is the compatibility of each precipitation step and the LbL-formation of a stable polyelectrolyte shell. Encapsulated macromolecules are trapped inside the capsule as long as the shell remains impermeable for these molecules. This situation could be utilized for the fabrication of enzymatic microreactors if small molecules, such as substrates and reaction products, could diffuse freely through the capsule wall and interact with the trapped enzyme. At the end of an enzymatic reaction, the encapsulated macromolecules could be released after a certain change in pH or salt concentration.

Precipitation of Dyes Inside Capsules – Model of Drug Encapsulation

The semipermeable properties of the capsule walls create different physico-chemical conditions of the capsule interior compared to the exterior, which can be used to conduct chemical or physical reactions. For instance, encapsulation of a polyanion inside a capsule will cause the pH value to decrease because protons will permeate into the capsule to compensate the negative charges and achieve electroneutrality of the inner solution. The pH will be close to the pK value of the polyanion but lower than the pH of the exterior. This pH gradient can be used to precipitate small organic molecules inside the capsules, creating a concentration gradient of dissolved molecules inside and outside the capsule. As a consequence, more molecules will permeate into the capsule. *(23)*

This pH-dependent loading/precipitation approach could be utilized for drug encapsulation. The dye carboxytetramethylrhodamine (CR) has been used as a model compound to study the feasibility of this approach. CR has a pH-dependent solubility and becomes insoluble at pH < 3.5. In the presence of capsules filled with the polyanion PSS, maintaining an inner pH near 2.5, CR molecules will migrate into the capsules, be subjected to the low pH, and begin to precipitate. *(24)* Figure 10 displays a SEM image of capsules filled with CR precipitates.

The same loading/precipitation principle can be applied by establishing a polarity gradient across the capsule walls by encapsulation of hydrophilic polymers. Immersed in a water/organic solvent mixture, these capsules will keep a higher water content inside the capsules than outside, as demonstrated using a fluorescent polarity marker. *(25)* Many poorly water soluble molecules, i.e. drugs, can be dissolved in water/organic solvent mixtures (i.e. water/acetone mixtures) with an overall high ratio of the organic solvent. After migration into the water-rich interior of a capsule, these molecules will precipitate. This process can be supported by controlled evaporation of the organic solvent from the bulk, forcing even more molecules to migrate into the capsules and, eventually, precipitate, resulting in an aqueous suspension of capsules containing precipitated organic molecules. Interestingly, these precipitates did not produce X-ray diffraction signals unless they were annealed. This observation indicates that the precipitates are either amorphous or exist of nanocrystallites too small to be captured by the X-ray beam. *(25)* An amorphous or nanocrystalline morphology could be a highly desirable feature for many drug applications since it facilitates dissolution and hence bioavailability.

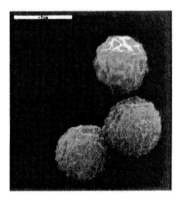

Figure 10. Scanning electron micrograph of CR precipitates formed in capsules loaded with PSS. Scale bar is 5 μm.

Conclusions

Uniformity, simplicity, and versatility are major advantages of the LBL polyelectrolyte capsule formation technology. The particular aspects of this approach are summarized in Figure 11. A colloidal particle serves as the initial template. Seemingly any colloidal particle ranging in size from 50 nm to tens of microns can be used as a template to fabricate the shell, i.e. organic and inorganic particles, drug nanocrystals, biological cells, protein aggregates, and condensed DNA. The shell can be composed of a variety of materials, depending on the desired application, stability, comparability, or other specific requirements.

Selective shell permeability facilitates trapping macromolecules inside the capsules. These macromolecules can be encapsulated following different approaches, i.e. by precipation from solution or precipitation on the surface of colloidal particles *prior* to formation of the encapsulating shell. Alternatively, the polyelectrolyte shells can be reversibly opened and closed by changes of the pH and ionic strength of the solution or by solvent exchange, allowing encapsulation of macromolecules *after* formation of the shells. These different loading approaches result in different capsule sizes, monodispersities, macromolecule concentrations inside the capsules, encapsulation efficiencies, and possibilities to incorporate several substances in one capsule. Incorporation of appropriate (bio)degradable macromolecules into the shell walls would allow the release of the capsule content at a desired timescale. Enzyme trapping into capsules whose shells are impermeable for the enzyme but permeable for small molecules, i.e. reactants and products, will allow fabrication of microreactors.

264

The enzyme is protected against high molecular weight inhibitors and proteolytic agents, while preserving most of its initial activity. Products of one or multi-step enzymatic reactions in the capsules could be released from or remain inside the capsules. The capsules themselves could be easily removed from solution by filtration, centrifugation, or by application of a magnetic field if magnetic particles were used as layer constituents. Chemical treatment of the capsules after their formation has not been discussed in this contribution. However, further modifications, i.e. cross-linking of the preformed capsules, could significantly change capsule properties, such as permeability or stability. Research on this topic is under way.

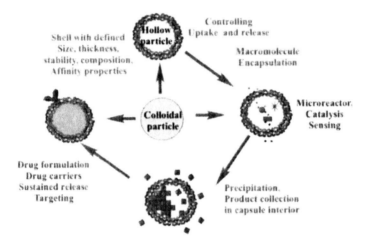

Figure 11. Comprehensive illustration of applications of the step-wise shell formation on colloidal particles. (See page 7 of color insert.)

Acknowledgements

The author thanks the Sofia Kovalevskaya Program of the Alexander von Humboldt Foundation, and the German Ministry of Education and Research. Professor H. Möhwald is gratefully acknowledged for continuous support and stimulating discussions, as well as Professor E. Donath, Professor N. I. Larionova, A. A. Antipov, I. L. Radtchenko, and N. Balabushevich for fruitfull collaborations over the years.

265

References

1. 1. Iler, R.K. *J. Colloid Interface Sci.* **1966**, *21*, 569.
2. Lee, H.; Kepley, L.J.; Hong, H.G.; Akhter, S.; Mallouk, T.E. *J. Phys. Chem.,* **1988**, *92*, 2597.
3. Decher, G.; Hong, J.-D. *Macromol. Chem., Macromol. Symp.* **1991**, *46*. 321.
4. Sukhorukov, G. B.; Donath, E.; Lichtenfeld , H.; Knippel, E.; Knippel, M; Budde, A.; Möhwald, H. *Colloids & Surfaces A* **1998**, *137*, 253.
5. Donath, E.; Sukhorukov, G.B.; Caruso, F.; Davis, S.; Möhwald. H. *Angew. Chemie, Inter. Ed. Eng.* **1998**, *37*, 2201.
6. Voigt, A.; Lichtenfeld, H.; Zastrow, H.; Sukhorukov, G.B.; Donath E.; Möhwald, H. *Industrial & Engineering Chemistry Research* **1999**, *38*, 4037.
7. Bobreshova, M.E.; Sukhorukov, G.B.; Saburova, E.A.; Elfimova, L.I.; Sukhorukov, B.I.; Sharabchina, L.I. *Biophysics* **1999**, *44*, 813.
8. Balabushevitch, N.G.; Sukhorukov, G.B; Moroz, N.A.; Larionova, N.I.; Donath, E.; Möhwald H. *Biotechnology & Bioengineering* **2001**, *76*, 207.
9. Caruso, F.; Trau, D.; Möhwald H.; Renneberg, R. *Langmuir* **2000**, *16*, 1485.
10. Trubetskoy, V.S.; Loomis, A.; Hagstrom, J.E.; Budker, V.G.; Wolff, J.A. *Nucleic Acids Research* **1999**, *27*, 3090.
11. Finsinger, D.; Remy, J.S.; Erbacher, P., Koch, C.; Plank, C. *Gene Therapy* **2000**, *7*, 1183.
12. Dallüge, R.; Haberland, A.; Zaitsev, S.; Schneider, M.; Zastrow, H.; Sukhorukov, G.B.; Böttger, M. *Biochim. Biophys. Acta,* **2002**, *1576*, 45.
13. Antipov, A.A.; Sukhorukov, G.B.; Leporatti, S.; Radtchenko, I.L.; Donath, E.; Möhwald, H. *Colloids & Surfaces A* **2002**, *198-200*, 535.
14. Caruso, F.; Wenjun, Y.W.; Trau D.; Renneberg, R. *Langmuir* **2000**, *16*, 8932.
15. Neu, B.; Voigt, A.; Mitlöhner, R.; Leporatti, S.; Donath, E.; Gao, C.Y.; Kiesewetter, H.; Möhwald, H.; Meiselman, H.J.; Bäumler, H. *J. Microencapsulation* **2001**, *18*, 385.
16. Antipov, A.A, Sukhorukov, G.B, Donath, E, Möhwald, H. *J. Phys. Chem. B* **2001**, *105*, 2281.
17. Klitzing, R. v.; Möhwald, H. *Macromolecules* **1996**; *29*, 6901.
18. Kabanov, V.; Zezin, A. *Pure Appl. Chem.* **1984**, *56*, 343.
19. Sukhorukov, G.B.; Antipov, A.A.; Voigt, A.; Donath, E.; Möhwald, H. *Macromol. Rapid Com.* **2001**, *22*, 44.
20. Tiourina, O.P.; Antipov, A.A.; Sukhorukov, G.B.; Larionova, N.L.; Lvov, Y; Möhwald, H. *Macromol. Biosci.* **2001**, *1*, 209.
21. Lvov, Y.; Antipov, A. A.; Mamedov, A.; Möhwald, H.; Sukhorukov, G. B. *Nano Lett.* **2001**, *1*, 125.

22. Radtchenko, I.L.; Sukhorukov, G.B.; Möhwald, H. *Colloids & Surfaces A* **2002**, *202*, 127.
23. Sukhorukov, G.B.; Donath, E.; Brumen, M; Möhwald, H. *J. Phys. Chem. B* **1999**, *103*, 6434.
24. Sukhorukov, G.B. In *Microspheres, Microcapsules & Liposomes*; Arshady, R.; Guyot, A., Eds.; *Dendrimers, Assemblies, Nanocomposites;* Citus Books: London, UK, 2002, Vol. 5, pp 111-147.
25. Radtchenko, I.L.; Sukhorukov, G.B.; Möhwald, H. *Int. J. Pharmaceutics* **2002**, *in press.*
26. Ibarz, G.; Dähne, L.; Donath, E.; Möhwald, H. *Macromol. Rap. Com.* **2002**, *23*, 474.

Chapter 19

The Cost of Optimal Drug Delivery: Reducing and Preventing the Burst Effect in Matrix Systems

Christopher S. Brazel* and Xiao Huang

Department of Chemical Engineering, The University of Alabama,
Tuscaloosa, AL 35487-0203
*Corresponding author: email: cbrazel@coe.eng.ua.edu

The burst effect is a major consideration in designing controlled release systems. In most pharmaceutical applications, the burst effect is regarded as an event to be avoided, even at the cost of using an overcoat to reduce the initial burst. At minimum, burst release leads to a loss in treatment efficacy, as drug is lost in an uncontrolled and unpredictable pattern. We used an experimental system to study the underlying mechanisms of burst release, focusing on small molecular weight solutes embedded in poly(vinyl alcohol), PVA, matrices. Surface desorption and pore diffusion were included in a mathematical model to predict the influence of system parameters on the early portion of the release process (which is considerably more sophisticated than the often used time-independent burst release term). The model parameters led us to investigate economically feasible methods to treat the matrices and minimize the burst effect. These methods include surface extraction and surface-preferential cross-linking, which have both been shown to reduce the burst effect in PVA systems.

Introduction

The burst effect is a major detrimental side effect of many controlled release systems, carrying the risk of exposing the patient to a local or temporal drug overdose. Besides being adverse to the patient, the burst effect is economically inefficient, as much of the often costly pharmaceutical agent is lost from a controlled release device and first-pass metabolized without thera-peutic effect. As a consequence, the effective lifetime of a drug formulation often decreases as illustrated in Figure 1.

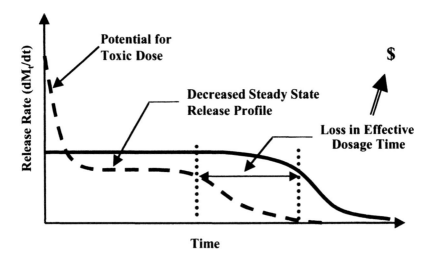

Figure 1. Potential impact of the burst effect on sustained release formulations (dashed curve) compared to a desired steady release profile (solid curve).

The burst effect continues to be a challenge in developing successful controlled release formulations, especially in hydrogel-based systems, where the burst related drug loss often accounts for a significant percentage of the total drug released. (*1-3*) Several diverse and often expensive methods have been applied to prevent the burst effect, i.e. encapsulation, surface coating of tablets, surface extraction, creation of devices with non-uniform drug distributions, and the use of two-part gelatin capsules. (*4-8*)

The burst effect has been noted primarily in systems with large surface area-to-volume ratio such as microspheres, carriers with large pores, and during the release of hydrophilic drugs and proteins with small molecular weights. The potential causes of the burst effect and some techniques preventing it have been reviewed in detail. (*2*) No one technique is a perfect solution to prevent burst in all types of controlled release devices, but many techniques add substantial cost due to additional processing or the requirement for additional excipients in the final pharmaceutical formulation. Because the burst effect is related to surface concentrations of drug in a solid formulation, methods used to control the burst are generally surface-related.

Surface coating is a widely-accepted approach to control the initial stages of drug release, with the coating thickness and material properties introducing a lag time that is almost invariably used to counteract the burst effect. (*9,10*) While the lag time can be desired in some oral drug delivery formulations, it is often undesired and actually prolongs the time it takes for drugs to be released and benefit the patient. A coating must be uniform and free of imperfections, thus a high level of quality control is required for this step, which is often conducted using fluidized-bed coating.

Surface extraction, an alternative approach to reduce the burst effect in matrix systems, was first reported by Lee. (*7*) This approach focused on removing the drug from the surface and concentrating it in the center of the controlled release device to create a sigmoidal drug distribution profile. The degree of burst was varied by varying the surface extraction time, resulting in drug release profiles with reduced burst effects. A major disadvantage of this technique is the often significant loss of loaded drug from the carrier, which has an economic impact on the pharmaceutical process, even if the extracted drug can be recycled. Nevertheless, surface extraction is being applied to reduce the initial burst. (*6,11,12*)

A number of researchers have investigated the effects of different physical parameters on sustained release. (*13-15*) However, the influence of parameters such as crosslinking ratio, drug loading concentration, and drug properties on the burst effect when using matrix controlled release devices has not been studied. Drug release from hydrogels is largely controlled by the difference between the molecular size of the drug and the mesh space within the matrix available for diffusion. Therefore it is conceivable that hydrogel design factors, i.e. the easily tunable parameters mentioned above, could be used to minimize the burst effect. We examined the burst effect in hydrogel systems based on poly(vinyl alcohol), PVA, focusing on small molecular weight hydrophilic solutes, which would be likely to release rapidly from porous hydrogel networks. Our goal was to develop an effective method to reduce the burst effect without influencing the overall release behavior. We also sought a technique that would minimize additional processing cost necessary to eliminate the burst effect.

Materials and Methods

The studies were performed using a drug delivery system based on a PVA hydrogel, crosslinked with glutaraldehyde as described elsewhere. (*16*) Briefly, linear PVA chains (MW 88,000; purchased from Acros Organics, Fairlawn, NJ) were dissolved in deionized water by heating at 90 °C for 24 hours before adding a crosslinking solution consisting of glutaraldehyde and small amounts of dilute methanol, acetic acid, and sulfuric acid solutions. Model solutes, including methylene blue, proxyphylline, and theophylline (all small molecular weight hydrophilic drugs), were incorporated at known concentrations during the crosslinking step. Crosslinked gels were formed as thin films by cross-linking the viscous solution between siliconized glass plates separated by Teflon spacers, kept at 37 °C for 24 hours. Disc-shaped samples of approxi-mately 15 mm in diameter by 0.9 mm in thickness were cut from the films using a cork borer. The release mechanism was swelling-controlled, which yields zero-order release kinetics as long as the polymer's relaxation time and solvent diffusion rate are on the same time scale. (*17*) Drug release was monitored using USP Type II dissolution cells (Distek Model 2100C) with deionized water at 37 °C as the release medium. The release solution was continuously circulated to a UV/vis spectrometer (Shimadzu Model UV-2401 PC), where the absorption at the peak band was measured using flow-through quartz cuvettes.

Surface extraction and surface-preferential crosslinking were used to reduce the burst effect in this hydrogel system.

Surface extraction. To remove excess drug from the outer layers of the delivery device, drug-filled dry samples were placed in deionized water for periods of time ranging from 1 to 10 minutes and thoroughly dried. The extracted quantity was measured using UV/vis spectroscopy. The dry drug samples were used for the release experiments.

Surface-Preferential Crosslinking. Following the initial, bulk crosslinking step to create the drug-loaded hydrogels, PVA can be crosslinked further at the surface by applying glutaraldehyde in acidic solution. (*18*) For example, the surface of a dry drug delivery device containing proxyphylline was dipped very briefly into a solution of glutaraldehyde and sulfuric acid. The exposure time was kept at about one second to restrict penetration of the aldehyde beyond a very thin surface layer. Additionally, the brief exposure to a solution was de-signed to minimize loss of proxyphylline during this procedure.

Results and Discussion

The burst effect is not easily observed in standard presentations displaying amount of drug released versus time curves (Figure 2). In contrast, graphs showing normalized drug release rate versus time curves clearly reveal the initial drug release behavior in PVA hydrogel systems (Figure 3). These figures also depict the importance of inter- and intramolecular crosslinking on the burst effect. Different concentrations of PVA in water were crosslinked in the presence of equivalent amounts of glutaraldehyde and proxyphylline to form hydrogels with the same crosslinking ratio and drug loading. The likelihood of intermolecular glutaraldehyde crosslinkages increases with the concentration of PVA, while more dilute solutions have a greater tendency to form intramolecular crosslinkages and, therefore, are generally less effective in creating a uniform three-dimensional network. These more loosely crosslinked networks lead to higher burst effects and overall release rates. Notably, the ratio of initial to sustained release rate did not change significantly by changing the PVA concentration.

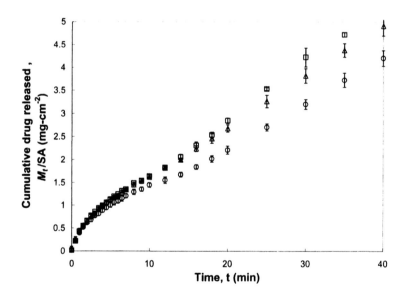

Figure 2. Effect of PVA concentration during crosslinking on proxyphylline release into DI Water at 37 °C. PVA concentrations during the crosslinking reaction were 5.5 (□), 7.0 (Δ) and 8.5 (○) wt%. All samples had a theoretical crosslinking ration of 1.5 mol%. Proxyphylline was loaded at 30 wt% of the PVA carrier. Error bars represent the standard deviation for three experiments.

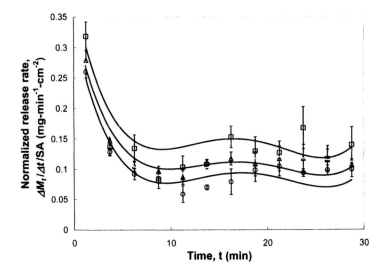

Figure 3. Data from Figure 2, replotted as release rate versus time. The release rate is normalized by the sample surface area exposed to the release media. Error bars represent standard deviations for three experiments. Lines shown are guides for the eyes.

To evaluate whether the burst effect can be altered by modifications in the physical properties of the release device, the ratio of initial release rate to sustained release rate, was defined as degree of burst (DB)

$$DB = \frac{\left(\dfrac{dM_t}{dt}\right)_{t<2.5\,\text{min}}}{\left(\dfrac{dM_t}{dt}\right)_{SS}} \qquad (1)$$

where M_t represents the mass of drug released in time t. In this equation, the numerator represents the initial or burst release rate, and the denominator represents the sustained release rate after the burst effect has diminished and the rate reaches steady state. Thus, an ideal system would have a DB value of 1 for no burst release, greater than 1 for the burst effect, and less than 1 if lag release was observed. The 2.5-minute time period was defined for the PVA system used since this was the time required for the release rate to drop to a steady state. The prescribed time interval would change for different release systems but is a good comparator for the parameters tested in this work.

Design Parameter Evaluation

Table 1 summarizes the degree of burst measured for three drugs at varying experimental parameters, including drug loading concentration, PVA crosslinking ratio, and PVA concentration prior to crosslinking. The degree of burst increased with the drug loading concentration for theophylline, but either decreased or gave inconclusive trends with the two other drugs. Increasing the bulk crosslinking ratio resulted in some reduction of the burst effect as shown in Table 1 for the release of methylene blue. However, this trend was not observed for proxyphylline and other drugs (data not shown). The final design factor tested was the PVA concentration used in the crosslinking reactions (see Figures 2 and 3). For the range studied (5.5 to 8.5 wt% PVA), there was no statistical difference in DB for proxyphylline release, although there may be a minimum concentration required to avoid a highly porous macrostructure and the related burst.

Table 1. Degree of burst for drug release from PVA hydrogels as a function of physical parameters of the drug/carrier system. Errors represent standard deviations for three to four experiments.

Model drug	Loading concn. (wt% drug)	PVA crosslinking ratio (mol glutar-aldehyde/mol vinyl alcohol)	PVA concn. during cross-linking (wt%)	Degree of burst, DB
Theo-phylline	5	1.5	7	2.40 ± 0.00
	10	1.5	7	2.97 ± 0.05
Proxy-phylline	5	1.5	7	2.87 ± 0.38
	10	1.5	7	2.81 ± 0.26
	15	1.5	7	2.40 ± 0.23
	20	1.5	7	2.89 ± 0.22
	30	1.5	5.5	2.55 ± 0.09
	30	1.5	7	2.50 ± 0.13
	30	1.5	8.5	2.67 ± 0.08
Methylene Blue	5	1.5	7	1.62 ± 0.21
	10	1	7	2.17 ± 0.15
	10	1.5	7	1.56 ± 0.51
	10	2	7	1.55 ± 0.02

The degree of burst displayed in Table 1 ranged from as low as 1.5 to about 3, but none of the design parameters showed significant improvement in reducing the burst effect on its own. The greatest factor influencing the degree of burst was the drug used in the respective experiments. Unfortunately for designing controlled release systems, the drug to be used is not a variable. The results indicate that the burst effect is especially prominent for low molecular weight, highly water-soluble drugs with low partition coefficient in the polymer matrix, such as proxyphylline. None of the parameters studied have shown potential to control the delivery of a drug at a specified rate without a burst effect at approximately twice the sustained rate. Thus, for these experimental parameters the burst release rate can be decreased only at the expense of decreasing the overall release rate.

Developing a Model to Represent the Burst Effect

Little work has been done to model the initial portion of drug release, partly because burst effects only a small portion of the drug release profile, and partly because burst is thought to be unpreventable in many cases. (3) A convection-diffusion model has been used to model the burst effect, adjusted to include phenomena thought to be responsible for the effect. (19,20) The model accounts for one-dimensional axial diffusion (as would be expected from thin disc-shaped samples with an aspect ratio of greater than 15), and assumes no drug-polymer interactions, which was verified experimentally by infrared spectroscopy. The convection-diffusion model is based on two complementary equations, modeling water (subscript 1) diffusion into polymer hydrogels (subscript 2), and simultaneously describing drug (subscript 3) diffusion through and out of the polymer network. Water absorption is related to convection and polymer relaxation through Equation 2

$$\frac{\partial C_1}{\partial t} = \frac{\partial}{\partial x}\left(D_{1,2}\frac{\partial C_1}{\partial x} - vC_1\right) \tag{2}$$

and the boundary and initial conditions

$$C_1(t > 0, x = \pm\delta) = C_{1,e}(1 - e^{-t/\lambda}) \tag{3}$$

$$C_1(t = 0, x) = 0 \tag{4}$$

$$\frac{\partial C_1}{\partial x}(t, x = 0) = 0 \qquad (5)$$

Here, C_1 is the solvent concentration in the gel; t is time; x is the axial coordinate through which the diffusion occurs; $D_{1,2}$ is the diffusion coefficient of the solvent in the hydrogel; v is the moving velocity of the solvent front in the swelling gel; δ is the position of the gel surface relative to the center, which is a function of time; $C_{1,e}$ represents the equilibrium solvent concentration; and λ the characteristic relaxation time of the polymer. Moving boundary con-ditions are used to solve this equation, as the network swells significantly during the water sorption process.

The other portion of the convection-diffusion model is used to describe diffusion and release of drug dispersed in the polymer network. This is described by Fick's law for the one-dimensional transport in a slab sample with thickness, 2δ,

$$\frac{\partial C_3}{\partial t} = \frac{\partial}{\partial x}(D_{3,21}\frac{\partial C_3}{\partial x}) \qquad (6)$$

with boundary and initial conditions

$$C_3(t = 0, x) = C_3^0 \qquad (7)$$

$$\frac{\partial C_3}{\partial x}(t, x = 0) = 0 \qquad (8)$$

$$C_3(t, x = \pm\delta) = 0 \qquad (9)$$

where C_3 is the drug concentration in the polymer matrix; $D_{3,21}$ is the drug diffusivity in the swelling gel; C_3^0 is the initial drug concentration. Diffusivities for both water and drug were estimated to be functions of concentration as described by Fujita. *(21)*

Without modifying Equations (2-9), the polymer relaxation time, λ, is the only system-modifiable parameter in the convection-diffusion equations that has a significant effect on the burst effect. This was confirmed experimentally and led to further investigation of surface-crosslinked hydrogels with a gradient in polymer relaxation to control the initial period of drug release as is described later.

Two modifications were made to the convection-diffusion model to more accurately describe the burst effect in hydrogel systems. First, the front velocity, v, was modified to reflect pore diffusion at the beginning of water uptake, which occurs at a faster rate than diffusion between the polymer chains within the mesh. The front velocity was modeled in three stages.

(i) An early stage, where front velocity is a function of time

$$v = v_o \exp(-t/\alpha) \tag{10}$$

where α is the time constant for pore diffusion;

(ii) a middle stage, where front velocity is constant, and less than the initial velocity by a factor, b,

$$v = \frac{v_o}{b} \tag{11}$$

(iii) and the final stage, after fronts meet in the center of the sample,

$$v = 0 \tag{12}$$

Using the non-constant front velocity term to account for pore diffusion, modeled water uptake data had a more closely fit to experimental data than with the original convection-diffusion model (Figure 4). Here, the convection model showed a modest lag at the beginning of the swelling process, which was removed when the front velocity was changed. The new term provides a better, though still imperfect, model of the initial behavior of hydrogel-based controlled release systems when hydrated.

To incorporate the surface desorption into the transport model, the perfect sink boundary condition, Equation (9), was replaced by the surface desorption kinetics

$$\frac{\partial C_3}{\partial t}(t, x = \delta) = k_d C_3 \tag{13}$$

$$C_3(t, x = \pm\delta) = C_3^0 \exp(-k_d t).$$ (14)

Here, k_d is the desorption constant for drug on the surface of the hydrogel leaving the network. This modification takes into consideration that drug initially located on the surface may be rapidly released, as the only release barrier is the desorption process.

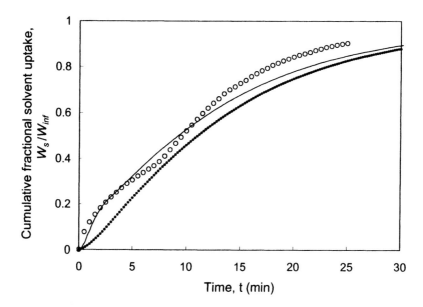

Figure 4. Model results for water uptake using the convection-diffusion model with constant (dotted line) and changing (solid line) front velocity, compared to experimental swelling data of 10 wt% theophylline-loaded PVA samples in 37°C DI water. Samples were made from 7 wt% aqueous solutions of PVA and crosslinked at 1.5 mol% (o). Model parameters used were: $\delta_0 = 0.062$ cm; $D_1^0 = 7.00\times10^{-5}$ cm²/min; $\lambda = 2.5$ min; $v_0 = 0.042$ cm/min; and $b = 14$ for the pore diffusion time constant.

After incorporating both the non-constant front velocity behavior and the desorption boundary condition into the model, prediction of the early stages of water uptake and drug release were sufficiently accurate (Figure 5).

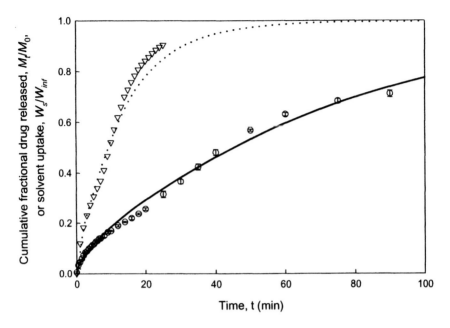

Figure 5. Comparison of model results for drug release (solid line) and solvent uptake (dotted line) to experimental data for drug release (o) and water uptake (▽). Experimental results were for release from 10 wt% theophylline-loaded PVA samples in 37°C DI water. Samples were made from 7 wt% aqueous solutions of PVA and crosslinked at 1.5 mol%. Model parameters were: $\delta_0 = 0.062cm$; $D_1^0 = 7.00\times10^{-5}\ cm^2/min$; $D_3^0 = 7.00\times10^{-5}\ cm^2/min$; $\lambda = 2.5\ min$, $k_d = 8min^{-1}$; $v_0 = 0.042\ cm/min$; $b = 14$.

Minimization of the Burst Effect

The potential of surface extraction to reduce the burst effect in hydrogels was confirmed experimentally using proxyphylline-loaded PVA hydrogels. At first glance, this technique is highly effective in burst reduction (Table 2). For example, a 2-minute extraction effectively reduced the burst effect (DB = 1.27) without significantly altering the long-term release profile. However, surface extraction has an inherent flaw in that much of the drug is removed from the device and must be recycled (if possible) to aid in economical processing. As shown in Table 2, over 8 wt% of loaded proxyphylline was extracted from the hydrogels within the 2-minute extraction. This amount increased to 22 wt% after a 10-minute extraction, and would be even more pronounced in micro-sphere systems where the surface area-to-volume ratio is significantly higher.

Furthermore, extraction times longer than 2 minutes were shown to decrease the steady state release rate. In summary, surface extraction is a simple tech-nique to minimize the burst effect but it may not be the most economical method.

Table 2. Degree of burst and amount of drug extracted for proxyphylline release from surface-extracted PVA hydrogel samples.

Extraction time (min)	Degree of burst, DB	Amount of drug extracted (% of drug load)
0	2.50 ± 0.13	0
1	1.57 ± 0.17	4.74 ± 0.47
2	1.27 ± 0.08	8.13 ± 0.26
5	1.33 ± 0.11	14.08 ± 0.93
10	1.49 ± 0.30	22.33 ± 1.91

Surface-preferential crosslinking, on the other hand, offers numerous advantages in processing and optimizing drug release profiles. This technique can be applied in the order of seconds and is less expensive than the well-utilized method of adding a coating layer to the release device to prevent burst. PVA hydrogel samples that were placed in a crosslinking solution of glutar-aldehyde showed a significant drop in the initial release rate (Table 3).

Table 3. Degree of burst and amount of drug extracted for proxyphylline release from surface preferential crosslinked PVA hydrogel samples.

Glutaraldehyde concn. in surface crosslinking soln. (wt%)	Degree of burst, DB	Amount of drug extracted (% of drug load)	Lag time in release profile (min)
0	2.50 ± 0.13	0	0
3.3	1.08 ± 0.09	0.02	0
10.0	0.09 ± 0.07	0.02	30

Perhaps even more important, the long term release rate was kept at nearly the same level as found for systems with no further treatment (Figure 4). The degree of burst for proxyphylline released from PVA samples surface-crosslinked in 3.3 wt% glutaraldehyde solutions dropped to 1.0 within statistical error, reducing the burst release without reducing the steady state release rate. Increasing the concentration of the surface crosslinking solution resulted in a lag profile, tunable by the concentration of glutaraldehyde used and the length of time a hydrogel is exposed to this solution. Because the sur-face layers on these samples are highly crosslinked, the mesh space available for diffusion at the early stages of release is diminished. Another significant finding using this technique was that less than 0.2 wt% of the loaded proxy-phylline (compared to 8 wt% using surface extraction) was removed from the sample due to the brief contact between the dry drug-loaded hydrogel and the crosslinking solution.

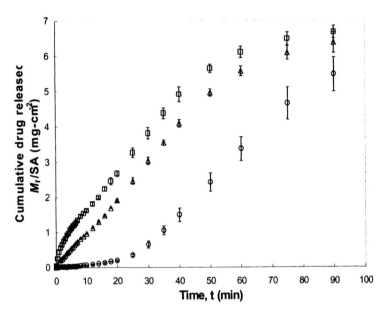

Figure 6. Proxyphylline release profiles after surface-preferential crosslinking using glutaraldehyde at concentrations of 3.3 (Δ) and 10.0 (○) wt%, and a control of untreated PVA hydrogels (□). Hydrogels were formed from 7 wt% aqueous PVA solutions, with a nominal crosslinking ratio of 1.5 mol%. Proxy-phylline was loaded at 30 wt%. Error bars represent standard deviations for three experiments.

Conclusions

The burst effect is a significant problem in many drug delivery strategies, and has not been adequately modeled for hydrogel systems. By incorporating two new phenomenological behaviors (non-constant glassy/rubbery front velo-city, and surface desorption) into the convection-diffusion model for water uptake and drug release, the model can predict drug release profiles, including the burst effect, more accurately.

Surface-preferential crosslinking was found to reproducibly alter the initial drug release profile, diminishing the burst, or even creating a controllable lag time. This technique can be easily applied to oral drug delivery systems, for any crosslinkable polymer-based material in geometries ranging from micro-spheres to tablets. Surface-preferential crosslinking has several advantages over other techniques used to reduce the burst effect:

- Minimal addition to processing (especially compared to fluidized-bed coating);
- Successful prevention of the burst effect without reduction in post-burst sustained release rates;
- Economical use of drug, as a minimal amount of drug was removed during treatment;
- Applicability to systems of all geometries and sizes;
- Reproducible, predictable behavior; and
- Ability to tune burst, eliminate burst, or create a lag release profile.

Other methods used to modify the burst release in PVA hydrogel systems included hydrogel design parameters and surface-extraction. While none of the design factors (crosslink ratio, drug loading concentration, or PVA concentration) were successful at reducing the degree of burst, surface extraction reduced the initial release rates, though at the expense of significant drug lost in the extraction.

The surface-preferential crosslinking technique can be used in existing process equipment such as a fluidized-bed coater for microspheres, or spray-coating systems for tablets. The process can be adapted for systems beyond PVA, and can also be applied to a number of pharmaceutical formulations with both therapeutic and economic advantages.

References

1. Batycky, R.P.; Hanes, J.; Langer, R.; Edwards, D.A. *J. Pharm. Sci.* **1997**, *86*, 1464-1477.
2. Patil, N.S.; Dordick, J.S.; Rethwisch, D.G. *Biomater.* **1996**, *17*, 2343-2350.
3. Huang, X.; Brazel, C.S. *J. Control. Rel.* **2001**, *73*, 121-136.
4. Pekarek, K.J.; Jacob, J.S.; Mathiowitz, E. *Mat. Res. Soc. Symp. Proc.* **1994**, *331*, 97-101.
5. Conte, U.; Maggi, L.; Colombo, P.; La Manna, A. *J. Control. Rel.* **1993**, *26*, 39-47.
6. Mallapragada, S.K.; Peppas, N.A.; Colombo, P. *J. Biomed. Mat. Res.* **1997**, *36*, 125-30.

7. Lee, P.I. *Polymer* **1984**, *25*, 973-978.
8. Lee, P.I., *J. Control. Rel.* **1986**, *4*, 1-7.
9. Lu, S.; Ramirez, W.F.; Anseth, K.S. *AIChE J.* **1998**, *44*, 1689-1696.
10. Wheatley, M.A.; Chang, M.; Park, E.; Langer, R. *J. Appl. Polym. Sci.* **1991**, *43*, 2123-2135.
11. Wang, H.T.; Schmitt, E.; Flanagan, D.R.; Linhart, R.J. *J. Control. Rel.* **1991**, *17*, 23-32.
12. Jameela, S.R.; Suma, N.; Jayakrishnan, A. *J. Biomater. Sci. Polym. Edn.* **1997**, *8*, 457-466.
13. Brazel, C.S.; Peppas, N.A. *STP Pharma Sci.* **1999**, *9*, 473-485.
14. Davidson, G.W.R. III; Peppas, N.A. *J. Control. Rel.* **1986**, *3*, 243-258.
15. Domb, A.; Davidson, G.W.R. III; Sanders, L.M. *J. Control. Rel.* **1990**, *14*, 133-144.
16. Huang, X.; Brazel, C.S. *Chem. Eng. Comm.* **2003**, *In press.*
17. Brazel, C.S.; Peppas, N.A. *Polymer* **1999**, *40*, 3383-3398.
18. Evangelista, R.A.; Sefton, M.V. *Biomaterials* **1986**, *7*, 206-211.
19. Narasimhan, B. In *Handbook of Pharmaceutical Controlled Release Technology*; Wise, D.L. et al., Eds.; Marcel Dekker: New York, 2000.
20. Brazel, C.S.; Peppas, N.A. *Eur. J. Pharm. and Biopharm.* **2000**, *49*, 47-58.
21. Fujita, H. *Fortschr. Hochpolym.-Forsch.* **1961**, *3*, 1-47.

Chapter 20

Biodegradable Nanoparticles as New Transmucosal Drug Carriers

María J. Alonso* and Alejandro Sánchez

**Department of Pharmacy and Pharmaceutical Technology, Faculty of Pharmacy, University of Santiago de Compostela, Santiago de Compostela, 15782 Spain
*Corresponding author: email: ffmjalon@usc.es**

This review describes a number of colloidal drug carriers designed specifically to overcome mucosal barriers and transport bioactive compounds across mucosae. Despite the broadly accepted view that hydrophobic particles are preferred to hydrophilic particles in terms of their ability to enter the intestinal mucosa, some hydrophilic polymers have demonstrated a positive effect on the transport of colloidal particles across mucosal surfaces. More specifically, nanoparticles made of polymers such as poly(ethylene glycol)-poly(lactic acid), PEG-PLA, chitosan, and glucomannan are able to cross the epithelia, thereby acting as true carriers for the transport of bioactive compounds. This overview describes methodological approaches for producing these carriers, their drug association efficiency and capability for controlling the drug release, and finally their ability to overcome barriers such as the nasal, intestinal and ocular mucosae.

Introduction

For a long time it was assumed that the transport of particles across mucosal surfaces was an exceptional event that occurred rarely and to a very low extent. At the end of the 80's, however, it was observed that hydrophobic microparticles were transported across the M-cells overlaying the lymphoid tissues. As a consequence, the use of these microparticles for the delivery of vaccines to the immune system became quite popular. *(1,2)* This observation was soon taken as a general statement since it corroborated the fact that hydrophobic bacteria are internalized more easily than those with a more hydrophilic character are. Hence, many studies focused on loading vaccines into hydrophobic microparticles and investigating their ability to elicit mucosal and systemic immune responses following mucosal administration. Microparticles made of poly(lactide-co-glycolide) copolymers, for example, have widely been used, and results of these studies have been reviewed recently. (3)

The influence of particle size on transmucosal transport became an important research object, motivated by prior observations that small polystyrene particles were able to overcome the intestinal barrier. *(4,5)* A general conclusion from these studies was a more favorable transport across epithelia for nanoparticles than for microparticles. *(6)* Consequently, nanoparticles made of biodegradable polymers were developed and bioactive molecules associated to them, with the final goal of improving their transport across the intestinal and nasal mucosae. Interesting results have been reported for poly (alkylcyanoacrylate) nanoparticles and nanocapsules in terms of their ability to enhance the bioavailability of associated compounds. *(7-9)* Most recent attention, however, has been focused on the use of PLA and PLGA nanoparticles as carriers for transmucosal transport. *(10-14)* Two main approaches have been adopted for the association of bioactive macromolecules to these nanoparticles: (i) the adsorption onto preformed nanoparticles, *(15,16)* and (ii) the encapsulation within nanoparticles. *(17)* The adsorption approach has the advantage of not exposing the associated macromolecules to the often harmful conditions required for producing the nanoparticles. Disadvantages are masking the surface properties of the nanoparticles by the macromolecules, a low protection level for the adsorbed macromolecules, and a less predictable release rate. The major disadvantage of the encapsulation approach is the exposure of the macromolecules (i.e. proteins) to deleterious emulsification conditions, requiring special precaution in terms of emulsification energy and formulation conditions.

Over the last few years our group has taken on the challenge of designing different types of nanoparticles, all of them being formed of or coated by hydrophilic polymers. Among these polymers, we have chosen the synthetic polymer poly(ethylene glycol), PEG, and two polysaccharides, chitosan and glucomannan. We have investigated their interaction with cells and mucosal surfaces, and loaded them with a variety of bioactive compounds. The present article is aimed at reviewing the characteristics and potential of these particles as carriers for transmucosal drug transport.

Materials and Methods

Materials and methods for the preparation, characterization, and *in-vivo* evaluation of PLA-PEG, chitosan, and chitosan-coated nanoparticles have been described in detail in the respective references given in the text.

The visualization of PLA-PEG nanoparticles in rat nasal mucosa was achieved using the fluorescent label rhodamine 6G. A total polymer dose of 10 mg per rat was given in six separated fractions at 4-minute time intervals (each time a volume of 10 μL was dropped into each nostril). Four minutes after the last administration, the rats were sacrificed and 5 mL of 4 % aqueous formaline (vol./vol.) were injected into their traquea. The rat nasal epithelia were excised, fixed, frozen, and sectioning (12 μm) with a cryostat (Leica) for further observation by fluorescence microscopy (Olympus AX70, 60 A).

Results and Discussions

PEG-based Nanoparticles

Despite the evidence for transport of PLA and PLGA nanoparticles across the intestinal epithelia, two major obstacles have been identified as limiting steps for this process: (i) the instability of these nanoparticles in intestinal fluids, and (ii) the low internalization of the particles in the intestinal epithelium. *(12-14)* The nanoparticles' instability is mainly driven by their interaction with proteins and enzymes present in the mucosal fluids. *(18)* The low internalization could be a consequence of particle agglomeration in the biological environment and/or their inability to interact with epithelial cells.

Coating nanoparticles with a hydrophilic PEG layer is a promising approach for reducing the interaction with serum proteins, as demonstrated recently by prolonged circulation times of PEGylated nanoparticles ("stealth" nanoparticles) following intravenous administration. *(19)* We hypothesized, therefore, that a protective PEG coating could enhance the stability of nano-particles in other biological fluids and mucosal surfaces as well. An additional advantage of using PEG for mucosal drug administration is related to its mucoadhesion-promoting effect, which should improve the interaction of nanoparticles with mucosal surfaces. *(20)* We were able to verify the key role of PEG in preserving the stability of PLA nanoparticles in simulated gastrointestinal fluids as well as in the presence of mucosal proteins such as lysozyme and mucin *(21,22).* PLA nanoparticles aggregated massively upon incubation with lysozyme, whereas those coated with PEG (PLA-PEG nanoparticles) remained stable for at least two hours. *(22)* Besides the stability improvement, these particles have the capacity of encapsulating either hydrophilic or lipophilic compounds. Hydrophilic proteins such as bovine serum albumin, and hydrophobic peptides such as cyclosporin A could be encapsulated using emulsification solvent evaporation techniques. *(23,24)*

In order to elucidate the potential impact of PEG on the ability of PLA-PEG nanoparticles to carry bioactive macromolecules across mucosal surfaces, we loaded them with the radiolabeled protein ^{125}I-tetanus toxoid and followed its absorption and biodistribution after either nasal administration. The protein was encapsulated rather than adsorbed in order to avoid masking the surface properties of the particles and to control its release from the particles. The presence of a PEG coating around the nanoparticles significantly enhanced the transport of encapsulated toxoid across the nasal mucosa (Figure 1). *(25)*

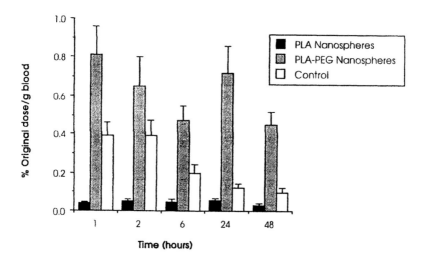

Figure 1. Blood levels of ^{125}I-Tetanus toxoid following nasal administration of ^{125}I-Tetanus toxoid-loaded PLA-PEG nanospheres. (Reproduced from Ref. (25). Copyright 1998 Kluwer Academic/Plenum Publishers.)

Notably, the concentration of the radioactive protein in lymph nodes and other relevant tissues was significantly higher for PEG-coated particles than for hydrophobic PLA nanoparticles. Similar observations were made following oral administration of the nanoparticles. *(21)*

These results suggested that PLA-PEG nanoparticles could work as carriers for transporting encapsulated antigen across the nasal and intestinal mucosae. Clear evidence for this carrier capacity is illustrated in Figure 2, which shows a cross-section of a rat nasal mucosa that was excised at 4 minutes post-nasal instillation of rhodamine-labeled PLA-PEG particles. The presence of the particles in the form of fluorescent round spots can be noted in the nasal epithelium and also in the sub-mucosal space. In contrast, the appearance of the mucosa was radically different displaying only the inherent tissue diffuse fluorescence following administration of non-coated PLA nanoparticles (results not shown).

Recently, we have assessed the efficacy of PEG-coated PLA particles versus non-coated particles for nasal immunization. Interestingly, the systemic and mucosal immune responses obtained for tetanus toxoid loaded into PLA-PEG particles were significantly higher than those corresponding to PLA particles. Furthermore, the IgG antibody responses elicited by the PLA-PEG nanoencapsulated vaccine increased over time for up to 6 months. *(26)* These results suggested that the particles were able to cross the nasal mucosa, reach the antigen presenting cells, and deliver the encapsulated vaccine in a controlled manner to the immunocompetent cells.

To further explore the potential of these new nanoparticles as carriers for the transport of more complex molecules such as plasmid DNA, model plasmids such as luciferase and β-galactosidase reporter genes were chosen and nanoencapsulation techniques were developed allowing the encapsulation of these plasmids either in the free form or associated with non-condensing polymers such as poly(vinylpyrrolidone) and poly(vinyl alcohol). *(27)* By judiciously adjusting the preparation conditions, particles of 100-200 nm in size with encapsulation efficiencies of 60-80% could be produced. The plasmids could be released for up to several weeks, either very rapidly or in a controlled manner. Plasmid DNA-loaded nanoparticles were administered to mice, and the immune response to the protein β-galactosidase encoded by the plasmid was determined. The response elicited by encapsulated plasmid was significantly greater than that of the corresponding control plasmid solution. *(28)* Notably, the response achieved for encapsulated plasmid following nasal administration was comparable to that elicited by the plasmid control solution following intramuscular injection. *(29)* These results provided further evidence for the ability of PLA-PEG nanoparticles to act as carriers for the transport of complex molecules across mucosal surfaces.

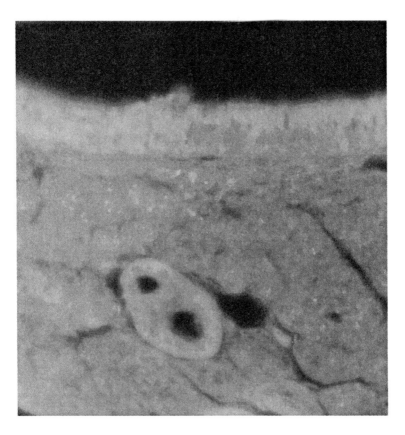

Figure 2. Fluorescent micrograph of a cross section of nasal mucosa from rat administered intranasaly with a suspension of PLA-PEG nanoparticles (mean size 1 μm). Fluorescent spots corresponding to the nanoparticles can be seen crossing the epithelium and reaching the submucosal space.
(See page 8 of color insert.)

Polysaccharide-based Nanoparticles

The polysaccharide chitosan is receiving increasing attention as a drug delivery material because of its beneficial properties such as biodegradability, mucoadhesion, and permeability enhancement. *(30-32)* For example, a chitosan-based nasal formulation containing influenza vaccine is undergoing clinical trials. *(33)* We took advantage of the hydrophilicity and positive charge of this polymer and developed different colloidal carriers useful for the encapsulation of hydrophobic and hydrophilic compounds. These systems could be divided into two classes: (i) nanoparticles made of either pure chitosan or chitosan mixed with other hydrophilic polymers, and (ii) colloidal systems consisting of a hydrophobic core, formed by an oil droplet or a hydrophobic polymer, coated by chitosan. Chitosan nanoparticles could be obtained by a very mild ionic crosslinking process, based on the interaction of chitosan with sodium tripolyphosphate. *(34)* Using this technique, it was possible to associate other hydrophilic polymers such as Poloxamers or PEG to the nanoparticle structure. *(35)* Alternatively, the formation of nanoparticles in aqueous media could be achieved by a controlled ionic interaction between chitosan and another, negatively charged, polysaccharide such as glucomannan. *(36)* The introduction of these secondary polymers allowed modulation of the surface charge of the particles and, consequently, their interaction with biological media.

A number of bioactive compounds with different physicochemical properties have been loaded into these nanoparticles by adjusting the formulation conditions appropriately. The highest loading achieved to date has been for insulin (50% loading). *(37)* This high loading capacity is caused, at least in part, by the acidic character of this peptide and its ability to strongly interact with the positively charged chitosan. Other hydrophobic peptides such as cyclosporin A and low molecular weight drugs such as doxorubicin could be loaded as well using specific strategies. *(38,39)*

A different approach was adopted for the preparation of chitosan-coated colloidal systems. This approach was based on complex-formation between a negatively charged phospholipid, i.e. lecithin, and the positively charged chitosan. *(40)* This complex can be formed at the interface of oil/water emulsions, either leading to the formation of chitosan-coated nanoparticles (the inner phase of the emulsion is a solution of a hydrophobic polymer, i.e. PLGA) or chitosan-coated nanocapsules (the inner phase of the emulsion is an oil or a mixture of an oil with a hydrophobic polymer). These techniques are mainly useful for the encapsulation of hydrophobic molecules that easily can be dissolved in the inner phase of an o/w emulsion. Examples of molecules that have been encapsulated into chitosan-coated nanocapsules include diazepam and indomethacin. *(40,41)* Nevertheless, hydrophilic proteins such as tetanus toxoid, could also be encapsulated in to chitosan-coated PLGA nanoparticles by adding an aqueous solution of the toxoid to the polymer solution. *(22)*

The release behavior from chitosan nanoparticles mainly depends on the interaction between the drug and chitosan, the chitosan molecular weight, and its degree of deacetylation. *(42)* In some cases, the drug-chitosan interaction can be adjusted by selecting suitable preparation conditions. For example, the interaction between insulin and chitosan and, hence, the release rate of insulin from the nanoparticles could be modulated by changing the pH of the chitosan solution. *(43)* This versatility renders these nanoparticles useful for the delivery of an array of drugs and vaccines following different modalities of administration. For example, a fast release would be desirable in case of insulin, whereas a sustained release would be more appropriate for achieving a long lasting response in the case of a vaccine such as tetanus toxoid. The release from chitosan nanocapsules, on the other hand, is typically rapid since the process is not controlled by the chitosan coating but mainly driven by the partition coefficient of the drug between the oily core and the release medium. *(40)*

Besides their versatility in terms of the type of drugs that can be associated with them, chitosan nanoparticles have the major advantage of being widely applicable to different modalities of administration. For example, insulin–loaded chitosan nanoparticles administered intranasal to rabbits led to a significant decrease of the plasma glucose levels compared to controls such as insulin solutions in the presence and absence of chitosan thus suggesting the impact of nanoparticles on the transport rate of insulin (Figure 3). *(37)* Similarly, a very high and long lasting immunogenic response in mice was observed following administration of tetanus vaccine-loaded nanoparticles by intranasal instillation. *(44)* This prolonged response led us to hypothesize that the nanoparticles cross the nasal mucosa and reach the antigen presenting cells. In this particular environment, the particles might deliver the associated antigen for extended periods of time. Chitosan nanoparticles also have a potential application for delivering drugs to the ocular mucosa. In a recent study carried out in rabbits, it was found that fluorescein-labeled chitosan nanoparticles remained associated to the cornea and conjunctiva for more than 24 hours. *(45)* This enhanced retention time could explain an earlier observation of enhanced retention of cyclosporin A associated to nanoparticles in the ocular mucosa following topical instillation to rabbits, compared to control formulations (Figure 4). *(38)* As seen here and in the earlier experiment (Figure 3), the presence of chitosan as nanoparticles is advantageous compared to chitosan in solution. It has been argued that this prolonged surface retention could be beneficial for the treatment of eye surface diseases such as dry eye.

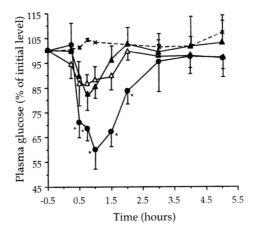

*Figure 3. Plasma glucose levels achieved in rabbits following nasal adminis-tration at pH 4.3 of acetate buffer (×); insulin acetate buffer (Δ); insulin-chitosan 210 Cl acetate buffer (▲); insulin-loaded chitosan 210 Cl nano-particles suspended in acetate buffer (●). (Mean ±SD, n=6). *Statistically significant differences from control insulin solution (p < 0.05). (Reproduced from Ref. (37). Copyright 1999 Kluwer Academic/Plenum Publishers.)*

CyA concentration in the conjunctiva
(ng CyA/g conjunctiva)

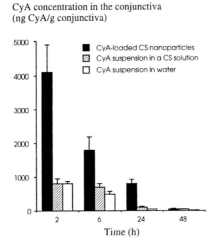

Figure 4. Cyclosporin A concentrations in the conjunctiva of rabbits after topical administration of cyclosporin A-loaded nanoparticles and control formulations. (Reproduced from Ref. (38). Copyright 2001 Elsevier Science.)

Chitosan nanocapsules, containing an oily core, as well displayed an interesting behavior when applied topically onto the eye. For example, the chitosan coating of these nanocapsules led to a significant improvement of the ocular bioavailability of indomethacin, a result attributed to the mucoadhesive properties of chitosan. *(41)*

Very recently, we have been able to produced chitosan-glucomannan nanoparticles intended for oral administration of proteins. *(36)* The rationale behind this idea was that glucomannan would improve the interaction of the particles with the mannose receptors in epithelial cells. The combination of these two polysaccharides resulted in the formation of composite nanoparticles that are stable in gastric fluids. Furthermore, fluorescence images of cross-sections of rat intestinal mucosa revealed the ability of these composite nanoparticles to overcome the intestinal mucosa. Chitosan-glucomannan nano-particles, therefore, can be proposed as an intestinal drug carrier. *(36)*

Based on these positive *in-vivo* results, it seemed a study of the mechanism underlying the interaction between chitosan nanoparticles and different cell lines was of primary importance. The bioactivity and internalization of doxo-rubicin-loaded nanoparticles in human melanoma A375 cells were tested using confocal microcopy. *(39)* The images suggested that the particles entered the cells and that this internalization process occurred over an extended period of time. Additionally, the persistence of fluorescent doxorubicin around the nucleus of the cells, following overnight incubation, gave an indication of the sustained release properties of these nanoparticles. An internalization process was also observed following incubation of chitosan nanoparticles with normal human conjunctival cell cultures. *(46)* The confocal images revealed an increasing amount of particles entering the cells over time (maximum incubation time: 2 hours), depending on the nanoparticle concentration. Using concentrations as high as 1 mg/mL, a large number of particles could be found in the cytoplasm. Notably, the particles exhibit very low toxicity even at high concentrations.

The internalization process for different types of nanoparticles was studied recently, using two cell model cultures, enterocyte-like Caco-2 cells, and the mucus secreting MTX-E12 cells. The results suggested rapid internalization of chitosan nanoparticles by these cells, and a significant increase of this transport intensity in the presence of mucus. This observation could be explained by the ability of chitosan to interact with mucus. In addition, these results suggested chitosan nanoparticle transport by adsorptive transcytosis, and that this transport was saturable as well as energy dependent. *(47)* From these various cell culture studies it seems reasonable to conclude that chitosan nanoparticles are indeed able to enter cells, however, intensity, rate, and transport mechanism vary depending on the cells characteristics.

Conclusions

In summary, the studies covered in this chapter corroborate the potential of polymer nanoparticles as carriers for transmucosal drug delivery. Additionally, they show that the use of hydrophilic polymers such as PEG, chitosan, or glucomannan is beneficial for improving the stability of these particles in biological media and for their transport across mucosal surfaces. The positive effects of these hydrophilic polymers provide some arguments against the classical believe that hydrophobic particles are preferable over hydrophilic particles as transmucosal carriers. However, no general statements should be made in terms of the physicochemical properties (hydrophobicity, zeta potential) affecting this transport. Indeed, the chemical composition of the carrier surface may have a profound effect on its behavior in biological environments.

References

1. O'Hagan, D.T. *Adv. Drug. Deliv. Rev.* **1990**, *5*, 265-285.
2. Eldridge, J.H.; Hammond, C.J.; Meulbroek, J.A.; Staas, J.K.; Gilley. R.M.; Tice, T.R. *J. Control. Rel.* **1990**, *11*, 205-214.
3. O'Hagan, D.T. *Adv. Drug. Deliv. Rev.* **1998**, *34*, 305-320.
4. Jani, P.; Halbert, G.W.; Langridge, J.; Florence, A.T. *J. Pharm. Pharmacol.* **1989**, *41*, 809-812.
5. Sanders, E.; Ashworth, C.T. *Exp. Cell. Res.* **1961**, *22*, 137-145.
6. Florence, A.T. *Pharm. Res.* **1997**, *14*, 259-266.
7. Maincent, P.; Le Vege, R.; Sado, P.; Couvreur, P; Devissaguet, J.P. *J. Pharm. Sci.* **1986**, *75*, 955-958.
8. Damgé, C.; Michel, C.; Aprahamian, M.; Couvreur, P. *Diabetes* **1988**, *37*, 246-251.
9. Hillery, A.M.; Toth, I.; Florence, A.T. *J. Control. Rel.* **1996**, *42*, 65-73.
10. Desai, M.P.; Labhasetwar, V.; Amidon. G.L.; Levy, R.J. *Pharm. Res.* **1996**, *13*, 1838-1845.
11. Carino, G.P.; Jacob, J.S.; Mathiowitz, E. *J. Control. Rel.* **2000**, *65*, 261-269.
12. Le Ray, A.M.; Vert, M.; Gautier, J.C.; Benoit, J.P. *Int. J. Pharm,.* **1994**, *106*, 201-211.
13. Desai, M.P.; Labhasetwar, V.; Walter, E.; Levy, R.J.; Amidon. G.L. *Pharm. Res.* **1997**, *14*, 1568-1573.
14. McClean S.; Prosser, E.; Meehan, E.; O'Malley, D.; Clarke. N.; Ramtoola. Z.; Brayden, D. *Eur. J. Pharm. Sci.* **1998**, *6*, 153-163.
15. Almeida, A.; Alpar, H.O.; Brown, R.H. *J. Pharm. Pharmacol.* **1993**, *15*, 198-203.

16. Jung, T; Kamm, W., Breitenbach, A.; Hungerer, K.D.; Hundt, E.; Kissel, T. *Pharm. Res.* **2001**, *18*, 352-360.
17. Blanco, M.D.; Alonso, M.J. *J. Pharm. Biopharm.* **1997**, *43*, 287-294.
18. Landry, F.B.; Bazile, D.V.; Spenlehauer, G.; Veillard, M.; Kreuter. J. *S.T.P. Pharm. Sci.* **1996**, *6*, 195-202.
19. Gref, R; Minamitake, Y.; Peracchia, M.T.; Trubetskoy, V.; Torchilin, V.; Langer, R. *Science* **1994**, *263*, 1600-1603.
20. De Ascentis, A.; Grazia, J.L.; Bowman, C.N.; Colombo, P.; Peppas, N.A. *J. Control. Rel.* **1995**, *33*, 197-201.
21. Tobío, M.; Sánchez, A.; Vila, J.L.; Soriano, I.; Evora, C.; Vila-Jato, J.L.; Alonso, M.J. *Colloid. and Surf. B: Biointerf.* **2000**, *18*, 315-323.
22. Vila, A.; Sánchez, A.; Tobío, M; Calvo. P.; Alonso, M.J. *J. Control. Rel.* **2002**, *78*, 15-24.
23. Quellec, P.; Gref, R.; Dellacheric, E.; Sommer, F., Tran. M.D.; Alonso, M.J. *J. Biomed. Mater. Res.* **1999**, 47, 388-395.
24. Gref, R.; Quellec, P.; Sánchez, A.; Calvo, P.; Dellacherie, E.; Alonso, M.J. *Eur. J. Pharm. Biopharm.* **2001**, *51*, 111-118.
25. Tobío, M.; Gref, R.; Sánchez, A.; Langer, R.; Alonso, M.J. *Pharm. Res.* **1998**, *15*, 270-275.
26. Vila, A.; Sánchez, A.; Soriano, I.; Evora, C.; McCallion, O.; Alonso, M.J. *Proceedings of the 29th International Symposium on Controlled Release of Bioactive Materials* **2002**, 287.
27. Pérez, C.; Sánchez, A.; Putnam, D.; Ting, D.; Langer, R.; Alonso, M.J. *J. Control. Rel.* **2001**, *75*, 211-224.
28. Vila, A.; Sánchez, A.; Perez, C.; Alonso, M.J. *PAT*, **2002**, *13*, 1-8.
29. Pérez. C.; Sánchez, A.; Alonso, M.J. University of Santiago de Compostela, Spain, *Unpublished.*
30. Hirano, S.; Seino, H.; Akiyama, I.; Nonaka, I.; In *Progress in Biomedical Polymers*; Gebelein, C.G.; Dunn, R.L., Eds.; Plenum Press: New York, 1990, pp 283-289.
31. Borchard, C.; Lueβen, H.L.; De Boer, G.A.; Coos Verhoef, J.; Lehr, C.M.; Junginger, H.E. *J. Control. Rel.* **1996**, *339*, 131-138.
32. Artursson, P.; Lindmark, T.; Davis, S.S.; Illum, L. *Pharm. Resv.* **1994**, *11*, 1358-1361.
33. Illum, L.; Jabbal-Gill, I.; Hinchcliffe, M.; Fisher, A.N.; Davis, S.S. *Adv. Drug. Del. Rev.* **2001**, *51*, 81-96.
34. Calvo, P.; Remuñan-López, C.; Vila-Jato, J.L.; Alonso, M.J. *Appl. Pol. Sci.* **1997**, *63*, 125-132.
35. Calvo, P.; Remuñan-López, C.; Vila-Jato, J.L.; Alonso, M.J. *Pharm. Res.* **1997**, *14*, 1431-1436.
36. Cuña, M.; Alonso-Sande, M.; Remuñan-López, C; Alonso-Lembrero, J.L.; J.P. Pivel; Alonso, M.J. *Proceedings of the 29th International Symposium on Controlled Release of' Bioactive Materials* **2002**, 136.
37. Fernández-Urrusuno, R.; Calvo, P.; Remuñan-López, C.; Vila-Jato, J.L.; Alonso, M.J. *Pharm. Res.* **1999**, *16*, 1576-1581.

38. De Campos, A.; Sánchez, A.; Alonso, M.J. *Int. J. Pharm.* **2001**, *224,* 159-168.
39. Janes, K.A.; Fresneau, M.P., Mazaruela, A.; Fabra, A.; Alonso, M.J. *J. Control. Rel.* **2001**, *73,* 255-267.
40. Calvo, P.; Remuñan-López, C; Vila-Jato, J.L.; Alonso, M.J. *Colloid. Polym. Sci.* **1997**, *275,* 46-53.
41. Calvo, P.; Vila-Jato, J.L.; Alonso, M.J. *Int. J. Pharm.* **1997**, *153*, 41-50.
42. Kevin, J.; Alonso, M.J. *J. Appl. Pol. Sci.* **2003**, *In press.*
43. Ma Z.; Yeoh, H.H.; Lim, L.Y. *J. Pharm. Sci.* **2002**, *91,* 1396-1404.
44. Vila A.; Sánchez. A.; Alonso, M.J. *Proceedings of the* 29th *International Symposium on Controlled Release of Bioactive Materials* **2002**, 275.
45. De Campos, A.; Alonso, M.J. University of Santiago de Compostela, Spain, *Unpublished.*
46. Enriquez de Salamanca, A.; Biehold, Y.; Callejo, S.; Jarrin, M.; Vila, A.; Alonso, M.J. *4*[th] *Int. Symposium on Ocular Pharmocology and Pharmaceutics* **2002**, 38.
47. Behrens I.; Vila Pena, A.I.; Alonso, M.J.; Kissel, T. *Pharm. Res.* **2002**, *19,* 1185-1193.

Chapter 21

A Novel Peroral Peptide Drug Delivery System Based on Superporous Hydrogel Polymers

G. Borchard[1,3], F. A. Dorkoosh[1,4], J. C. Verhoef[1],
M. Rafiee-Tehrani[2], and H. E. Junginger[1]

[1]Division of Pharmaceutical Technology, Leiden/Amsterdam Center
for Drug Research, Leiden, The Netherlands
[2]College of Pharmacy, Tehran University of Medical Sciences, Tehran, Iran
[3]Current address: Enzon Pharmaceuticals, 20 Kingbridge Road,
Piscataway, NJ 08854
[4]Current address: N.V. Organon, Postbus 20, 5340 BH Oss, The
Netherlands

We report here the development and testing of a drug
carrier system for the peroral delivery of peptide drugs.
The carrier system is based on superporous hydrogel
(SPH) and SPH composite (SPHC) polymers. Their fast
swelling properties result in opening of tight epithelial
junctions, allowing for the paracellular route of transport
of macromolecular compounds, and the increase of
retention time of the delivery system at the site of
absorption in the intestine. Both properties were shown to
increase the absorption of the somatostatin-analog octreotide after peroral application in pigs. We therefore
suggest this delivery system as an alternative approach for
peroral peptide drug delivery.

Introduction

The design of novel delivery systems, aiming at increasing the peroral bioavailability especially for hydrophilic and macromolecular drugs such as peptides and proteins, is a main focus of pharmaceutical research and development. The increasing number of therapeutic peptides and proteins supplied by means of modern biotechnology renders the development of such delivery systems mandatory. The majority of existing peptide and protein drugs have yet to be administered via parenteral injection routes, which are inconvenient, time and money consuming and occasionally dangerous. Since oral administration is connected to a good patient compliance, this route attracts the greatest interest. *(1)* Several obstacles, however, have to be overcome when designing an effective delivery system for these drugs. This includes site-specific drug delivery to guarantee the absorption of a predictable and reproducible therapeutic dose, and the improvement of poor peroral bioavailability of these drugs by overcoming both intestinal metabolic barriers as well as the physical barrier of the tight intestinal epithelium. *(2,3)* The poor bioavailability of these drugs after oral administration results from low membrane permeability characteristics, rapid degradation by proteolytic enzymes in the gastrointestinal tract, and clearance mechanisms such as first-pass effect and excretion in the bile. *(4,5)*

Up to now, several approaches have been employed for site-specific peptide drug delivery such as using magnetic systems, unfoldable or expandable systems, and mucoadhesive systems. To this range of delivery concepts we added a new system based on the concept of mechanical fixation at the site of drug absorption. This new concept is different from mucoadhesive systems and overcomes their shortcomings. *(6)* In contrast to mechanical attachment, mucoadhesive dosage forms will stay attached to the mucosal layer for a short period of time at a specific site of the intestine. In addition, by using this novel system we realised an appropriate time-controlled release profile, which is necessary for the intestinal absorption of peptide drugs. For a normal release profile from the dosage form, drug release will be started from time zero, indicating that from the moment the dosage form is in the intestinal lumen the drug release is started. However, for delivery of peptide drugs a lag time of 20-30 min is necessary to inactivate proteolytic enzymes and to open the tight junctions to allow for paracellular transport of the peptide drugs. Thereafter a burst release is required in which the whole amount of peptide drug should be released from the dosage form in a short period of time. This type of drug release is called time-controlled release profile.

In order to achieve mechanical interaction of this novel drug delivery system with the intestinal wall, superporous hydrogel (SPH) and SPH composite (SPHC) polymers were used. Superporous hydrogels are a new generation of hydrogels, which are able to swell very quickly due to their highly porous structure. *(7,8)* The difference between SPH and SPHC is their swelling ratio and mechanical stability. SPH swells more quickly, but is mechanically less stable, whereas SPHC is swelling less, but is mechanically more stable. In this chapter, the developmental procedure of this system and successive *in vitro* and *in vivo* studies are described.

Materials and Methods

Preparation of Superporous Hydrogels. The swelling properties of hydrogels are mainly related to the elasticity of the network, the presence of hydrophilic functional groups (such as -OH, -COOH, -CONH$_2$, -SO$_3$H) in the polymer chains, the extent of cross-linking, and porosity of the polymer. Additionally, the physical characteristics of hydrogels including their swelling ratio also depend on the balance between attractive and repulsive ionic interactions and solvent mediated effects. *(9,10)* Because of their rigid crystalline structure and low elasticity in the polymer chains, conventional hydrogels swell very slowly and, correspondingly, the time for absorbing water is long, ranging from a few hours to even days. Although such slow swelling is beneficial for many applications, there are many situations where fast swelling of the polymer is more desirable. Therefore, a new generation of hydrogels, which swell and absorb water very rapidly, has been developed. Examples of this new generation are Superporous Hydrogels (SPH) and SPH composites (SPHC), which swell to equilibrium size in a short period of time. *(11)* The fast swelling of these polymers can not only be related to the above mentioned factors, but also to capillary wetting of interconnected open pores. In the case, when the swelling ratio of this category of polymers exceeds 100, it is obvious that during the synthesis of these polymers a large internal surface by a large number of interconnected pores is formed; therefore, water can be rapidly absorbed by capillary attracttion forces within the pores, and these polymers swell to their maximum volume very quickly. *(12,13)*

The method reported by Chen *et al.* was adapted to prepare SPH and SPHC polymers. *(11)* Monomeric acrylic acid (AA) and acrylamide (AM) were used for the synthesis of SPH (Figure 1). N,N′-methylenebis acrylamide (Bis) was used as a cross-linker, and Pluronic® F127 was used as a stabilizer for the foam, which is formed by carbon dioxide produced during the synthesis. Pluronic® F127 does not contribute to the chemical structure of the polymer, but is very important as a surface active agent to create a highly porous hydrogel. The foam should be stable for a few minutes in order to introduce the desired large number of pores during the synthesis of the SPH polymer. Ammonium persulfate (APS) is used as an initiator and N,N,N′,N′-tetramethylethylenediamine (TMEDA) as a catalyst.

The synthesis of SPHC was done in the same way as described for SPH. However, in one of the SPH composites the potassium salt of 3-sulfopropyl acrylate (SPAK) was used as a monomer instead of acrylic acid, and crosscarmellose sodium (Ac-Di-Sol) was used as the stabilizer to introduce additional mechanical stability of the polymer by physical entanglement with the polymer chains. Ac-Di-Sol does not contribute to the chemical structure of the polymer, but is applied to enhance mechanical stability of the polymer.

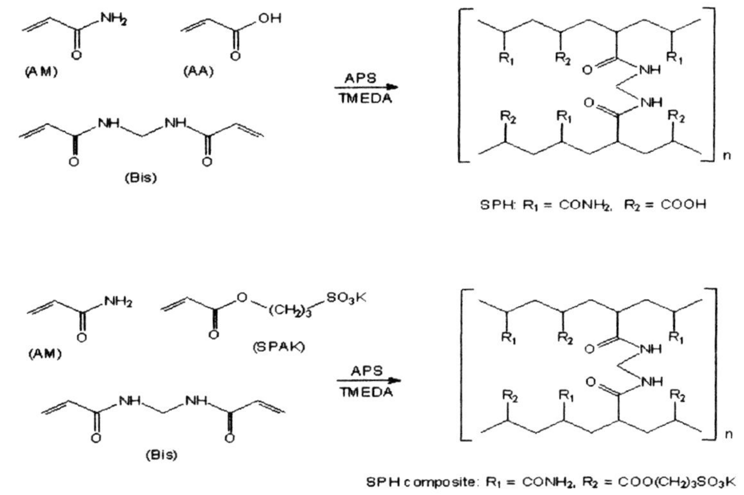

Figure 1. Synthesis of superporous hydrogels (SPH) and SPH composites: Acrylic acid (AA); Acrylamide (AM); N,N'-methylenebis acrylamide (Bis); ammonium persulphate (APS); N,N,N',N'-tetramethylethylenediamine (TMEDA); Potassium salt of 3-sulphopropyl acrylate (SPAK).

The following reaction mechanism is proposed for the synthesis of SPH and SPH composite (Figure 1), based on solid-state ^{13}C-NMR spectra of the polymers. *(7)* The combination of APS/TMEDA will initiate the radical polymerization. The formed radicals will attack the double bonds of acrylic acid (AA) and acrylamide (AM) and, to a lesser extent, the double bond of N,N'-methylenebis acrylamide (Bis). Subsequently, the double bonds will be opened and the monomers will covalently bind to each other and form a long aliphatic chain. These chains are subsequently cross-linked by the added cross-linker. The cross-linking density between the polymer back-bone chains is related to the concentration of the cross-linker used during the polymerization. This concentration influences the swelling ratio of the polymer, because the two polymer chains will attach to each other more strongly with increasing amounts of cross-linker and, therefore, reduce the swelling capacity of the polymer. Consequently, a reduced swelling ratio results in the formation of smaller pore sizes during foam formation. A correlation between viscosity of the initial polymer solution and pore sizes of the resulting hydrogel was not observed.

The synthesis of SPH composite follows the same general scheme as SPH, only that SPAK instead of AA was used as a monomer. Therefore, the sequence of AM and SPAK monomers (instead of the AM and AA monomers) is initiated with the same cross-linker (Figure 1) in the proposed radical polymerization.

Characterization of Superporous Hydrogels. Since the SPH polymers are very porous as observed by SEM (Figure 2), the measured density is related to the porosity of these polymers and can be defined as apparent density. As shown in Table I, the apparent density of SPH polymers obtained by freeze-drying for two days is substantially lower than SPH dried by organic solvents or by freeze-drying for one day. Therefore, it is very likely that SPH freeze-dried for two days contains more pores and can swell more rapidly as already shown in swelling ratio studies (Figure 4). The apparent densities of the polymers dried by organic solvents and by one-day freeze-drying are higher, indicating a reduced amount of free space of pores. These results are in accordance with the present swelling ratio studies. The apparent density of SPH composite is 0.91 ± 0.12 g/cm^3 and is higher than the apparent density of SPH.

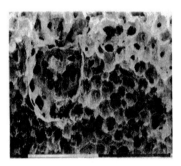 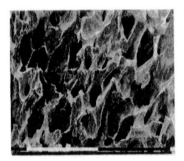

Figure 2. Scanning electron microscopy (SEM) images of SPH (left) and SPHC(right) hydrogels. The SPH polymer has a higher porosity, which is in accordance with apparent density results. The number of pores is smaller in the structure of SPH composite, which explains the lower swelling ratio and higher apparent density for SPH composites. Bar is 1000 μm.

Table I. Apparent density of SPH after different drying procedures.

Drying procedure	Apparent Density (g/cm^3)
Absolute ethanol	0.53 ± 0.08
Acetone	0.49 ± 0.07
Diethyl ether	0.65 ± 0.09
Freeze-drying for 1 day	0.74 ± 0.07
Freeze-drying for 2 days	0.39 ± 0.05

Data are expressed as the mean ± standard deviation (S.D.) of three experiments.

Results and Discussion

In Vitro Studies on Drug Carrier Systems based on SPH/SPHC Polymers for Peroral DrugDelivery

Transport Studies in Caco-2 Cell Monolayers. The intestinal absorption of peptide drugs is mainly limited by enzymatic degradation by lumenal and membrane-bound enzymes and low permeability of the intestinal epithelium. The intestinal epithelium regulates the passage of natural compounds such as nutrients and foods, and serves as a barrier for paracellular passive transport of large hydrophilic molecules. The intestine is lined with a single layer of columnar epithelial cells joined at the apical surface by the tight junctional complex. (14,15) The junctional complex forms a continuous seal, which segregates the apical and basolateral membrane compounds, causes cell differentiation, and conveys size and charge selectivity properties due to the fixed negative charges located at the tight junction. Moreover, the stereochemical structure of hydrophilic compounds contributes to their selectivity for paracellular permeability. (16,17) In order to improve the absorption of these poor permeability hydrophilic compounds, the junctional complex has to be altered in order to open the intestinal paracellular barrier. Co-administration of drugs with an absorption enhancer is believed to improve the transport of hydrophilic macromolecules via the paracellular pathway. There are three major criteria for evaluating absorption enhancers: (1) effectiveness of the enhancers, (2) cytotoxicity effects, and (3) mechanism(s) by which drug absorption is enhanced. *(18)*

Several classes of absorption enhancers, such as surfactants (e.g., sodium lauryl sulphate), chelating agents (e.g., EDTA, salicylates), bile salts (e.g., sodium deoxycholate), fatty acids (e.g., oleic acid), non-surfactants (e.g., unsaturated cyclic urea), and polymers (e.g., polyacrylates, chitosans) have been investigated. *(19-22)* However, in some cases application of enhancers causes cytotoxicity *in vitro* and *in vivo*, suggesting that the improved permeability is mediated by mucosal membrane damage. For instance, sodium dodecyl sulphate (SDS), a well-known pharmaceutical wetting agent, could enhance the permeability of hydrophilic markers. However, SDS causes severe damage in Caco-2 cell monolayers. *(23)* Chitosan, with a low degree of acetylation, was shown to be an effective drug absorption enhancer at low and high molecular weights, exerting no toxic side effects. *(24)* Carbomer (0.5%) is also used as an absorption enhancer and opens the tight junctions by lowering the extracellular calcium concentration. *(22)* Consequently, the ideal absorption enhancer must improve the intestinal absorption of drugs without causing cell membrane damage. *(25)*

Superporous hydrogels (SPH) and SPH composite (SPHC) are a new class of hydrogels which swell very quickly due to their highly porous structure. Although mucoadhesive properties of SPH/SPHC polymers can not entirely be ruled out, the mechanism of increasing the retention of these systems depends on the mechanical fixation by swelling of the polymers. *(6)* Mechanical pressure produced by swelling of SPH and SPHC polymers is suggested to cause the opening of intercellular tight junctions. *(26)* The potential of SPH and SPHC polymers to open the tight junctions was evaluated by monitoring the transepithelial electrical resistance (TEER) and quantifying the permeability of hydrophilic model compounds (^{14}C-mannitol and fluorescently labelled dextrans) across Caco-2 cell monolayers, a well-established model of the intestinal epithelium. *(15,27)* Carbomer was used in these studies as a positive control due to the fact that the chemical structure of carbomer resembles superporous hydrogel polymers. *(7,22)* As shown in Figure 3, both SPH and SPHC polymers were able to decrease TEER significantly (compared to the control and 0.5% carbomer) by their swelling and applied mechanical pressure on monolayers.

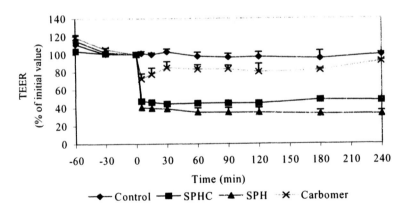

Figure 3. Effects of polymers on TEER of Caco-2 cell monolayers. Data are expressed as mean ± SD of 3 to 5 experiments.

The observed reduction in TEER was associated with an increase in the flux of ^{14}C-mannitol across Caco-2 cell monolayers, indicating the capability of SPH and SPHC polymers for opening of tight junctions and modulating the paracellular permeability of the monolayers. This increased permeability might be caused by affecting the cell membrane integrity. Therefore, the reversibility of this effect is an important issue when screening these polymers as penetration enhancers. It was observed that after removal of the polymers from the monolayers, TEER values recovered to almost initial values within two days, indicating that the effects of SPH and SPHC polymers on tight junctions were reversible (Figure 4).

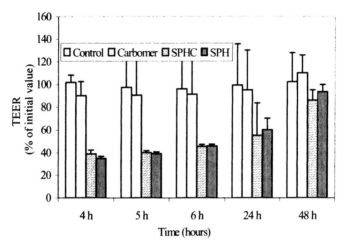

Figure 4. TEER recovery of Caco-2 cell monolayers after removal of the polymers. Data are expressed as mean ±SD of 3 to 5 experiments.

SPH and SPHC polymers were also evaluated for their effects on enhancing paracellular transport of fluorescein isothiocyanate-labelled dextrans with molecular weights of 4,400 Da (FD4) and 19,900 Da (FD20). The reason for using FD4 and FD20 as model compounds for evaluation of SPH and SPHC polymers in Caco-2 cell monolayers was their hydrophilicity and high molecular weight. Therefore, the transport route of these compounds is restricted to the paracellular pathway. *(22,28)* When SPH and SPHC polymers were apically added to Caco-2 cell monolayers, they started to swell and to exert mechanical pressure on the cells which caused the opening of the tight junctions. As is evident from Figure 5, both SPH and SPHC polymers improved markedly the cumulative transport of FD4 compared to carbomer and the negative control. As observed in Figure 6, the cumulative transport of FD20 across the Caco-2 cell monolayers was lower than found with FD4. Comparing the apparent permeability (P_{app}) values of FD4 and FD20, it is obvious that the total transport of FD20 across the Caco-2 cell monolayers is less than FD4. However, the enhancement ratios for SPH and SPHC polymers compared to the negative controls are quite similar. In addition, we had already established in earlier studies that SPH and SPHC polymers are able to enhance the transport of FD4 across porcine intestine *ex vivo* by exerting mechanical pressure on the intestinal epithelium. *(29)*

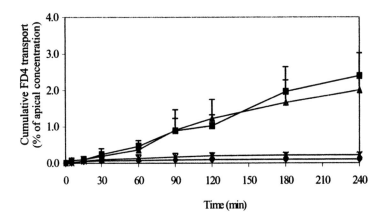

Figure 5. Cumulative transport of FD4 (MW 4,400 Da) across Caco-2 cell monolayers; (■) 20 mg SPHC, (▲) 10 mg SPH, (♦) control, (✗) 0.5% carbomer. Data are expressed as mean ± SD of 3 to 5 experiments.

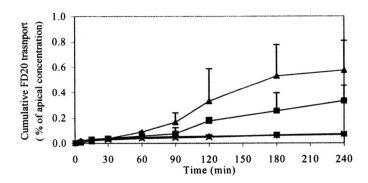

Figure 6. Cumulative transport of FD20 (MW 19,600 Da) across Caco-2 cell monolayers; (■) 20 mg SPHC, (▲) 10 mg SPH, (♦) control, (✗) 0.5% carbomer. Data are expressed as mean ± SD of 3 to 5 experiments.

Cytotoxicity Studies in Caco-2 Cell Monolayers. Assessment of eventual Caco-2 cell toxicity of SPH and SPHC polymers was performed by nuclear staining with propidium iodide and successive visualization using confocal laser scanning microscopy (CLSM). In case of polymer applications (Figure 7A,B), the monolayers appeared to exclude propidium iodide and showed no differences with the control group. However, when 0.1% sodium dodecylsulfate (SDS) was applied to the cells, propidium iodide was taken up by the cells, indicatiing severe cell damage (Figure 7C). Comparison of SPH- and SPHC-treated cells with SDS-treated cells revealed that the number of dead cells was substantially less in case of polymer applications, which demonstrates the safety of SPH and SPHC polymers for mucosal application.

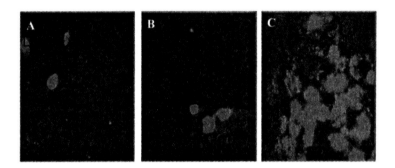

Figure 7. CLSM image of Caco-2 cell monolayers using propidium iodide as impermeable dead cell staining probe; (A) cells incubated with SPH polymer, (B) cells incubated with SPHC polymer, (C) cells treated with 0.1% SDS for 10 min. (See page 8 of color insert.)

Preparation of SPH- and SPHC-Based Delivery Systems. Drug delivery systems based on superporous hydrogels (SPH) and SPH composites (SPHC) were developed for the peroral administration of peptide drugs. In this case, the somatostatin-analogue octreotide was used. Octreotide is a synthetic octapeptide, which has retained the essential pharmacophoric part of the native molecule somatostatin. Octreotide is more potent than somatostatin and clinically used for the treatment of acute variceal bleeding in cirrhotic patients, insulin-dependent diabetes, and inhibition of gall bladder contraction during continuous jejunal feeding in patients with pancreatic pseudocyst. *(30-32)* The currently available delivery system for octreotide is an injectable dosage form, which is not ideal for long-term drug administration in cirrhotic and diabetic patients.

Our delivery systems were developed for site specific mechanical fixation at the gut wall and showed specific release patterns. Each of these systems was made of two parts, (1) the conveyor system made of SPHC which is used for keeping the dosage form at specific site(s) of the GI tract by mechanical interaction of the dosage form with the intestinal membranes, and (2) the core containing the active ingredient incorporated · in the conveyor system. The core was either inserted into the conveyor system (core inside, c.i.) or attached to its surface (core outside, c.o.).

For the preparation of the conveyor systems, SPH and SPH composite polymers were synthesized as described above. For the c.i. system, a hole was made in the center of SPHC polymer as a body and a piece of SPH polymer was used as a cap of the conveyor system (Figure 8A). For the c.o. system, two holes were made on the surface of the SPHC polymer as the conveyor system (Figure 8B). The core component of the c.i. delivery system consisted of octreotide microparticles. These microparticles were prepared by dispersing 15 mg octreotide in melted PEG 6000. The cooled mass was then crushed using a mortar and sieved through sieve mesh size 400 µm. Microparticles smaller than 400 µm were used as a core formulation. These microparticles were filled in the hole inside the SPH composite and the hole was closed with a piece of SPH as a cap. The reason for using SPH as a cap is that the swelling ratio of SPH is higher than SPH composite, and that the cap is ejected, allowing a burst release of the peptide drug. (6) The core component for c.o. delivery system contained a mixture of 7.5 mg octreotide and 92.5 mg lactose, which were pressed as minitablets (4 mm diameter). Two tablets were attached to the conveyor system using a biodegradable glue (Histoacryl®). In another formulation for the core component of the c.o. delivery system, 20 mg N-trimethyl chitosan chloride (TMC) was added as an additional absorption enhancer to the c.o. formulation. (34) However, since TMC is a sticky powder, 20 mg Explotab had to be added as well to the tablet formulation as a disintegrant in order to achieve a burst release profile. In the following, this formulation is referred to as c.o.t. delivery system. All peroral formulations were placed in gelatin capsules (size 000), and the capsules were enteric-coated with 6% Eudragit S100 solution. As a negative control only 15 mg octreotide without any polymer (o.o.) was filled in a gelatin capsule and enteric-coated.

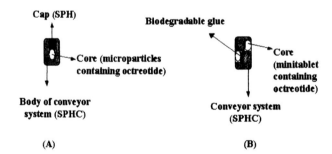

Figure 8. Schematic figures of SPH and SPHC delivery systems; (A) core inside delivery system (c.i.), (B) core attached to surface of delivery system (c.o.).

The release of octreotide from both types of delivery systems was almost complete after 150 minutes. Another peptide drug, buserelin, incorporated in the delivery systems in the same way, was released in a similar manner (Table II).

Table II. Amount of peptide drugs released from the two different delivery systems after 150 minutes.

| | % of released peptide drugs | |
	Buserelin	Octreotide
Core inside (microparticles)	99.1 ± 0.9	98.1 ± 1.2
Core outside (tablets)	98.3 ± 1.2	97.9 ± 1.1

Data are expressed as a mean ± S.D. of 3 experiments.

In Vivo Studies on Drug Carrier Systems based on SPH/SPHC Polymers for Peroral DrugDelivery

The three different formulations (c.i.; c.o.; and c.o.t.) were tested *in vivo* in female pigs (body weight 23.5 ± 4.0 kg). *(33)* These studies were performed in cooperation with the Central Laboratory Animal Institute (Utrecht University, Utrecht, The Netherlands). One week before the start of experiments, all animals were anesthetized and a silicone cannula inserted into their jugular veins for blood sampling. One week after surgery, the pigs received different octreotide administrations according to a randomized cross-over setup. Animals were fasted overnight before each administration, but had access to water *ad libitum*. The formulations were administered to the animals every other day at 48-hours intervals between administrations as a wash-out period. Before administration, the animals were sedated to facilitate peroral and i.v. administrations. Each capsule was administered via the mouth into the stomach using a plunger applicator during the sedation period. For i.v. administration, 5 ml of an octreotide solution (100 µg/ml) were given via the cannulated jugular vein. Blood samples were withdrawn at pre-determined intervals. All animals were fed 6 hours post-dosing. At the end of all experiments the pigs were euthanized by an overdose of pentobarbital and the GI tract was inspected macroscopically for possible damage. No abnormalities or lesions were observed in the intestinal tract of these animals.

Pharmacokinetic parameters, including total area under the plasma concentration-time curve (AUC), peak plasma concentration (C_{max}) and time to reach peak plasma concentration (t_{max}), for all peroral administrations were calculated directly from the plasma octreotide concentrations. The AUCs for the individual plasma profiles were calculated with the linear trapezoidal rule. Plasma concentration-time profiles were fitted according to:

$$C_t = A_1 e^{-\alpha_1 t} + A_2 e^{-\alpha_2 t}$$

in which C_t represents the plasma concentration of octreotide at time t, and A_1, A_2, α_1, α_2 are the coefficients and exponents of this equation. Absolute bioavailability values after peroral administrations of octreotide were calcualted according to:

$$F = \frac{AUC_{peroral} \times D_{i.v.}}{AUC_{i.v.} \times D_{peroral}} \times 100\%$$

in which F is the absolute bioavailability and D is the administered dose.

The pharmacokinetic parameters after i.v. administration of 500 µg octreotide in pigs are summarized in Table III. The octreotide plasma profiles were fitted to a 2-compartment model, resulting in a short distribution half-life of about 7 minutes and a long elimination half-life of 52 minutes, quite similar to previously reported values in pigs. *(34)*

Table III. Pharmacokinetic parameters after i.v. administration of octreotide.

Parameters	Mean $\pm$ SEM; n = 6
t½dist. (min)	6.9 ± 1.5
t½elim. (min)	51.7 ± 8.1
V_d (ml/pig)	423 ± 54
Cl (ml/min/pig)	23.4 ± 2.4
AUC (ng/ml*min)	5621 ± 549

t½dist., distribution half-life; t½elim., elimination half-life; V_d, volume of distribution; Cl, clearance; AUC, area under curve.

The plasma octreotide concentration versus time profiles obtained for each one of the peroral administrations, including c.o., c.i., o.o. and c.o.t., are shown for two of the six pigs (subject no. 2 and 6) in Figures 9 and 10. Since these drug delivery systems based on SPH and SPHC polymers were placed in enteric-coated gelatin capsules size 000, the passage of capsules from the stomach to the intestine varied in each subject and also after each administration. It has been well established that dosage forms up to about 3 mm in size pass through the contracted pylorus within 30 to 120 minutes. However, if the size of dosage forms is increased to more than 3 mm they may reside in the stomach from 1 to 10 hours. *(36,37)* Therefore, the gastric emptying-time for enteric-coated capsules size 000 can vary from 2 to 6 hours, as clearly observed in Figures 9 and 10. As a result, the t_{max} for each administration is different, which can be due to the natural contraction of the pylorus or anatomy and physiology of the animals with respect to gastric emptying-time.

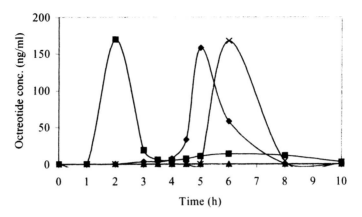

Figure 9. Blood plasma profiles of octreotide after peroral administration of 15 mg/pig: subject 2. (♦) c.o. (core outside); (■) c.i. (core inside); (▲) o.o. (only octreotide without any polymer); (✗) c.o.t. (c.o. with TMC).

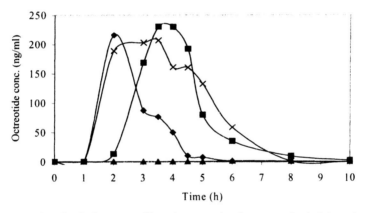

Figure 10. Blood plasma profiles of octreotide after peroral administration of 15 mg/pig: subject 6. (♦) c.o. (core outside); (■) c.i. (core inside); (▲) o.o. (only octreotide without any polymer); (✗) c.o.t. (c.o. with TMC).

The plasma octreotide levels for the negative control (octreotide without SPH/SPHC polymers) was the lowest compared to the other peroral administrations. This indicates that, after the enteric-coated capsules have reached the intestine and the enteric-coat and gelatin layers have been dissolved, the SPHC conveyor systems swelled rapidly and attached mechanically at the absorption site in the intestine. This mechanical fixation to the gut wall enhances the absorption of octreotide due to increased residence time of the delivery system in the intestine and to opening of tight junctions by mechanical pressure and water influx from the intestinal mucosa into the polymers. *(6,26)* This water influx forced the intestinal epithelial cells to maintain their homeostatic pressure by compensating the water loss by opening of the tight junctions, in order to facilitate a rapid uptake of water together with octreotide molecules and to maintain the homeostasis of the intestinal cells and thereby also enhancing plasma octreotide levels.

It is well-known that, for the absorption of hydrophilic and macro-molecular drugs such as peptides and proteins, initially the tight junctions should be opened and then a burst release of such drugs is necessary. *(4,6)* This so-called "time-controlled burst release profile" can be achieved using the present SPH- and SPHC-based delivery systems, since a rapid increase in plasma octreotide levels was observed after peroral administration of these systems in all three formulations (c.o., c.i. and c.o.t.). Moreover, the absorption and elimination of octreotide in some of the pigs (e.g., subject no. 2; Figure 9) were very fast, showing plasma octreotide profiles between two time point measurements with rather sharp peaks and probably resulting in underestimated bioavailability values. If the time points between measurements would have been shorter, it might have caused broader octreotide absorption peaks and higher bioavailability values.

The pharmacokinetics of octreotide in each pig after peroral administration of the different formulations are given in Table IV. T_{max} appeared to vary between two and six hours in most of the administrations in different subjects, except for the c.i. administration in subject no. 3 in which the capsule did not pass the pylorus and thus no octreotide absorption was observed. Therefore, this administration was omitted from bioavailability calculations. Mean C_{max} values ($\pm$ SEM) for c.o., c.i. and c.o.t. administrations were 152.0 $\pm$ 14.7, 175.9 $\pm$ 15.9 and 157.9 $\pm$ 15.4 ng/ml, respectively, which were significantly higher than C_{max} for o.o. administrations (17.8 $\pm$ 11.5 ng/ml). This observation demonstrates that the present SPH- and SPHC-based delivery systems are able to increase the intestinal absorption of octreotide substantially, by mechanisms discussed above. When the chitosan-derivative TMC was added to the c.o. formulations (c.o.t.), the octreotide absorption profile was observed to be broader. TMC, as a sticky powder, obviously prolongs the absorption time of octreotide.

The average absolute bioavailabilities of octreotide after each administration are also presented in Table IV. Peroral administration of octreotide without polymers (o.o.) resulted in a significantly lower (P<0.05) bioavailability then obtained by using SPH and SPHC polymers in c.i. and c.o. administrations. The addition of TMC to the c.o. formulation resulted in an even higher bioavailability of octreotide. It has already been reported that TMC was shown to substantially increase the intestinal absorption of octreotide in rats and pigs. *(34,35)* TMC is well soluble at neutral pH values and can interact with epithelial tight junctions, thereby facilitating the transport of hydrophilic molecules like octreotide by the paracellular pathway.

Table IV. Pharmacokinetic parameters of octreotide after peroral administration in pigs.

Pig no.	c.o.				c.i.				o.o.				c.o.t.			
	t_{max} [h]	C_{max} [ng/ml]	AUC [ng/ml*min]	F [%]	t_{max} [h]	C_{max} [ng/ml]	AUC [ng/ml*min]	F[b] [%]	t_{max} [h]	C_{max} [ng/ml]	AUC [ng/ml*min]	F [%]	t_{max} [h]	C_{max} [ng/ml]	AUC [ng/ml*min]	F [%]
1	3.5	138.8	5249	3.1	4.5	171.1	6277	3.7	5	70.5	4996	3.0	5	100.04	9442	5.6
2	5	157.9	13832	8.2	2	169.6	14817	8.8	4	0.1	3.0	0.01	6	167.5	15603	9.3
3	6	120.7	13022	7.7	0	0	0	—	3	29.8	4571	2.7	6	177.3	28539	16.9
4	4	160.8	30282	18.0	6	178.3	35789	21.2	3	0.2	14	0.01	3	129.4	36291	21.5
5	4.5	117.9	4566	2.7	5	130.8	14570	8.6	3.5	5.2	157	0.1	5	166.3	25336	15.0
6	2	215.8	21390	12.7	3.5	230.1	36003	21.4	6	1.3	211	0.1	3.5	206.8	47644	28.3
Mean (SEM)				8.7 (2.4)[a]				12.7 (3.6)[a]				1.0 (0.6)				16.1 (3.3)[a]

c.o., core outside delivery system; c.i., core inside delivery system; o.o., only octreotide (negative control); c.o.t. core outside delivery system including TMC. t_{max}, time to reach plasma peak concentration; C_{max}, plasma peak concentration; AUC, area under curve; F, absolute bioavailability.
[a] c.o., c.i. and c.o.t. are significantly different from o.o. at $P < 0.05$.
[b] mean of 5 pigs.

Conclusions

In conclusion, drug delivery systems based on superporous hydrogels are able to enhance the peroral absorption of peptide drugs due to their swelling properties and mechanical attachment to the intestinal wall. This mechanical fixation increases the residence time of the delivery systems in the intestine and also opens the tight junctions. The increased peroral bio-availability of octreotide using SPH- and SPHC-based delivery systems indicates that effective peroral absorption of peptide drugs requires appropriate delivery systems containing different absorption enhancers and excipients for disruption of the the the intestinal tight junctional barrier.

Acknowledgments

The financial support of Aventis Research & Technology (Frankfurt, Germany) is kindly appreciated.

References

1. Fix, J.A. Oral controlled release technology for peptides: status and future prospects. *Pharm. Res.* **1996**, *13*, 1760.
2. Bai, J.P.; Chang, L.L.; Guo, J.H. Targeting of peptide and protein drugs to specific sites in the oral route. *Crit. Rev. Ther. Drug Carrier Syst.* **1995**, *12*, 339.
3. Fix, J.A. Strategies for delivery of peptides utilizing absorption-enhancing agents. *J. Pharm. Sci.* **1996**, *85*, 1282.
4. Davis, S.S. Delivery systems for biopharmaceuticals. *J. Pharm. Pharmacol.* **1992**, *44*, 186.
5. Bai, J.P. Distribution of brush-border membrane peptidases along the rabbit intestine: implication for oral delivery of peptide drugs. *Life Sci.* **1993**, *52*, 941.
6. Dorkoosh, F.A.; Verhoef, J.C.; Borchard, G.; Rafiee-Tehrani, M.; Junginger, H.E. Development and characterization of a novel peroral peptide drug delivery system. *J. Control. Rel.* **2001**, *71*, 307.
7. Dorkoosh, F.A.; Brussee, J.; Verhoef, J.C.; Borchard, G.; Rafiee-Tehrani, M.; Junginger, H.E. Preparation and NMR characterisation of superporous hydrogels (SPH) and SPH composites. *Polymer* **2000**, *41*, 8213.
8. Chen, J.; Park, K. Synthesis and characterization of superporous hydrogel composites. *J. Control. Rel.* **2000**, *65*, 73.
9. Barbieri, R.; Quaglia, M.; Delfini, M.; Brosio, E. Investigation of water dynamic behaviour in poly(HEMA) and poly(HEMA-co-DHPMA) hydrogels by proton T2 relaxation time and self-diffusion coefficient n.m.r. measurements. *Polymer* **1998**, *39*, 1059.

10. Bhalerao, V.S.; Varghese, S.; Lele, A.K.; Badiger, M.V. Thermoreversible hydrogel based on radiation induced copolymerisation of poly(N-isopropyl acrylamide) and poly(ethylene oxide). *Polymer* **1998**, *39*, 2255.

11. Chen, J.; Park, H.; Park, K. Synthesis of superporous hydrogels: Hydrogels with fast swelling and superabsorbent properties. *J. Biomed. Mater. Res.* **1999**, *44*, 53.

12. Van Dijk-Wolthuis, W.N.E.; Tsang, S.K.Y.; Kettenes-van den Bosch, J.J.; Hennink, W.E. A new class of polymerizable dextrans with hydrolyzable groups: hydroxyethyl methacrylated dextran with and without oligolactate spacer. *Polymer* **1997**, *38*, 6235.

13. Peniche, C.; Cohen, M.; Vazquez, B.; San Roman, J. Water sorption of flexible networks based on 2-hydroxyethyl methacrylate-triethylenglycol dimethacrylate copolymers. *Polymer* **1997**, *38*, 5977.

14. Sakai, M.; Imai, T.; Ohtake, H.; Azuma, H.; Otagiri, M. Effects of absorption enhancers on the transport of model compounds in Caco-2 cell monolayers: assessment by confocal laser scanning microscopy. *J. Pharm. Sci.* **1997**, *86*, 779.

15. Artursson, P. Epithelial transport of drugs in cell culture: A model for studying the passive diffusion of drugs over intestinal absorptive (Caco-2) cells. *J. Pharm. Sci.* **1990**, *79*, 476.

16. Daugherty, A.L.; Mrsny, R.J. Regulation of the intestinal epithelial paracellular barrier. *Pharm. Sci. Technol. Today* **1999**, *2*, 281.

17. Pauletti, G.M.; Gangwar, S.; Knipp, G.T.; Nerurkar, M.M.; Okumu, F.W.; Tamura, K.; Siahaan T.J.; Borchardt, R.T. Structural requirements for intestinal absorption of peptide drugs. *J. Control. Rel.* **1996**, *41*, 3.

18. Aungst, B.J.; Saitoh, H.; Burcham, D.L.; Huang, S.-M.; Mousa, S.A.; Hussain, M.A. Enhancement of the intestinal absorption of peptides and nonpeptides. *J. Control. Rel.*, **1996**, *41*, 19.

19. Meaney, C.M.; O'Driscoll, C.M.. A comparison of the permeation enhancement potential of simple bile salt and mixed bile salt: fatty acid micellar systems using the Caco-2 cell culture model. *Int. J. Pharm.* **2000**, *207*, 21.

20. Lee, V.H.L.; Yamamoto, A.; Kompella, U.B. Mucosal penetration enhancer for facilitating of peptide and protein drug absorption. *Crit. Rev. Ther. Drug Carrier Syst.* **1991**, *8*, 91.

21. Lindmark, T.; Schipper, N.; Lazorova, L.; de Boer, A.G.; Artursson, P. Absorption enhancement in intestinal epithelial Caco-2 monolayers by sodium caprate: assessment of molecular weight dependence and demonstration of transport routes. *J. Drug Target.* **1998**, *5*, 215.

22. Borchard, G.; Luessen, H.L.; De Boer, A.G.; Verhoef, J.C.; Lehr, C.-M.; Junginger, H.E. The potential of mucoadhesive polymers in enhancing intestinal peptide drug absorption. III: Effects of chitosan-glutamate and carbomer on epithelial tight junctions in vitro. *J. Control. Rel.* **1996**, *39*, 131.

23. Anderberg, E.K.; Artursson, P. Epithelial transport of drugs in cell culture. VIII: Effects of sodium dodecyl sulfate on cell membrane and tight junction permeability in human intestinal epithelial (Caco-2) cells. *J. Pharm. Sci.* **1993**, *82*, 392.

24. Schipper, N.G.M.; Olsson, S.; Hoogstraate, J.A.; de Boer, A.G.; Vårum, K.M.; Artursson, P. Chitosans as absorption enhancers for poorly absorbable drugs 2: Mechanism of absorption enhancement. *Pharm. Res.* **1997**, *14*, 923.

25. Quan, Y.-S.; Hattori, K.; Lundborg, E.; Fujita, T.; Murakami, M.; Muranishi, S.; Yamamoto, A. Effectiveness and toxicity screening of various absorption enhancers using Caco-2 cell monolayers. *Biol. Pharm. Bull.* **1998**, *21*, 615.

26. Dorkoosh, F.A.; Borchard, G.; Rafiee-Tehrani, M.; Verhoef, J.C.; Junginger, H.E. Evaluation of superporous hydrogel (SPH) and SPH composite in porcine intestine ex-vivo: assessment of drug transport, morphology effect, and mechanical fixation to intestinal wall. *Eur. J. Pharm. Biopharm.* **2002**, *53*, 161.

27. Delie, F.; Rubas, W. A human colonic cell line sharing similarities with enterocytes as a model to examine oral absorption: advantages and limitations of the Caco-2 model. *Crit. Rev. Ther. Drug Carrier Syst.* **1997**, *14*, 221.

28. Hosoya, K.-I.; Kubo, H.; Natsume, H.; Sugibayashi, K.; Morimoto, Y.; Yamashita, S. The structural barrier of absorptive mucosae: site difference of the permeability of fluorescein isothiocyanate-labelled dextran in rabbits. *Biopharm. Drug Disp.* **1993**, *14*, 685.

29. Dorkoosh, F.A.; Setyaningsih, D.; Borchard, G.; Rafiee-Tehrani, M.; Verhoef, J.C.; Junginger, H.E. Effects of superporous hydrogels on paracellular drug permeability and cytotoxicity studies in Caco-2 cell monolayers. *Int. J. Pharm.* **2002**, *241*, 35.

30. Ottesen, L.H.; Aagaard, N.K.; Kiszka-Kanowitz, M.; Rehling, M.; Henriksen, J.H.; Pedersen, E.B.; Flyvbjerg, A.; Bendtsen, F. Effects of a long-acting formulation of octreotide on renal function and renal sodium handling in cirrhotic patients with portal hypertension: a randomized, double-blind, controlled trial. *Hepatology* **2001**, *34*, 471.

31. Harrigan, R.A.; Nathan, M.S.; Beattie, P. Oral agents for the treatment of type 2 diabetes mellitus: pharmacology, toxicity, and treatment. *Ann. Emerg. Med.* **2001**, *38*, 68.

32. Takacs, T.; Hajnal, F.; Nemeth, J.; Lonovics, J.; Pap, A. Stimulated gastrointestinal hormone release and gallbladder contraction during continuous jejunal feeding in patients with pancreatic pseudocyst is inhibited by octreotide. *Int. J. Pancreatol.* **2000**, *28*, 215.

33. Dorkoosh, F.A.; Verhoef, J.C.; Verheijden, J.H.M.; Rafiee-Tehrani, M.; Borchard, G.; Junginger, H.E. Peroral absorption of octreotide in pigs formulated in delivery systems based on superporous hydrogel polymers. *Pharm. Res.* **2002**, in print.

34. Thanou, M.; Verhoef, J.C.; Marbach, P.; Junginger, H. E. Intestinal absorption of octreotide: N-trimethyl chitosan chloride (TMC) ameliorates the permeability and absorption properties of the somatostatin analogue in vitro and in vivo. *J. Pharm. Sci.* **2000**, *89*, 951.

35. Thanou, M.; Verhoef, J.C.; Verheijden, J.H.M.; Junginger, H.E. Intestinal absorption of octreotide using trimethyl chitosan chloride: studies in pigs. *Pharm. Res.* **2001**, *18*, 823.

36. Digenis, G.A.; Sandefer, E.P.; Page, R.C.; Doll, W.J.; Gold, T.B.; Darwazeh, N.B. Bioequivalence study of stressed and nonstressed hard gelatin capsules using amoxicillin as a drug marker and gamma scintigraphy to confirm time and GI location of in vivo capsule rupture. *Pharm. Res.* **2000**, *17*, 572.

37. Parr, A.F.; Sandefer, E.P.; Wissel, P.; McCartney, M.; McClain, C.; Ryo, U.Y.; Digenis, G.A.. Evaluation of the feasibility and use of a prototype remote drug delivery capsule (RDDC) for non-invasive regional drug absorption studies in the GI tract of man and beagle dog. *Pharm. Res.* **1999**, *16*, 266.

38. Dorkoosh, F.A.; Verhoef, J.C.; Ambagts, M.H.C.; Rafiee-Tehrani, M.; Borchard, G.; Junginger, H.E. Peroral delivery systems based on superporous hydrogel polymers: release characteristics for the peptide drugs buserelin, octreotide and insulin. *Eur. J. Pharm. Sci.* **2002**, *15*, 433.

Indexes

Author Index

Subject Index

A

336

molecules stabilizing bilayer with,
62–63
See also Polymeric micelles
Phospholipids
bilayer lipid membranes (BLM),
5–6
pH-sensitive drug release, 8
stabilization of bilayers, 62–63
Phototriggering, drug release, 8, 52,
55
pH-sensitive systems
acid-catalyzed hydrolysis for release,
55–56
carboxytetramethylrhodamine (CR)
loading/precipitation, 262
drug release, 8
liposomes, 27–28
nanocontainers, 225
pH-dependent release of fluorescent
dye, 229, 231*f*
polymers, 28
schematic of, nanocontainers,
230*f*
selective gene delivery, 62–63
See also Neutral liposome packaging
system; Stimuli-responsive
liposome-polymer complexes
Piroxicam
comparing predictions to
experimental drug release profiles,
209*f*
duration of release, 207
effect of intrinsic viscosity of
poly(lactide-*co*-glycolide) (PLG)
on release rates from uniform
microspheres, 207*f*
effect of PLG microsphere size and
loading on release rates, 206*f*
encapsulation and release, 204, 207
in vitro release profiles, 206*f*
mathematical model of release from
PLG microspheres, 208–209
non-steroidal anti-inflammatory drug
(NSAID), 204
zero-order release from mixtures of
uniform microspheres, 209–210

See also Poly(lactide-*co*-glycolide)
(PLG); Precision particle
fabrication (PPF)
Plasmenyl-type liposomes
cleavage pathways, 53*f*
intracellular drug delivery, 60
key reactions for lipid synthesis, 54*f*
plasmenyl-type lipid synthesis, 52
triggering strategy, 51–52
See also Vinyl ether-based drug
delivery
Plasmid deoxyribonucleic acid (DNA)
dehydration/rehydration liposomes
(DRV) entrapping, 64–65
ethanol and divalent cations trapping,
65
liposome formation, 64
method for trapping into neutral
liposomes, 65
poly(ethylene glycol) (PEG)-coated
poly(lactic acid) particles, 287
unilamellar membranes, 65
See also Deoxyribonucleic acid
(DNA); Neutral liposome
packaging system; Nucleic acids
Pluronic® block copolymers
accumulation and permeability of P-
glycoprotein (Pgp)-dependent
drugs, 138
attachment of specific ligand, 145
biological response-modifying
agents, 131
brain microvessel endothelial cells
(BMVEC), 144
changes in microviscosity, 141
critical micelle concentration (CMC),
132–133
cytotoxicity in drug resistant cancer
cells, 138
dose-dependent behavior, 141–142
doxorubicin alone and in
compositions, 138
doxorubicin pharmacokinetics and
biodistribution, 137
drug encapsulation in micelles, 163
drug resistance phenomena, 139–140